CHARGE Syndrome

Genetic Syndromes and Communication Disorders Series

Robert J. Shprintzen, Ph.D.
Series Editor

Waardenburg Syndrome by Alice Kahn, Ph.D.

Educating Children with Velo-Cardio-Facial Syndrome
by Donna Cutler-Landsman, M.S., Editor

**Medical Genetics: Its Application to Speech, Hearing, and
Craniofacial Disorders** by Nathaniel H. Robin, M.D.

Velo-Cardio-Facial Syndrome, Volume 1, by Robert J. Shprintzen and
Karen J. Golding-Kushner

CHARGE Syndrome by Timothy S. Hartshorne, Margaret A. Hefner,
Sandra L. H. Davenport, and James W. Thelin

CHARGE Syndrome

A Volume in the
Genetics and Communication Disorders Series

Timothy S. Hartshorne, Margaret A. Hefner,
Sandra L. H. Davenport, and James W. Thelin

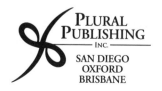

PLURAL
PUBLISHING
INC.

SAN DIEGO
OXFORD
BRISBANE

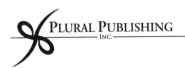

5521 Ruffin Road
San Diego, CA 92123

e-mail: info@pluralpublishing.com
Web site: http://www.pluralpublishing.com

49 Bath Street
Abingdon, Oxfordshire OX14 1EA
United Kingdom

FSC
www.fsc.org
MIX
Paper from
responsible sources
FSC® C011935

Typeset in 11/13 Garamond by Flanagan's Publishing Services, Inc.
Printed in the United States of America by McNaughton and Gunn
Second Printing February 2012

Library of Congress Cataloging-in-Publication Data:
CHARGE syndrome / [edited by] Timothy S. Hartshorne . . . [et al.].
    p. ; cm.—(Genetic syndromes and communication disorders series)
  Includes bibliographical references and index.
  ISBN-13: 978-1-59756-349-9 (alk. paper)
  ISBN-10: 1-59756-349-8 (alk. paper)
  1. Velocardiofacial syndrome. 2. Communicative disorders—Genetic aspects.
I. Hartshorne, Timothy S. II. Series: Genetic syndromes and communication
disorders series.
  [DNLM: 1. Abnormalities, Multiple–genetics. 2. Abnormalities, Multiple—
psychology. 3. Language Development. 4. Sensation Disorders—genetics.
QS 675 C472 2010]
  RB155.5.C43 2010
  616'.042–dc22
                                                    2010017039

Contents

Foreword

*I*t is a great honor for me as a clinical geneticist to write a foreword to a book that is dedicated to CHARGE syndrome. This is not because there is hardly any genetics in this book, but because in my experience, CHARGE syndrome is a very fascinating condition. Why this interest in CHARGE syndrome? Well, not just because our team in Nijmegen quite accidentally discovered the genetic cause of CHARGE syndrome, the *CHD7* gene. Or because it is amazing that a mutation in one single gene, out of approximately 30,000 genes, is able to cause such a complex and clinically highly variable disorder as CHARGE syndrome is. Or because unraveling the function of the gene and how mutations result in CHARGE syndrome is an exciting challenge. No, it is foremost because I admire patients with CHARGE syndrome and their parents. Most children are real fighters, adorably stubborn, and have a great sense of humor, all perfect coping strategies for the hurdles that they are faced with.

This book is not about genetics, embryology, and pathogenesis of CHARGE syndrome but, far more importantly, it is about what might happen and what needs to be done after the diagnosis has been made. The major focus is on communication with the child, but we shouldn't forget communication with the parents. When the *CHD7* gene was discovered in 2004, we invited all the families that were involved in the study, explained our discovery to them, and asked them what kind of research they wanted us to do now the cause of CHARGE syndrome was known. Their answer was only partly related to science; what they wanted was an expert clinic. We were told that they were tired of explaining to the ophthalmologist that not being able to walk was due not only to problems with vision, but also a balance problem. Or telling the cardiologist that the feeding problems were due not only to less powerful suckling but also problems with the cranial nerves. Or explaining to the urologist that a simple orchidopexy in children with CHARGE is not that simple at all. Five years ago, we started a national clinic that now has over 50 children with CHARGE syndrome in follow-up and in which 12 different medical specialists are involved all of whom experience a very steep learning curve. But the Netherlands is a very small, heavily crowded country with short distances. Such an expert clinic is not feasible in many countries, especially due to the enormous distances that most of them face. Therefore, it is such an important accomplishment that with this new book, everyone involved in the care for a child with CHARGE syndrome has an expert team close at hand. All the authors who contributed to this book are authorities in their own field and have dedicated part of or their entire career to CHARGE syndrome. Hopefully, this book not only will stimulate integrated care and better surveillance, and thus result in an optimal communication, motor, socioemotional, and cognitive development of the child, but will also assist parents in their communication with the 1,001 professionals in the maze that is educational and medical care.

This book nicely illustrates how complex CHARGE syndrome is. However, we should not forget that every child is unique and that the syndrome is highly variable. The book can be considered as a guideline that should help to establish integrated multidisciplinary, but also individualized care. Integrated multidisciplinary care does not necessarily mean on the same spot. It means, again, communication. Communication between all professionals involved in the care for a child with CHARGE syndrome. This book will help us to understand each other's professional languages. Therefore, I sincerely hope that all people who are involved in the medical, educational, and daily care of a child with CHARGE syndrome will take advantage of this book and read not only the chapters that concern their own profession, but all of it.

Conny M. A. van Ravenswaaij-Arts, M.D., Ph.D.
Associate Professor Clinical Genetics
University Medical Centre Groningen
The Netherlands

Introduction

*C*ommunication, communication, communication.

For 25 years, this has been our mantra when asked what it is that children with CHARGE syndrome need. CHARGE is a very complex syndrome encompassing a wide variety of medical, developmental, and personality traits. Many children struggle just to survive. However, the biggest barrier to ultimate success for individuals with CHARGE is communication. Those children who are able to establish abstract communication in childhood ultimately do far better than those who do not. The barriers to communication are legion: life-threatening medical issues; decreased hearing, vision, and balance; difficulty handling secretions and moving the face; plus an educational system that is ill-prepared to meet their diverse needs.

Each individual with CHARGE has a unique set of features, making generalizations difficult and not very useful. No "average" or "typical" child with CHARGE syndrome exists. However, many similarities can be seen. Experienced observers have learned a lot about these individuals and developed ways to assess the issues, the strengths, and the weaknesses of each individual child. It is necessary to understand the world of the child—how each child experiences and interacts with their environment—to be able to implement therapies and set up environments that will be conducive to the establishment of effective communication systems.

The purpose of this volume is to help allied health professionals (as well as families and educators) get a comprehensive picture of the sensory, physical, and psychological issues that challenge children with CHARGE syndrome and to explore a variety of ways to overcome the challenges in assessment of each involved organ system and of the child as a whole. In spite of our goal of making each chapter very reader friendly, much technical information is presented, which we believe is critical to include for those professionals who are deeply involved with particular issues. We hope that readers will find that the information most critical to their work with CHARGE will be readily accessible in these chapters.

WHERE DID THE NAME COME FROM?

CHARGE is an acronym coined in 1981, which stood for the following: C = coloboma, H = heart, A = atresia of the choanae, R= retardation of growth and development, G = genitourinary, and E = ear anomalies and hearing loss (Pagon, Graham, Zonana, & Yong, 1981). The condition was designated as an "association," which meant a group of anomalies that are not associated just by chance. At that time, it was felt that not enough evidence existed for the term "syndrome" to be used. Several authors with extensive experience felt that the syndrome designation was appropriate since a nonrandom pattern of malformations was present and because the children often had similar outward appearances. When the *CHD7* gene was discovered in 2004, CHARGE universally was accepted as a syndrome and is no longer described as an association.

HOW IS CHARGE DIAGNOSED?

The 1981 paper (Pagon, et al.) suggested that 4 of the 6 characteristics in the acronym were sufficient to make the diagnosis. The diagnostic criteria were revised in 1998 (Blake, et al.) and in 2007 (Sanlaville; Verloes). Tables 1 and 2 show the revised major and minor criteria with the estimated percentage of people affected with each condition. As many of these features (as well as the "occasional findings") have an impact on language and other developmental skills, they are discussed in detail in this volume. It is important to note that no one cardinal feature of CHARGE can be found among affected individuals. Every characteristic ranges from absent to present and, when present, can vary from mild to severe. However, the most common features are the inner ear malformations.

CHARGE syndrome is caused by at least one gene (*CHD7*), which works very early in embryonic development (Vissers, van Ravenswaaij, Admiraal, Hurst, de Vries, Janssen, et al., 2004; Adams, Hurd, Beyer, Swiderski, Raphael, & Martin, 2007). Because this gene affects the so-called neural crest, many of the 12 cranial nerves that supply the head and neck are often affected (Blake, Hartshorne, Lawand, Dailor, & Thelin, 2008). These control vision, hearing, and smell as well as the muscles of the eyes, face, mouth, throat, and neck. As a consequence, more than 90% of individuals with CHARGE have both vision loss and hearing loss (classified as deafblindness). Most spend the first 2–3 years of life in and out of hospitals and clinics because of airway, heart, and feeding problems. Since medical issues can have a profound impact on growth and development, the medical section provides detailed descriptions and references for each affected system. Because the focus in the early years for these children is on overcoming life-threatening medical challenges, scant attention often is paid to development and communication. An extensive review of the medical features and management issues can be found in the GeneReview of CHARGE syndrome at http://genetests.org (Lalani, Hefner, Belmont, & Davenport, 2009).

TABLE 1. Major Diagnostic Characteristics of CHARGE Syndrome

Characteristic	Manifestations	Frequency
Coloboma of the eye	Coloboma of the iris, retina, choroid, disc; microphthalmos	80–90%
Choanal atresia or stenosis[1,2]	Unilateral/bilateral: bony/membranous, atresia/stenosis	50–60%
Cranial nerve dysfunction or anomaly	I: Hyposmia or anosmia/arhinencephaly	>90%
	VII: Facial palsy (unilateral or bilateral)	40%
	VIII: hypoplasia of auditory nerve	>80%
	IX/X: Swallowing problems with aspiration	70–90%
Characteristic CHARGE outer ear	Short, wide ear with little or no lobe, "snipped off" helix, prominent antihelix which is often discontinuous with tragus, triangular concha, decreased cartilage, often protrude, usually asymmetric	>50%
Characteristic CHARGE middle or inner ear	Ossicular malformations	>80%
	Mondini defect of the cochlea	>80%
	Absent or hypoplastic semicircular canals	>90%

[1]Choanae are passages in the back of the nose which are blocked (atretic) or narrowed (stenotic)

[2]Cleft palate may substitute for this characteristic in some cases

Establishment of an adequate communication system is crucial to living a meaningful life. Research on hearing impairment demonstrates that some mode of communication needs to be established in the first few months of life for development of symbolic language (Vohr, Jodoin-Krauzyk, Tucker, Johnson, Topol, & Ahlgren, 2008). Due to the complexities of cochlear malformations, tracheostomies preventing verbal output, and visual impairment, standard speech therapy and sign language methods need to be modified. Some of these children may never attain easily recognizable verbal speech despite best efforts. Creative approaches utilizing all available modes of communication often are required. It is important to understand, however, that ALL BEHAVIOR IS COMMUNICATION. Families and professionals should document and shape behavior while still striving for a formal communication system.

CHARGE may be the only disorder that presents with deficits of all of the senses [Part I]. These deficits alone make many aspects of life a challenge. Throughout this book we use the term "deafblind" rather than the older term "deaf-blind" to reflect that the impact is more than hearing impairment plus visual impairment. The combination of the two results in much more profound disability than the simple addition of the two would imply. And with CHARGE all of the senses may be affected! However, an even greater issue is

TABLE 2. Minor Diagnostic Characteristics of CHARGE Syndrome

Characteristic	Manifestations	Frequency
Genital hypoplasia	Males: Micropenis, cryptorchidism; Females: Hypoplastic labia	50%
	Both: Delayed puberty	>50%, 90% in males
Cardiovascular malformation	Especially conotruncal defects (e.g., tetralogy of Fallot), aortic arch anomalies	75–85%
Growth deficiency	Short stature	70%
	Growth hormone deficiency	15%
Orofacial cleft	Cleft lip and/or palate	15–20%
Tracheoesophageal (T-E) fistula	T-E defects of all types	15–20%
Renal anomalies	Ectopic or solitary or duplex kidney, UPJ obstruction, reflux, hydronephrosis	30–40%
Distinctive facial features	Square face with broad prominent forehead, prominent nasal bridge and columella, flat midface, small chin which gets larger with age	70–80%
Palmar crease	Hockey-stick palmar crease	50%
CHARGE behavioral profile	OCD or other perseverative behavior	>50%

the combined consequences of sensory issues superimposed on a distinctive constellation of medical and physiologic disorders [Part II] that give rise to a unique course of individual development [Part III] and result in restricted forms of communication (that are uncommon) [Part IV]. The sum of the individual challenges governs the resulting patterns of behavior as well as factors that are critical in parenting and social interaction [Part V].

CHARGE syndrome is highly complex, highly variable, and has a profound impact on those with the syndrome and their families. It is our hope that this volume will be a valuable tool in working toward the goals of understanding the multiple interconnected challenges that CHARGE syndrome presents and maximizing all aspects of development.

Timothy S. Hartshorne, Ph.D.
Margaret A. Hefner, M.S.
Sandra L. H. Davenport, M.D.
James W. Thelin, Ph.D.

REFERENCES

Adams, M. E., Hurd, E. A., Beyer, L. A., Swiderski, D. L., Raphael, Y., & Martin, D. M. (2007). Defects in vestibular sensory epithelia and innervation in mice with loss of Chd7 function: implications for human CHARGE syndrome. *Journal of Comparative Neurology, 504,* 519–532.

Blake, K. D., Davenport, S. L., Hall, B. D., Hefner, M.A., Pagon, R. A., Williams, M. S., & Graham, J. M. Jr. (1998). CHARGE association: an update and review for the primary pediatrician. *Clinical Pediatrics, 37,* 159–174.

Blake, K. D., Hartshorne, T. S., Lawand, C., Dailor, A. N., & Thelin, J. W. (2008). Cranial nerve manifestations in CHARGE syndrome. *American Journal of Medical Genetics, 146A,* 585–592.

Lalani, S. R., Hefner, M. A., Belmont, J. W., & Davenport, S. L. H. (2009). *Gene Review: CHARGE Syndrome.* Retrieved December 16, 2009, from http://www.ncbi.nlm .nih.gov/bookshelf/br.fcgi?book=gene&part=charge

Pagon, R. A., Graham, J. M., Jr., Zonana, J., & Yong, S. L. (1981). Coloboma, congenital heart disease, and choanal atresia with multiple anomalies: CHARGE association. *Journal of Pediatrics, 99,* 223–227.

Sanlaville, S., & Verloes, A. (2007). CHARGE syndrome: An update. *European Journal of Human Genetics, 15,* 389–399.

Vissers, L. E., van Ravenswaaij, C. M., Admiraal, R., Hurst, J. A., de Vries, B. B., Janssen, I. M., . . . van Kessel, A. G. (2004). Mutations in a new member of the chromodomain gene family cause CHARGE syndrome. *Nature Genetics, 36,* 955–957.

Vohr, B., Jodoin-Krauzyk, J., Tucker, R., Johnson, M. J., Topol, D., & Ahlgren, M. (2008). Early language outcomes of early-identified infants with permanent hearing loss at 12 to 16 months of age. *Pediatrics, 122,* 535–544.

Acknowledgments

*T*he editors thank all of the families and the children and adults with CHARGE syndrome who have taught us much of what we know and helped us focus on what further questions need to be addressed. A special thanks to everyone who provided photographs of themselves and/or their children for the book—many more than we were able to use. We also would like to acknowledge our chapter authors: we approached the top people in many fields who understand CHARGE, and in spite of complicated schedules and commitments, they agreed to write chapters and to allow our editing. Three individuals who read, edited, and commented on chapter drafts deserve individual thanks: Valerie Weber, Rachel Jones, and Ellen Shumka. The first editor would like to express his appreciation to his son, Jacob Hartshorne, who has CHARGE and has been the inspiration for his father's work. Finally, the editors would like to recognize Marion Norbury, the founder of the CHARGE Syndrome Foundation, who brought us all together and made this collaboration possible.

This book is dedicated to the families who have the urgent need for information to help their children with CHARGE syndrome and to the professionals who make the special effort to understand this rare syndrome.

Contributors

Véronique Abadie, M.D., Ph.D.
Hôpital NECKER: 149 rue de Sèvres, 75015 Paris, France
Faculté PARIS DESCARTES, 15 rue de l'école de Médecine, 75006
Paris, France
Chapter 7

Joan C. Arvedson, Ph.D.
Program Coordinator of Feeding and Swallowing Services
Children's Hospital of Wisconsin—Milwaukee
Clinical Professor in the Division of Gastroenterology,
Department of Pediatrics, Medical College of Wisconsin
Milwaukee, Wisconsin
Chapter 12

Susan M. Bashinski, Ed.D.
Associate Professor, Special Education
East Carolina University
Greenville, North Carolina
Chapter 26

Daniela Baumgartner, M.D.
Department of Pediatric Cardiology
Innsbruck Medical University
Innsbruck, Austria
Chapter 14

Kim D. Blake, M.D.
Professor, General Pediatrics
Department of Pediatrics
Dalhousie University
Halifax, Nova Scotia, Canada
Chapters 19 & 24

Pierre Bonfils, M.D., Ph.D.
Department of Otolaryngology Head Neck Surgery,
Unité Centre National de la Recherche Scientifique UPRESSA 7060,
Hôpital Europeen Georges Pompidou,
Paris, France
Chapter 7

David M. Brown, M.A., D.Sc. (Hon)
Consultant teacher of the deafblind
California Deaf-Blind Services
San Francisco State University
San Francisco, California
Chapter 5

Christel Chalouhi, M.D.
General Pediatrics
Hôpital NECKER: 149 rue de Sèvres, 75015
Paris, France
Chapter 7

Swapna K. Chandran, M.D.
Assistant Professor
Pediatric Otolaryngology
Laryngology
University of Louisville School of Medicine
Louisville, Kentucky
Chapter 8

Sarah E. Curtis, Au.D.
Audiologist
Central Florida Speech and Hearing Center
Lakeland, Florida
Chapter 6

Sandra L. H. Davenport, M.D.
Clinical Genetics and Pediatrics
Owner/Director Sensory Genetics/Neurodevelopment
Bloomington, Minnesota
Chapters 1, 17, 24

Laurie S. Denno, Doctoral Candidate
Behavior Analyst
Perkins School for the Blind, Deafblind Program
Waterford, MA

Doctoral Candidate in Applied Behavior Analysis
Simmons College
Boston, Massachusetts
Chapter 22

Patrick Faulcon, M.D.
Department of Otolaryngology Head Neck Surgery,
Unité Centre National de la Recherche Scientifique UPRESSA 7060,
Hôpital Europeen Georges Pompidou,
Paris, France
Chapter 7

Elizabeth E. Gilles, M.D.
Assistant Professor of Pediatrics
University of Minnesota
Medical Director, Pediatric Neurology
Children's Hospitals and Clinics
Minneapolis, Minnesota
Chapter 13

Christopher R. Grindle, M.D.
Dept of Otolaryngology-Head & Neck Surgery,
Thomas Jefferson University
Philadelphia, Pennsylvania
Chapter 10

Joshua K. Hartshorne, Doctoral Candidate
Department of Psychology
Harvard College
Cambridge, Massachusetts
Chapter 24

Timothy S. Hartshorne, Ph.D.
Professor of Psychology
Central Michigan University
Mount Pleasant, Michigan
Chapters 21, 24, 28, 31, 32

Nancy Salem-Hartshorne, Ph.D.
Assistant Professor
Department of Psychology
Central Michigan University
Mount Pleasant, Michigan
Chapters 19, 20, 21, 24

Margaret A. Hefner, M.S.
Clinical Associate Professor
Division of Medical Genetics
Department of Pediatrics
Saint Louis University School of Medicine
St. Louis, Missouri
Chapter 1

Helen S. Heussler, MB BS FRACP DM
Staff Specialist and Senior Lecturer University of Queensland Level 2
Mater Children's Hospital
South Brisbane, Queensland, Australia
Chapter 23

Lea Hyvärinen, M.D.
Professor, Rehabilitation Sciences
University of Dortmund, Germany
Senior Lecturer, Developmental Neuropsychology
University of Helsinki, Finland
Chapter 2

Emily King Miller, M.A., CF-SLP
Clinical Fellow in Speech-Language Pathology
Blount Memorial Total Rehabilitation
Alcoa, Tennessee
Chapter 27

Jeremy Kirk, M.D., FRCPCH
Department of Endocrinology
Birmingham Children's Hospital
Birmingham, England
Chapter 16

Angela E. Lin, M.D.
Associate Clinical Professor of Pediatrics
Harvard Medical School
Cambridge, Massachusetts
Chapter 14

Jill F. Maddox, Au.D.
Pediatric Audiologist
Children's Healthcare of Atlanta
Atlanta, Georgia
Chapter 6

Claes Möller, M.D., Ph.D.
Professor of Medical Disability Research
Professor of Audiology
Örebro University Hospital
Örebro, Sweden
Chapter 4

Jude Nicholas, Psy.D.
Clinical Neuropsychologist
Vestlandet Resource Center
Bergen, Norway
Chapter 30

Jeremy D. Prager, M.D.
Clinical Fellow
Pediatric Otolaryngology Head & Neck Surgery
Cincinnati Children's Hospital Medical Center
Cincinnati, Ohio
Chapter 11

Evan J. Propst, M.D., M.Sc., FRCSC
Clinical Fellow
Pediatric Otolaryngology—Head and Neck Surgery
Cincinnati Children's Hospital Medical Center
Cincinnati, Ohio
Chapter 11

Michael J. Rutter, M.D., FRACS, FRCS
Pediatric Otolaryngologist and Director of Clinical Research
Cincinnati Children's Hospital Medical Center
Associate Professor, University of Cincinnati College of Medicine
Cincinnati, Ohio
Chapter 11

Udayan K. Shah, M.D., FAAP, FACS
Associate Professor
Department of Otolaryngology-Head and Neck Surgery
Thomas Jefferson University
Director, Fellow & Resident Education
Nemours/Alfred I DuPont Hospital for Children
Philadelphia, Pennsylvania
Chapters 8 & 10

Kasee K. Stratton, Doctoral Candidate
Department of Psychology
Central Michigan University
Mount Pleasant, Michigan
Chapters 24 & 31

Nancy K. Steele, M.Ed.,
Technical Assistance Specialist
National Consortium on Deaf-Blindness
Knoxville, Tennessee
Chapter 27

Lori Ann Swanson, Ph.D., CCC-SLP
Assistant Professor
Department of Communicative Disorders
University of Wisconsin—River Falls
River Falls, Wisconsin
Chapters 25 & 27

James W. Thelin, Ph.D.
Associate Professor Emeritus
Department of Audiology and Speech Pathology
University of Tennessee—Knoxville
Knoxville, Tennessee
Chapters 3, 6, & 27

Sara J. Thelin, M.A. CCC-SLP
Speech-Language Pathologist (Retired)
Knoxville, Tennessee
Chapter 27

N. Wendell Todd, M.D., MPH
Professor, Otolaryngology and Pediatrics
Emory University
Atlanta, Georgia
Chapter 9

Lori S. Travis, Au.D., CCC-A, F-AAA
Clinical Audiologist
Wolf and Yun, PSC & Affordable Hearing Aids
Elizabethtown, Kentucky
Chapter 6

Lee Elizabeth Wachtel, M.D.
Medical Director, Neurobehavioral Unit
Kennedy Krieger Institute
Assistant Professor of Psychiatry
Johns Hopkins School of Medicine
Baltimore, Maryland
Chapter 29

Marc S. Williams, M.D., FAAP, FACMG
Director, Intermountain Healthcare Clinical Genetics Institute
Clinical Professor, Department of Pedatrics,
Divison of Medical Genetics,
University of Utah
Salt Lake City, Utah
Chapters 15 & 18

PART I

Sensory Issues in CHARGE

*C*HARGE syndrome has features that overlap with a multitude of other genetic conditions. What is unique about CHARGE is the multisensory impairment. Among genetic conditions, CHARGE is the leading cause of congenital deafblindness (dualsensory impairment). Individuals with CHARGE have disturbances not only in hearing and vision, but in all seven senses (hearing, vision, smell, taste, touch, proprioception, and inner ear balance). The impact of multisensory impairment is not additive, but multiplicative. First and foremost, understanding CHARGE requires an understanding of sensory impairment.

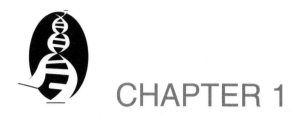

CHAPTER 1

Overview and Sensory Issues

SANDRA L. H. DAVENPORT, M.D. AND
MARGARET A. HEFNER, M.S.

*H*umans have receptors for five "input" senses, which allow access to external stimuli, namely vision, hearing, smell, touch, and taste. In addition, the body has other receptors that allow the body to recognize its position in space and in relation to itself, namely vestibular and proprioceptive senses. In CHARGE syndrome, all seven of these senses may be affected.

Vision, hearing, smell, and balance are usually all affected in individuals with CHARGE syndrome. This means a child with CHARGE may not see you unless you are at a specific distance and in the individual child's visual field, or the child may see only parts of you and not as a person. These children also may not hear your natural voice, or they may not hear you at all. These same children may not smell properly in order to identify food, perfumes, or other common odors and may not have enough balance to attain normal motor milestones. These children are *input impaired*.

Most children with CHARGE have normal brain-imaging studies and, therefore, must be presumed to have normal brain function until proven otherwise. Before a child with CHARGE can be said to have anything other than normal intelligence, that child must have been in settings with appropriate adaptations that address the multiple sensory issues for a number of years. Most adaptations for people who are hearing impaired use visual enforcers; however, a visually impaired individual with hearing loss may not see or understand these enforcers. Likewise, most adaptations for visually impaired individuals are auditory and are completely lost to those who are hearing impaired in addition to visually impaired. Dual sensory loss (*deafblindness*, see Sidebar 1–1) requires unique adaptations. Hearing, vision, and smell

Sidebar 1
Definition of Deafblindness

One might assume defining *deafblindness* is straightforward. Actually many definitions exist, and although most states have put a definition into regulations, they are not all identical. Although all definitions indicate that deafblindness involves both hearing and vision impairment, some specify the degree of impairment that must exist; whereas others allow "functional" definitions. Some state deafblind projects automatically serve children with CHARGE, but others require that the child have specific vision and auditory losses before they may receive services.

Following is the federal definition of deafblindness:

Deafblindness means concomitant hearing and vision impairments, the combination of which causes such severe communication and other developmental and educational needs that they cannot be accommodated in special education programs solely for children with deafness or children with blindness. 34 CFR 300.8 (c) (2).

The U.S. Code, Title 29–Labor, Chapter 21–Sec. 1905 also has a definition, established when funding was authorized for the Helen Keller National Center:

(2) the term "individual who is deaf-blind" means any individual—

   (A) (i) who has a central visual acuity of 20/200 or less in the better eye with corrective lenses, or a field defect such that the peripheral diameter of visual field subtends an angular distance no greater than 20 degrees, or a progressive visual loss having a prognosis leading to one or both these conditions;
   (ii) who has a chronic hearing impairment so severe that most speech cannot be understood with optimum amplification, or a progressive hearing loss having a prognosis leading to this condition; and
   (iii) for whom the combination of impairments described in clauses (i) and (ii) cause extreme difficulty in attaining independence in daily life activities, achieving psychosocial adjustment, or obtaining a vocation;

   (B) who despite the inability to be measured accurately for hearing and vision loss due to cognitive or behavioral constraints, or both, can be determined through functional and performance assessment to have severe hearing and visual disabilities that cause extreme difficulty in attaining independence in daily life activities, achieving psychosocial adjustment, or obtaining vocational objectives; or

(C) meets such other requirements as the Secretary may prescribe by regulation.

are the primary "distance" senses. In other words, sounds, sights, and smells orient a person to the setting and alert one to the approach or presence of a person, animal, or other object. If all three distance senses are decreased or absent, the person with CHARGE may not be aware of someone who is present until physical contact is made. This can be both startling and frightening, leading to the person with CHARGE being "jumpy" and sometimes having significant tactile and oral aversions.

Although hearing impairment leads primarily to delayed language acquisition, vision impairment combined with vestibular dysfunction leads to delayed motor milestones. Hartshorne, Nicholas, Grialou, and Russ (2007) reported that crawling in children with CHARGE occurred on average at 1 year, 8 months (range <1 to 5 years old, 88 participants) and walking on average occurred at 3 years, 1 month, (range 1 to 10 years, 95 participants). In addition to the sensory losses, some children have bilateral facial palsy, resulting in a complete lack of facial expression (Figure 1-1). If all of these

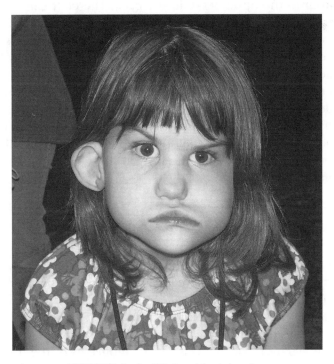

FIGURE 1–1. Bilateral facial palsy.

conditions are present, major developmental milestones are delayed significantly and intellectual disability often is presumed. Usually, this is a false assumption (see Chapter 20). If central vision is affected (as with a macular coloboma, see Chapter 2), the individual with CHARGE will not make direct eye contact. Lack of apparent eye contact combined with the lack of language development in the presence of unusual behaviors may lead to a diagnosis of autism. Usually, this is also an inaccurate assumption.

SPECIFIC ANOMALIES THAT AFFECT SENSORY FUNCTION

Eyes and Vision

The primary cause of visual impairment is a coloboma of the eye globe (see detailed discussion in Chapter 2). This congenital defect occurs when a cleft fails to close in the bottom of the retinal layer lining the inside of the eye. Since the retina contains the photoreceptor cells that detect light and images, the affected retina cannot process images coming from the upper visual field. Since glasses cannot correct this impairment, all visual gestures or materials must be presented within the individual's visual communication bubble, i.e., that space in front and to the sides of the person with CHARGE in which people, hands, or objects can be seen (Figure 1–2). The size and location of the coloboma has major implications for vision since the cleft can extend from the iris in front to the optic nerve in the back. The cleft can be tiny so that vision is hardly impaired at all or very large, in which case the eye may be small (microphthalmic) and vision severely impaired or even absent.

If the coloboma involves the macula, the central vision may be affected. This area allows one to see things clearly and is measured using standard eye charts. When the macula is affected, people and objects may be blurred or even completely missing when one looks directly at them. This causes the person to look above or to the right or left of the object in order to figure out what it is. If the coloboma is in the optic nerve, the effect may be similar to a moderately sized retinal coloboma in that the vision in that eye can be reduced significantly.

Auditory System and Hearing

All structures of the peripheral and central auditory systems may be involved (see Chapter 8). Some anomalies have little or no effect on hearing while others have large effects. Misshapen external ears or pinnas that are a very recognizable characteristic of CHARGE almost never cause hearing loss. Malformations of the ossicles of the middle ear typically cause conductive hearing loss that can be moderate to severe. Congenital anomalies of the inner ears typically cause cochlear or sensorineural hearing losses that are usually greatest

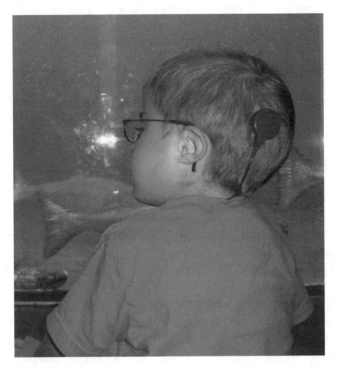

FIGURE 1–2. The communication bubble. Note how close the child is to the fish tank.

in the high frequencies, which are critical to understanding speech. The combined conductive and cochlear losses are often asymmetrical between the ears. About half of the losses are severe to profound mixed hearing losses. Even a mild hearing loss can have major developmental implications when combined with other sensory deficits.

The craniofacial anomalies in CHARGE often cause Eustachian tube dysfunction which, in turn, leads to middle-ear disease with recurrent ear infections and chronically draining ears. Most individuals with CHARGE have had several sets of tympanostomy tubes inserted surgically in the attempt to overcome middle-ear disease. By late childhood, ear infections become less frequent, but sinus infections become increasingly frequent, even chronic. Frequent infections (middle ear and sinus) result in pain, decreased stamina, and fluctuating hearing loss. Draining middle ears and floppy outer ears can complicate the use of amplification devices.

Olfactory System and Smell

The sense of smell is notoriously difficult to evaluate (see Chapter 7). However, one study in France was able to demonstrate that all 25 individuals with CHARGE evaluated had either a decreased or absent sense of smell (Chalouhi et al., 2005). Imaging of the brain also showed abnormal olfactory bulbs (Pinto et al., 2005). Since smell is a primary contributor to the enjoyment of food, the lack of smell may decrease the motivation to eat. Smell also is involved with memory and can be a powerful way to recognize people, pets, and different environments. In addition, if both hearing and vision are gone, smell is the remaining distance sense. If it is decreased or absent, then only touch, taste, and proprioception are available to communicate and learn about the environment.

Gustatory System and Taste

Taste buds detect sweet, sour, salty, bitter, and umani (savory) substances. To our knowledge these are not affected in CHARGE, but no studies have been done. The taste buds are partially supplied by the chorda tympani, a branch of the facial nerve (cranial nerve VII) that passes through the middle ear. Because the facial nerve in CHARGE often is in an unusual place, it can be damaged either in development or during surgery. Taste buds also are supplied by cranial nerve IX, the glossopharyngeal nerve, which is thought to be at least partially responsible for the swallowing problems prevalent in the first few years of life. In the absence of other sensory input, infants and toddlers with CHARGE may mouth objects longer than children with normal distance senses in order to learn more about them.

Touch, Pain, and Pressure

Touch is the primary venue for sensory input in many children with CHARGE because vision, hearing, and smell are impaired. Therefore, great respect for the type of touch and especially touching of the hands (Miles, 2003) is advisable. It is not known whether the perception of touch is altered in individuals with CHARGE. Often, children appreciate firm, deep touch or pressure and respond well to techniques of sensory integration. Children with CHARGE may be particularly sensitive to textures and may have preferences for or aversions to particular sensory experiences such as walking on grass or sand or being in water.

If touch is the major way to learn about what people and objects look like—or, more accurately, feel like—then great care must be taken to let them know not only what an object feels like but also where it is located and what happens to it when it is no longer in contact with the body. Using touch as the primary mode of communication can be slow and fatiguing since communication happens only with physical contact. Providing an immersion environment is difficult and time consuming.

Pain appears to be experienced differently in persons with CHARGE (see Chapter 30). Families frequently comment that children can sustain an injury with lacerations that seems to cause curiosity rather than pain. On the other hand, they may not like injections any more than any other child. Children with CHARGE experience many different sources of pain—from surgeries and other medical procedures to illnesses such as ear and sinus infections. Whether they have a higher pain threshold or have simply accommodated to the experience of pain is not known.

Balance and Mobility

Vestibular Mechanism

Vestibular dysfunction is nearly universal in individuals with CHARGE (see Chapter 4). It is a major cause of poor balance and delay in motor milestones. The vestibular portion of the inner ear usually is malformed, often with three nubbins rather than three complete semicircular canals. The effect of this is a predictable method of developing locomotion in which the child stays close to the ground. This means scooting on the back long enough to wear off a spot of hair combined with rolling and combat crawling for months before getting up into a crawl position. Even then, the child prefers to keep the head down in a "five-point" crawl (Figure 1–3). Children typically cruise for a very long time before walking independently. Gait may be unusual throughout life with the feet shuffling along the ground.

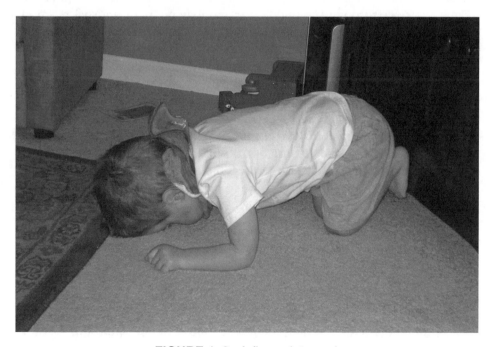

FIGURE 1–3. A five-point crawl.

Proprioception and Muscle Tone

Low muscle tone can be associated with vestibular, tactile, and proprioceptive sensory difficulties (Brown, 2005). Hypotonia, especially in the upper body, although not well studied, has been commented on by many parents. It probably contributes to the motor delay and exacerbates the fatigue seen in both children and adults with CHARGE.

The term *proprioception* was coined by C.S. Sherrington (1907) and refers to the sensation derived from movement of stretch receptors in muscles and tendons as well as movement of joints. Proprioception allows the individual to feel where their body and limbs are in space and in relation to each other (Brown, 2005). Brown describes a number of observations of individuals with CHARGE that imply poor proprioceptive abilities: avoidance of pushing up with hands and arms, problems with standing and bearing weight, a need for support when standing, heavy foot stomping, tip-toe walking, uncoordinated movements, use of excess force, and seeking strong pressure inputs.

OTHER PHYSICAL ISSUES AFFECTING COMMUNICATION

Cranial Nerve Anomalies

Anomalies of cranial nerve VII result in unilateral or bilateral facial palsy. Unilateral facial palsy is a frequent and major anomaly in CHARGE. Since the facial nerve goes through the middle ear and may be in an unusual position, surgery in the space behind the middle ear (e.g., for a cochlear implant) needs to be done with care. Facial nerve damage can cause problems with lip closure and with tongue function. Occasionally, it also may interfere significantly with eye lid closure. Bilateral facial palsy is much less common but has more of an impact on development since facial expression is a primary source of expressive communication, especially when formal language is lacking.

Dysfunction of cranial nerves IX and X results in uncoordinated movement of the soft palate and closure of the epiglottis. In addition, the cartilage of the trachea may be soft (see Chapters 11 and 12). These anomalies can affect phonation and swallowing.

Fatigue

Infections and surgeries plague children with CHARGE during the first few years of life. Choanal atresia, facial clefts, heart defects, or other anomalies also may be present and require multiple surgeries. Just these issues cause great expenditure of energy and result in fatigue, as well as interference with opportunities for typical joint interaction between the child and parents, impacting attachment as well as communication.

Deafblindness alone, however, is universally a source of fatigue. It takes great concentration to attend if you have either vision loss or hearing loss—even more so if you lack both. Constant touch may be desirable for communication but tiring for both parties.

Abnormal sleep patterns are common in CHARGE (Hartshorne et al., 2009) as is true in other deafblind conditions; lack of sleep results in fatigue and irritability in both the child and the parents. Keeping an upright posture (e.g., sitting in a classroom for several hours) also can be fatiguing because of the hypotonia.

OVERALL PICTURE

The age of walking is delayed in CHARGE. The inability to walk independently is related partially to vestibular anomalies but may be affected by a number of other physical or sensory factors. For those who provide communication and language services, it is important to note that a significant relationship exists between the ability to walk independently and the acquisition of symbolic language (Thelin & Fussner, 2005; see also Chapter 6).

The typical child with CHARGE is delayed significantly in all developmental areas usually assessed in the first few years of life: language, gross motor, fine motor, sensorimotor, and personal-social. These early assessment results suggest that the child may be disabled intellectually. However, at least three of the five input senses are usually impaired, although the brain imaging usually shows no malformations. Although some individuals with CHARGE will have significant mental challenges, many can function in the normal range if adequate accommodations are made to ensure understanding of input. Those individuals who are properly prepared can live independently, be gainfully employed, and even attend college. We are aware of at least one middle-aged adult with two master's degrees and many other professionals who have CHARGE syndrome.

The challenge is to assemble a team of professionals to assess the function of the senses and develop an adequate plan for communication, communication, communication.

REFERENCES

Brown, D. (2005). CHARGE syndrome "behaviors": Challenges or adaptations? *American Journal of Medical Genetics*, *133A*, 268–272.

Chalouhi, C., Faulcon, P., Le Bihan, C., Hertz-Pannier, L., Bonfils, P., & Abadie, V. (2005). Olfactory evaluation in children: Application to the CHARGE syndrome. *Pediatrics*, *116*(1), e81–88.

Hartshorne, T .S., Heussler, H. S., Dailor, A. N., Williams, G. L., Papadopoulos, D., & Brandt, K. K. (2009). Sleep disturbances in CHARGE syndrome: Types and relationships with behavior and caregiver well-being. *Developmental Medicine and Child Neurology, 51*, 143–150.

Hartshorne, T. S., Nicholas, J., Grialou, T. L., & Russ, J. M. (2007). Executive function in CHARGE syndrome. *Child Neuropsychology, 13*, 333–344.

Miles, B. (2003, October). Talking the language of the hands to the hands. *National Consortium on Deaf-Blindness.* Retrieved June 3, 2010, from http://www.national db.org/NCDBProducts.php?prodID=47.

Pinto, G., Abadie, V., Mesnage, R., Blustajn, J., Cabrol, S., Amiel, J., . . . Netchine, I. (2005). CHARGE syndrome includes hypogonadotropic hypogonadism and abnormal olfactory bulb development. *Journal of Clinical Endocrinology and Metabolism, 90*, 5621–5626.

Sherrington, C. S. (1907). On the proprioceptive system, especially in its reflex aspect. *Brain, 29*, 467–482.

Thelin, J. W., & Fussner, J. C. (2005). Factors related to the development of communication in CHARGE syndrome. *American Journal of Medical Genetics, 133A*, 282–290.

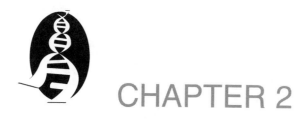

CHAPTER 2

The Eye and Vision

LEA HYVÄRINEN, M.D.

One of the cardinal features of CHARGE syndrome is ocular coloboma, which is a defect in the development of the eye between weeks 5 and 7 of gestation. Colobomas cause defects in the visual field and often lower than normal visual acuity.

EARLY DEVELOPMENT OF THE RETINA

The optic nerves and retina of the eyes are extensions of the brain. First, finger-like structures develop, one on each side of the neural tube (the embryonic precursor to the central nervous system). The tip of this extension then flattens and develops an indentation that becomes a bowl-shaped neural plate. This develops into the retina with an open furrow, the optic fissure, in the lower part of the bowl. At the same time, the immature retina induces development of the lens as a thickening of the epithelial layer next to it, later forming a vesicle to become the lens of the eye (Figure 2-1).

The lower part of the retinal bowl has a furrow, or fissure, where the vessels grow into the eye. During week 7, the edges of the furrow begin to fuse, first in the middle and then continuing forward and backward. If something goes wrong during the closure of the furrow, it stays partially or completely open (Color Plate 1), resulting in a coloboma. If the retinal coloboma extends to the disc, the posterior wall of the globe is irregular in its structure, and refractive error becomes very difficult to measure. Wherever there is a defect

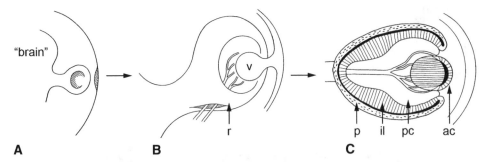

"brain"

r

p il pc ac

A   B   C

FIGURE 2–1. Simplified drawing of the early development of the eye. **A.** A finger-like extension of the neural tube section which becomes the brain with an indentation at its end and thickening of the epithelial tissue next to it. **B.** The bowl-shaped retina (r) is open in its lower part where vessels grow in the space between the retina and the lens vesicle (v). **C.** The outer layer of the retina develops into the pigment epithelial layer (p); the inner layer (il) develops into numerous specialized cells in several layers. The lens forms at the same time and gets its nutrition first via vessels that grow in the primitive posterior chamber (pc) from the optic nerve head toward the lens. The space between the lens and the cornea becomes the anterior chamber (ac) of the eye.

of the retina, there also will be a defect of the choroid (the vascular layer behind the retina) because the choroid is induced to grow by the developing retina. As a result, the lower part of the wall of the eye has only the outer layer of white sclera. The optic disc may not have formed at all or may have an unusual structure, with the incoming vessels entering at the edges of a deep central cup, the so-called "morning glory" disc.

Colobomas, thus, are caused by closure defects of the optic fissure of the eye during early fetal life. A coloboma can involve any of the lower eye structures, namely, the ciliary body, retina, optic nerve, or, less often, the iris. A coloboma also may extend all the way from the iris into the optic nerve. The functional effects of a coloboma are extremely variable and depend on which parts of the eye are involved. A small coloboma of the iris sometimes makes the pupil look like an old-fashioned keyhole, which gives the name to this condition, "keyhole pupil" (Color Plate 2). A coloboma of the retina will affect the visual field.

VISUAL FIELD

All infants with a suspected diagnosis of CHARGE and other midline defects should have a dilated exam by a pediatric ophthalmologist. The defects in the closure of the optic fissure may be small and not extend to the iris so the eyes may look normal. If the defect in the lower part of the eye is so large that it involves the optic disc (see Color Plate 1), the retina might look so severely involved that an ophthalmologist who has not assessed infants with coloboma before may describe the functional situation as much worse than it actually is.

Visual field (VF) testing measures sensitivity in the different parts of the retinas that receive visual signals from the environment. When light rays travelling from above go through the pupil and land on the coloboma, which has no sensory cells, no visual information is transmitted and thus there is field loss in the upper visual field. Often the eyes are small (microphthalmic), and only one eye may be used for looking.

If the coloboma is as large as shown in Color Plate 1, the macula is displaced higher up than normal, changing the location of central vision. Thus, the infant or child seems to look at the hairline of an adult person when actually looking at the eyes of the person. This needs to be explained to all caregivers so that the infant or child is not perceived to be avoiding eye contact. Lack of normal eye contact often is experienced as traumatic by the parents. Therefore, they should get support in communication and interaction until they become accustomed to the unusual eye contact.

Children whose eyes are of normal size and who use both eyes together are binocular, and their two visual fields support each other. A partial loss of the visual field in one eye may be partially filled in by the other eye's visual field (Figure 2–2).

Visual field testing can be challenging with young children or with individuals with limited communication skills. If thorough visual field testing is not feasible, some implications still can be drawn from the size and placement of the colobomas. It is important for the caretakers to describe the loss of the

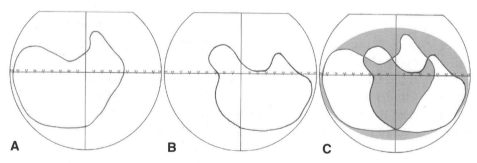

A   **B**   **C**

FIGURE 2–2. Coloboma of both retinas causes loss of visual field in its upper part, i.e., opposite to the location of the coloboma. If the child is binocular (uses both eyes together) and the losses of visual field are not symmetric, the functional visual field may be close to normal. The small losses in the uppermost part of the visual field do not disturb daily functioning. **A.** The visual field of the left eye; **B.** the visual field of the right eye; **C.** the visual fields drawn on top of each other. The gray area in the middle is the normal visual field covered by both eyes, the binocular field. The gray areas above and below depict the small losses of visual field.

upper visual field in cases where it affects the communication field. Adults need to kneel down to the level of the infant and child and not pretend communicating within the blind area of the visual field.

VISUAL ACUITY

Visual acuity (recognition VA) is the ability of a person to see the high contrast details when using optimal correction of refractive errors. Measurement of VA is done using eye charts and near cards with symbols or numbers for those who can respond appropriately. For those who cannot, but who will shift their gaze or follow a moving target, grating tests (which use alternating dark and light lines) are used for measurement of detection VA, which is different from recognition VA. The child's eye muscle (ocular motor) functions need to be tested for accommodation, fixation, saccades, and following.

Quite often, the visual functioning is much better than one might expect from the structure of the eye. Therefore, repeated evaluations of visual functioning during the first years of life are mandatory. If a refractive error shows high myopia (nearsightedness), corrective lenses need to be fitted early. They are not fitted for distance vision because the visual sphere of these infants (the space within which the child responds visually) is limited to the area within reach. This short distance requires undercorrection of minus lenses (for nearsightedness) so that the infant can see objects at close distances even if he or she is unable to accommodate or focus the lenses of the eyes. If the refractive error requires correction of the farsightedness, then a lens is an overcorrecting plus lens to make the image clear at near distance. All caregivers should try to observe the extent of the child's visual responses, noting how close various objects have to be and where they need to be placed within the visual sphere. These observations should be stressed when communicating with the ophthalmologist.

When the infant learns to sit, bifocal lenses are used. Again, the values of the correcting lenses need to correspond to the child's visual sphere: the upper part of the lens is corrected to one meter distance and the lower part of the lens to 10 cm or 20 cm distance, the distance where the infant explores objects visually. Eyeglasses often slip down on the nose and, therefore, need to have a large lower part (reading lens) placed higher than usual. Some children have less nystagmus when fixating at objects close by, either because they converge or turn their head to block nystagmus. A head tilt or turn is likely to improve the quality of the image but also may be due to *strabismus* (lack of eye coordination), so unusual head postures need to be reported to the ophthalmologist.

The effect of posture, a concern in CHARGE, often is significant. Therefore, measurements of visual acuity should be repeated in several postures to determine in which posture the infant or child can best use vision and which postures inhibit the use of vision. This information then should be communicated to the parents, educators, and other professionals working with the child. Children's therapists know the best postures for testing and the time of the day when the child is most alert. The tests also should be performed at times when the child is not functioning optimally to document the variation in visual functioning during the day.

If no reliable results can be obtained with the grating acuity test, the infant's responses to high-contrast toys can be observed during therapy sessions (Figure 2-3). Observation of the infant's functioning during therapies and in interaction with the parents and caregivers often are the most revealing situations for evaluation of visual functioning.

Visual acuity as recognition acuity matching pediatric symbols should be measured as early as possible. With training using the LEA 3D Puzzle (available from Good-Lite), visual acuity values sometimes can be measured with single symbol near test as early as 18–24 months of age. The values vary as a function of the size of the retinal coloboma between 20/20 and 20/1000; the larger the coloboma, the lower the visual acuity value.

CONTRAST SENSITIVITY

In addition to visual field and visual acuity, contrast sensitivity also should be assessed in children with CHARGE. Low-contrast vision is important in communication situations and in the exploration of low-contrast details in the environment. The Hiding Heidi test (available from Good-Lite) uses pictures of a smiling face at different contrast levels for observations on what is the lowest contrast to which the infant or child responds (Figure 2-4). If an infant responds to high-contrast pictures but not to the pictures at lower contrast levels, it is advisable to increase contrast on the faces of parents and all caretakers so that the infant can see the facial expressions.

Because high contrast can be helpful, some teachers and therapists use strong makeup (lipstick, eyeliner, eyebrow pencil) to encourage good eye contact and responses to expressions when communicating with children. Men can use brown contour pen instead of lipstick. Dark moustaches also add visual information on the face.

VISUAL BEHAVIORS

Children with CHARGE show large variation in the use of their vision and in the integration of sensory information from all modalities. In addition to the

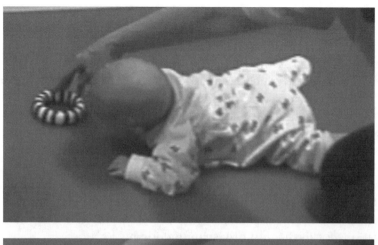

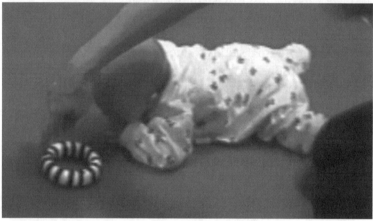

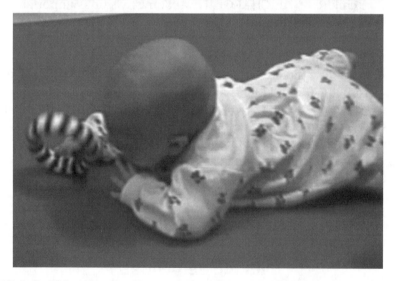

FIGURE 2–3. This infant had been diagnosed as totally blind the day before this therapy session. A young doctor described the situation to the father as, "Unfortunately, the changes in the retinas are so huge that this infant is never going to see." In a pleasant therapy situation, the infant followed the movement of the high-contrast grating pattern of the ring using head movements and grasped the ring.

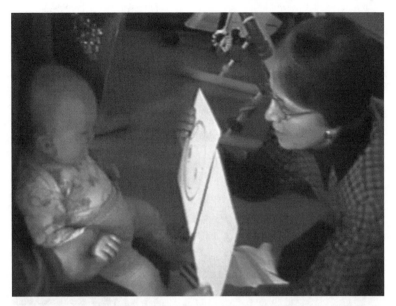

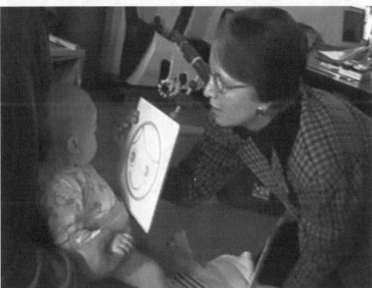

FIGURE 2–4. Testing low-contrast vision for communication with the Hiding Heidi test (Good-Lite, Chicago, IL). In this case, the infant responded to full-contrast (95%) and 25% contrast (dark gray) pictures but not to the lighter contrasts, which means that the infant is unlikely to perceive faint shadows on the faces.

impaired vision, hearing, and balance, they may have decreased sensitivity to tactile and proprioceptive information, which affects their ways of exploring (Figure 2-5). Infants may not bring their hands to the midline and from there into the mouth and, thus, do not learn to know their hands well enough to

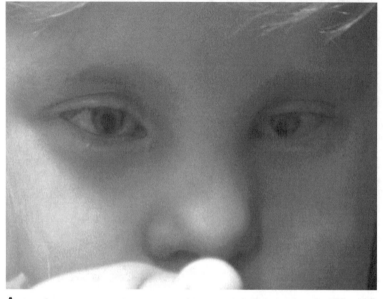

A

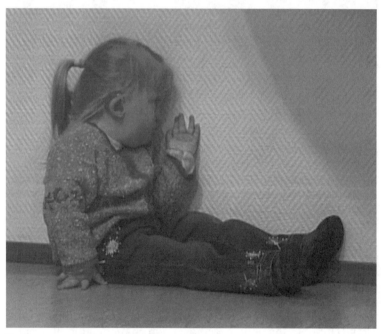

B

FIGURE 2–5. A. The right eye is slightly microphthalmic, the left more microphthalmic and strabismic, turned up and inward. **B.** The infant uses tactile information from the back of her hand and from her cheeks to explore the structure of the surface. This is a sign of too low sensitivity or hypersensitivity in the fingertips.

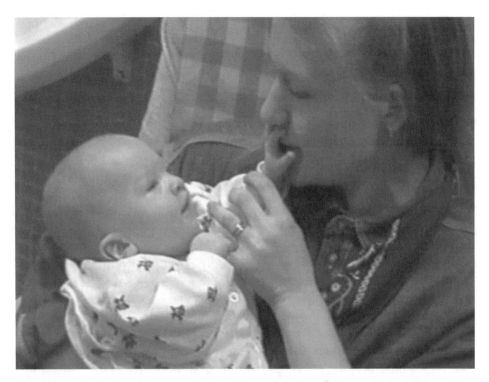

FIGURE 2–6. Infant Tadoma of a deaf infant with coloboma in both eyes. The mother helps the little hand to feel the movement of her lips and facial and neck muscles to convey the information that during communication something happens at and near the mouth.

use them when exploring details. The limited visual sphere is likely to result in specific delays in copying expressions and gestures most likely because they do not perceive this kind of visual information. Intensive training of communication and interaction as a part of early intervention activates these important functions.

If an infant has colobomas in both eyes, microphalmia, and severe vision loss, tactile information should be used from early on to support communication. Infants use modified Tadoma technique placing the little hand in turn on the lips and the neck to feel the movements related to speech (Figure 2-6).

COMPLICATIONS AND MANAGEMENT

Infants and children with coloboma are at risk for increased intraocular pressure (glaucoma) and/or detachment of the retina. If an infant or child presses on the eye ("eye poking") the risk of retinal detachment is high. Because the child does not know that the lights he or she sees are early symptoms of a retinal detachment, he or she does not report them. Any delay in the diagnosis of retinal detachment makes corrective surgery much more difficult. If the macula has been detached, central vision may remain poor. Any change in visual status should be treated as a medical emergency.

Children with an iris coloboma may be photophobic because the pupil cannot close to accommodate to varying light situations. They may be more comfortable with tinted lenses, even indoors.

Because retinal colobomas interfere with the upper visual field, children should be positioned so that they can use their lower visual field. Objects, face, and signs, should be placed within the visual field.

In preschool years, children can learn to sit still during eye exams, and the need for corrective lenses can be assessed more accurately. Depending on the child's cognitive level, use of magnifiers can be evaluated, eye-hand coordination tested in play situations, and perception of lip movements observed. If motion perception is poor at high speeds, lip movements may be so blurred that the lower part of the face disappears. This can be so unpleasant to look at that the child will look past the person who is talking but at the person's face when answering. This may be misinterpreted as an autistic feature.

Impaired vision affects all areas of development, especially the development of communication, social interaction, and motor functions. Therefore, early intervention should start without delay as an integral part of examinations and treatment. The infant should be carried well supported several hours a day. If the infant is in an intensive care unit, the parents should be allowed to have their hand on the infant as often as possible.

When the infant starts to move, the structure of the home should be explored systematically so that the child gets a good foundation for developing awareness of space and concepts related to directions and distances by measuring them with his own body.

In the day care, children need to have an intervener who is able to explain to other children how they can play with the child with CHARGE syndrome and let him learn to recognize other children using impaired sight and tactual information. Usually, all children of the small group are fond of tactual stories told on their bodies and thus learn to accept the communication of the "different child" who thus becomes less different.

In the kindergarten and at school, participating in the classroom activities can be demanding but usually is well arranged. The activities on the schoolyard often are more demanding than the classroom work. The child does not hear properly and worse-than-normal vision does not carry enough information for the child.

School age children with CHARGE should receive information about the structure of the eyes and the disorder that they have. Description of the structure of the normal eye requires good communication skills; description of the changes in the retina requires a three-dimensional model eye. It is important

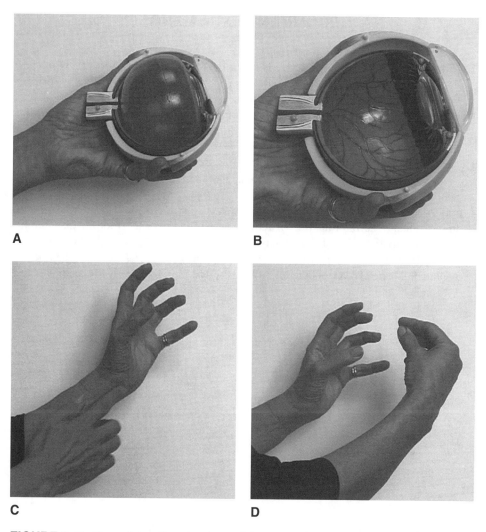

FIGURE 2–7. Describing the structure of the eyes. **A.** and **B.** The structures of the eyes are best described using a model eye. **C.** After that the hand can depict the eyeball, vessels coming in through the optic nerve head into the eye at the optic disc. **D.** Measurement of intraocular pressure with the applanation tonometry.

to describe how much normal looking retina is present rather than stress the losses of vision (Figure 2-7).

For a child his or her vision is perfect, the world seen as he or she sees it is the only known reality. It is important to explore with the child as many objects and environments as often as possible to build a bridge from the child's world to our world. It is surprising how much some children can learn if several people function as their eyes and ears supporting and interpreting the weak and distorted incoming information.

RECOMMENDED READINGS

Hyvärinen L. (1987). Assessment of vision of deaf-blind persons. In G. C. Woo (Ed.), *Low vision: Principles and applications* (pp. 386–395). New York, NY: Springer-Verlag.

Hyvärinen, L. (2007). Implications of deafblindness on visual assessment procedures: Considerations for audiologists, ophthalmologists, and interpreters. *Trends in Amplification, 11*, 227–232.

Hyvärinen, L., Gimble, L., & Sorri, M. (1990). *Assessment of vision and hearing of deaf-blind persons.* Burwood, Australia: Royal Victorian Institute for the Blind School.

Lahtinen, R. (2008). Haptices and haptemes. A case study of developmental process in social haptic communication of acquired deafblind people. Doctoral dissertation. Helsinki University, Faculty of Behavioural Sciences. Cityoffset Oy, Tampere.

Lahtinen, R. (2009). *Environmental description for visually and dual sensory impaired people.* Published by A1 Management UK. Printed by Art-Print Oy, Helsinki, Finland.

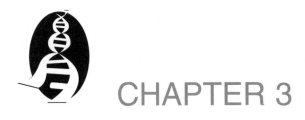

CHAPTER 3

Hearing

JAMES W. THELIN, Ph.D.

AUDIOLOGIC ISSUES

In CHARGE syndrome, hearing, balance, and mobility are related to patterns of structural anomalies of the auditory, vestibular, and visual systems. Some patterns of anomalies are common across individuals, but the group of deficits for an individual can be unique. It is of great value to an individual with CHARGE if the persons who provide care or services understand an individual's specific deficits and challenges. The purpose of the first section of this chapter is to provide information in three areas: (1) a listing of the conditions that have been reported for CHARGE with a description of how they affect individuals; (2) a description of the factors that affect audiologic measurements with notes on special adaptations of procedures that may be needed for individuals with CHARGE; and (3) examples of audiologic findings for individuals with CHARGE. Throughout this chapter, formal medical terms are used; the everyday term follows in parentheses.

Auditory Structures and Anomalies in CHARGE Syndrome

In CHARGE syndrome, every structure within the auditory system—from the external ears to the cortex of the brain—can be affected (Thelin, Mitchell, Hefner, & Davenport, 1986). From an audiologic standpoint, the most important question is, "How might these anomalies affect hearing and the development of communication?" The anomalies are listed here, and their potential consequences are discussed. Most individuals with CHARGE have some, not all, of these anomalies. It is important to know which anomalies are present for a particular individual.

External Ears

The external ear (tan color in Color Plate 3) is composed of the external ear (pinna or auricle), the external auditory canal (or ear canal), and the tympanic membrane (eardrum, purple in Color Plate 3). In CHARGE, the pinnas are nearly always malformed. The shapes of the malformed ears differ greatly, but the shapes are so distinctive that "characteristic CHARGE ear" is one of four major diagnostic criteria for the syndrome (see Chapter 8 and Color Plate 8).

The malformed pinnas and narrow ear canals rarely cause hearing loss, but they do pose problems in fitting air-conduction hearing aids. The shape of the pinna often is too irregular or shallow to fit an in-the-ear hearing aid and the cartilage that permits the pinna to maintain its position often is so soft that it will not support a behind-the-ear hearing aid. Behind-the-ear aids (the type used most often) often flop off the pinna and need to be secured with some type of device around the aid or held on the head with toupé tape. In very rare cases, the ear canal is occluded completely, and an air-conduction hearing aid cannot be used.

Middle Ears

The middle ear is an air-filled cavity (dark pink in Color Plate 3) whose lateral boundary is the tympanic membrane and that connects to the pharynx (back of the throat) though the Eustachian tube (dark pink in Color Plate 3). The eardrum is connected to the cochlea (inner ear, light brown in Color Plate 3) by three ossicles (small bones, light brown in Color Plate 3): malleus (hammer), incus (anvil), and stapes (stirrup). Movement of the tympanic membrane is transmitted through the ossicles to the footplate of the stapes, which is fitted into the oval window of the cochlea. The function of the Eustachian tube is to open nearly every time the jaw moves to equalize air pressure in the external auditory canal and inside the middle-ear cavity. If fluid exists in the middle-ear cavity, it should drain out the Eustachian tube.

The auditory purpose of the external and middle ears is to "conduct" sound from the environment to the inner ear. Hearing loss caused by either of these structures is called *conductive hearing loss*. Conductive hearing loss reduces the level of the sound reaching the inner ear. The amount of loss may be different at different sound frequencies. If the level of the sound is increased by the amount of the loss, the hearing loss is corrected.

In CHARGE, ossicular anomalies that cause conductive hearing loss are very common. The ossicular conductive losses can be very large (in the extreme, >70 dB), bilateral, but often very different in the two ears (Thelin, Mitchell,

Hefner, & Davenport, 1986). Ossicular conductive hearing loss typically is not corrected with surgical reconstruction because a significant risk of damaging the inner ear exists, which can lead to deafness in that ear. Eustachian tube dysfunction is a second cause of conductive hearing loss. If the Eustachian tube fails to ventilate the middle-ear cavity properly, a vacuum forms in the middle ear, the tympanic membrane retracts, and effusion (fluid) may accumulate in the middle-ear cavity. Tympanic membrane retraction and middle-ear effusion cause conductive hearing loss that progresses and fluctuates with middle-ear disease. This type of loss combines with ossicular conductive loss to create an even greater conductive hearing loss. Because of craniofacial anomalies and chronic respiratory problems typical of CHARGE, the vast majority of individuals with CHARGE experience Eustachian tube dysfunction. Many individuals have had multiple sets of tympanostomy tubes (PE or pressure equalization tubes) surgically inserted in the tympanic membranes to prevent middle-ear disease caused by the failure of the Eustachian tube to open the accumulation of middle-ear effusion, which can be infected and the conductive hearing loss caused by middle-ear disease.

Many individuals with CHARGE have chronic middle-ear disease that causes fluctuating hearing loss—sometimes with drainage through a perforated tympanic membrane into the ear canal. If air-conduction hearing aids are worn, the drainage may cause the hearing aid ear molds to clog and prevent the sound from reaching the ear. In some cases, drainage in the ear canals becomes a source of infection if hearing aids with ear molds are worn. With very large conductive losses, the gain must be so high that the hearing aid re-amplifies its own sound and causes a squealing sound called "feedback." Reducing hearing aid gain, to stop feedback, may result in inadequate amplification for the large hearing loss. Feedback also may occur if ear molds do not fit very snugly into the ear canals. In some cases, air-conduction hearing aids are not the best option, and bone-conduction aids are used to bypass the external and middle ears and vibrate the skull to stimulate the cochleas (if patients have normal or nearly normal function). Bone-conduction hearing aids can be worn with a head-band or surgically implanted in the skull behind the ear. ("Baha" is the brand name of the implantable bone-conduction device in current use.) (See Color Plate 4 and Figure 3–1).

Inner Ears

The inner ear is housed in the bony labyrinth (shown in light brown in Color Plate 3) in the temporal bone (shown in beige in Color Plate 3), which in turn houses membranous labyrinth (shown in light brown in Color Plate 3) that house the auditory and vestibular sense organs. These sense organs are hair cell structures that change motion, caused by sound or movement of the head, into neural activity that can be interpreted by the brain. The auditory section contains the inner ear (cochlea) that responds to sound and the vestibular section contains the structures that respond to motion. The saccule

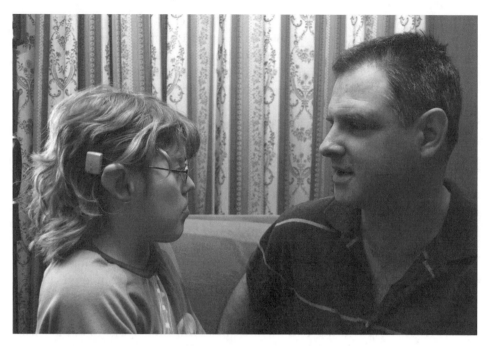

FIGURE 3–1. The Baha allows for bone conduction of sound.

and utricle respond to linear acceleration of the head, and the three semicircular canals respond to the angular acceleration of the head. The semicircular canals are linked through neural pathways in the brainstem to the eyes to form the vestibulo-ocular reflex (VOR) arc, which stabilizes visual images while the head is in motion (like a steady-cam on a video camera).

In CHARGE, it is common for the bony labyrinth to be underdeveloped, reducing the number of structures available for sensing sound and head motion (Morimoto, et al., 2006). The snail-shell shaped cochlea may have fewer turns than normal (Mondini defect is a common form of this anomaly), and, in nearly every individual with CHARGE, the semicircular canals are malformed significantly or absent (Satar, Mukherji, & Telian, 2003; Morimoto, et al., 2006). The number of hair cell sensory structures may be greatly reduced. In a vast majority of individuals with CHARGE, significant cochlear hearing loss (also called *sensorineural hearing loss*) exists, and the VOR is absent. The sensorineural losses usually are bilateral and often asymmetrical. In sensorineural hearing loss, not only are hearing thresholds elevated (as with conductive hearing loss), but the clarity of speech is reduced—and reduced the most with the largest sensorineural hearing losses. In the extreme, with severe-to-profound sensorineural loss, there may be no ability to understand speech even with the best hearing aids. In these cases, a cochlear implant is considered, in which electrodes placed in the cochlea stimulate the auditory nerve directly and bypass the nonfunctioning auditory sensory structures.

The most common form of hearing loss in CHARGE involves both senso-rineural and conductive losses, which is called *mixed hearing loss*. The distri-bution of hearing loss in CHARGE, by amount or degree of loss, is: 15% normal hearing, 38% mild-to-moderately severe loss, and 47% severe-to-profound loss (Dhooge, et al., 1998; Edwards, Van Riper, & Kileny, 1995; Shah et al., 1998; Thelin, et al., 1986).

Auditory Nerves

Cranial nerve VIII (dark yellow on the right side of Color Plate 3) is composed of auditory and vestibular sections. The nerves accept coded messages from the auditory and vestibular sensory structures and transmits them to the brainstem and then to the brain. They depart the bony labyrinth through a narrow bony channel—the internal auditory canal—and are in close proxim-ity to cranial nerve VII (the facial nerve).

In CHARGE, the auditory and vestibular nerves may be reduced in size or absent (Bamiou, Worth, Phelps, Sirimanna, & Rajput, 2001; Morimoto, et al., 2006). If the auditory nerve or the bony channel in which it is situated is narrow, opinions differ as to whether CI is acceptable or contraindicated (Morita, et al., 2004; Nadol, 1997; Nadol & Xu, 1992; Shelton, Luxford, Tonokawa, Lo, & House, 1989). The decision for use of a cochlear implant to overcome hearing loss is based on estimates of neural integrity of the auditory nerve based on anatomic images obtained with computerized tomography and magnetic resonance imaging. These images are used to show the presence or absence of neural fibers and of openings in the bone through which the neural fibers must pass. Cochlear implantation may be contraindicated if the auditory nerve does not appear to have an adequate diameter. Another factor in CHARGE is that the facial nerve may be located such that it is stim-ulated by a cochlear implant, which can result in contractions of facial muscles caused by acoustic stimulation (MacArdle, et al., 2002).

Central Auditory Nervous System

The auditory nerve divides and sends neural tracts to both sides of the brain-stem and both hemispheres of the cortex. At the cortical level, information can travel from the auditory cortex in one hemisphere to the other hemisphere via a crossing fiber tract called the *corpus callosum*. Much of the knowledge of the central auditory nervous system has been gained from physiologic tests of auditory function in which electrodes that are attached to the head meas-ure neural responses to sound. These are called auditory-evoked potentials; the most well-known is the auditory brainstem response (ABR or BAER). The ABR has the advantage that it can be measured while the individual is asleep or sedated. Other knowledge of central auditory processing (CAP) is obtained through complex behavioral testing in which the listener is required to sepa-rate or combine signals presented to the same or to opposite ears. These behavioral tests require the ability to use symbolic communication and the ability to understand instructions at the level of a typically developing child at age 6 or 7 years. Abnormal central auditory function does not cause hearing loss but rather results in the inability to process complex signals. Central auditory dysfunction cannot be overcome with a hearing aid or cochlear implant but can sometimes be assisted by FM auditory listening devices that improve the listening situation by suppressing background noise.

In CHARGE, the peripheral hearing loss (conductive and sensorineural) often is so great that it is difficult to obtain useful measurements of auditory-evoked potentials or behavioral tests of central auditory processing. Evidence from various sources demonstrates that central structures (brain) and function can be affected (see Table 13–2, Chapter 13). If central function is not normal, it would mean that the peripheral hearing loss is compounded by the diminished ability of the brain to process what has been heard.

Audiologic Assessment

The primary objectives of audiologic assessment is to obtain measurements of hearing or auditory function that can be used for two purposes: (1) to determine whether there is hearing loss that warrants the fitting of amplification and (2) to obtain a description of the hearing in each ear that will enable the selection of the appropriate hearing aid for each ear. Because individuals with CHARGE often are very difficult to test, audiologists may need to adapt their procedures and develop a strategy so that an adequate description of the hearing needs can be obtained in the shortest amount of time. This may require multiple test sessions in which limited goals are achieved in each session.

Reports have been received from some parents that the same basic audiologic procedures have been repeated without modification and without a special strategy, and the individual's hearing has not been specified after seven years of audiologic testing. In these cases, a modification of procedures may help to gain the needed results more rapidly The information provided here is an attempt to increase the likelihood of success in audiologic assessment for audiologists and others who care for and provide services to individuals with CHARGE. Individuals with CHARGE may have deficits in every sensory modality that can be so isolating and frustrating that the individual's only means of communication may be disruptive or self-destructive behavior. Hearing is an important sense that can be improved to open channels of communication with the world. Prompt and adequate audiologic assessment and treatment are very high priorities for individuals with CHARGE.

The most important audiologic results are thresholds of hearing for each ear obtained at different frequencies using pure-tone signals. The results are recorded on a *pure-tone audiogram*. The thresholds are obtained using earphones or insert earphones for air-conducted signals. (Results obtained using loudspeakers in the sound field are used to specify hearing in the better ear, but the hearing needs to be known in the two ears separately to fit hearing aids.) Pure-tone air-conduction thresholds indicate the *total* or *overall* hearing loss at test frequencies across the range of audible frequencies. Pure-tone bone-conduction thresholds indicate the amount of sensorineural hearing loss at each frequency. A bone-conduction vibrator placed on the skull is used to vibrate the cochlea directly. The difference between the air- and bone-conduction thresholds (air-bone gap) is the amount of conductive hearing loss. The most complete pure tone audiogram that can be obtained is the information that is needed to fit amplification in each ear. The information can be obtained with behavioral audiometry or with ABR tests.

Behavioral Tests of Hearing

Behavioral audiologic tests require the cooperation of the individual being tested, but the tests can be adapted to gain information when only minimal cooperation can be obtained. Pure-tone thresholds may be measured using a variety of responses: hand-button presses, hand-raises, conditioned play with small toys dropped into a bucket, or use of special response systems with big buttons and visual reinforcement for correct responses.

Speech thresholds and speech understanding may be measured using a variety of responses: spoken responses of words heard, pointing to pictures, and pointing to body parts. In one case, a 27-year-old male who was profoundly intellectually challenged communicated with the hearing examiner with utterances of "uh," "uh-uh," and "uh-uh-uh." Speech detection thresholds were obtained by air- and bone-conduction, and it was determined that this individual had a 60-dB hearing loss for speech that was composed of a 20-dB conductive loss and a 40-dB sensorineural loss.

A number of factors need to be considered that can pose obstacles to the behavioral evaluation of hearing:

Behavioral Issues. See also Chapter 28 for information on behavioral issues.

An individual with CHARGE may exhibit autistic-like behaviors, adaptive behaviors related to difficulties with sensory integration, obsessive compulsive behaviors, disruptive behaviors, and anxiety—all related to sensory and physical deficits that are specific to that individual. It is a great advantage to the audiologist if the individual is accompanied by a caregiver or professional who knows the individual well and can indicate the activities and conditions in which the individual with CHARGE can participate. In some cases, multiple visits may be required to familiarize the individual who has CHARGE with the test environment and tasks. Test procedures, such as putting on earphones, and behavioral responses can be practiced at home before the audiologic evaluation. In some cases, hearing test procedures are included with aural habilitation therapy, and the child with CHARGE benefits from working with a therapist with whom he or she is familiar.

Tactile Defensiveness. Children with CHARGE whose early lives are often a series of visits to physicians and hospitalizations for serious conditions are often resistant to contact with professionals.

Respiration. Individuals with respiratory problems may have difficulty listening at the threshold of hearing.

Symbolic Communication. See also Part IV. Communication development is almost universally delayed in CHARGE—often by years.

Ocular Colobomas. See Chapter 2. Colobomas create holes in the visual fields. For optimal vision, an individual may not look straight ahead but rather at some other angle to avoid a void in the visual field. This may change the interpretation of a head turn as a localizing response.

Communication Bubble. The auditory and visual deficits in CHARGE may restrict the distances and locations at which personal communication can be conducted optimally or even acceptably. The talker needs to be situated within a "communication bubble," in which the talker can be seen and heard. The size and configuration of the communication bubble will be dictated in part by voice levels, background noise, and ambient lighting.

Physiologic Tests of Auditory Function

Behavioral tests of hearing require a response that indicates that the listener heard the sound and interpreted it in a meaningful manner; the results of these tests are the best measures of hearing in its fullest sense. Physiologic tests of auditory function test aspects of activity in selected parts of the auditory system, but not hearing as a whole. The following is a list of auditory physiologic procedures that are commonly used in the clinical audiologic evaluation with comments issues related to CHARGE syndrome:

Auditory Brainstem Response. In ABR, electrical responses from the brainstem can be used to obtain frequency-specific and ear-specific estimates of hearing thresholds that are related closely to behavioral thresholds of hearing. ABR thresholds are used as estimates of hearing thresholds—especially when it is not possible to obtain valid behavioral thresholds of hearing. ABR threshold estimates can be used to fit hearing aids. ABR data does not indicate whether information is being processed in the brain. Two factors need to be considered if ABR tests are performed under sedation: (1) individuals with CHARGE are often medically fragile and (2) individuals with CHARGE can be resistant to sedation.

Electrocochleography (ECochG). This test is similar to ABR except that electrical activity is measured from the cochlea rather than the brainstem. ABR tests are used much more frequently.

Tympanometry and Acoustic Reflex Measurements. These are measurement in which sound reflected off the tympanic membrane is used to assess middle-ear function and sensory and neural structures in the lower part of the auditory system. If Eustachian tube dysfunction and middle-ear disease exists, as is so common in CHARGE, these measures often provide little useful information about hearing. Tympanometry is a test of middle-ear function that can be measured easily, but it is not a test of hearing.

Otoacoustic Emissions. With otoacoustic emissions (OAEs; transient evoked OAEs (TEOAEs); and or distortion product OAEs (DPOAEs), the function of the outer hair cells in the cochlea are assessed by passing a sound from the ear canal through the middle ear into the cochlea and measuring the sound that returns to the ear canal. Typically, OAEs have little value in the assessment of hearing in CHARGE because the responses are obliterated by middle-ear disease and sensorineural hearing loss.

Examples of Hearing Loss in CHARGE Syndrome

As with nearly every aspect of the disorders in CHARGE, no typical hearing loss can be determined. The purpose of the following section is to give examples of some audiologic findings that are common and some that are extraordinary. This information is expected to be of greatest value to audiologists.

Asymmetrical Mixed Hearing Losses

The pure tone thresholds are shown on the audiograms in Figure 3–2 for a 58-year-old female with CHARGE. The total loss is much greater in the right ear (severe) than in the left ear (mild–moderate). In the right ear, both the middle ear and the cochlea are affected more than in the right ear. The middle-ear or conductive losses are due to ossicular anomalies. This amount of asymmetry in hearing loss and types of hearing loss is not common and requires comprehensive test procedures to evaluate the status of the ears properly.

This is a rare case of familial CHARGE syndrome in which the affected individuals include the woman whose audiograms are shown, her mother, her brother (one of her four siblings), and at least three of her nine children (Mitchell, Giangiacomo, Hefner, Thelin, & Pickens, 1985). Among the affected individuals in this family, auditory anomalies were found in all, but the degree of hearing loss ranged from normal to profound.

Asymmetrical Mixed Hearing Losses with Special Challenges

In Figure 3–3, the audiometric results are shown for a 21-year-old female with CHARGE syndrome. In the right ear, there is a mild mixed loss in the lower frequencies (below 2000 Hz). This loss was caused by a combination of ossicular anomalies and a long history of chronic middle-ear disease that caused the

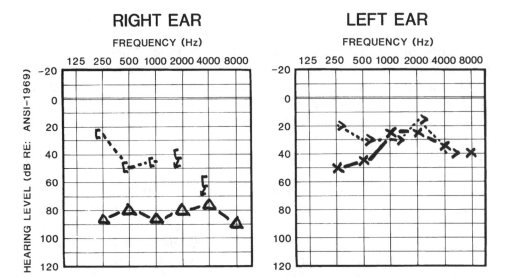

FIGURE 3–2. Pure-tone audiograms for a 58-year-old female with CHARGE syndrome. Right ear masked pure-tone thresholds: triangles are for conduction and brackets are for bone conduction. Left ear unmasked pure-tone thresholds: crosses are for air-conduction and "greater than" symbols are for bone conduction.

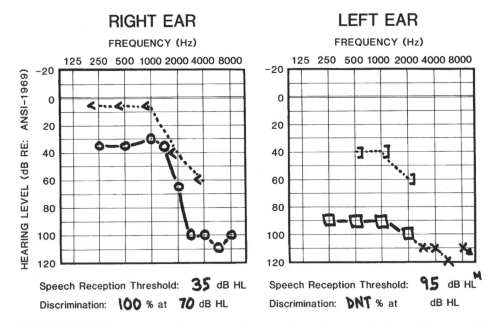

Speech Reception Threshold: **35** dB HL   Speech Reception Threshold: **95** dB HL^M

Discrimination: **100** % at **70** dB HL   Discrimination: **DNT** % at   dB HL

FIGURE 3–3. Pure-tone audiograms with speech testing results for a 21-year-old female with CHARGE syndrome. Right ear unmasked pure-tone thresholds: circles are for air-conduction thresholds and "less than" symbols are for bone-conduction thresholds. Left ear pure-tone thresholds: squares are for masked air-conduction thresholds; crosses are for unmasked air-conduction thresholds; right brackets are for masked bone-conduction thresholds.

ear to drain and interfere with hearing aid use. The cochlea was functioning normally, so no sensorineural hearing loss is experienced in this part of the frequency range. With the hearing in these lower frequencies in only the right ear, this young woman should have been able to do well understanding speech and in general communication while wearing a hearing aid.

In the higher frequencies (above 3000 Hz), the overall hearing loss is profound. Sounds in this frequency region cannot be adequately amplified with a hearing aid, and as a result, do not contribute to this individual's understanding of speech—especially for consonant sounds (e.g., "-s" and "-ed") that carry a great deal of information in spoken English. However, the results for the speech-reception threshold indicate a mild hearing loss (35 dB) and an excellent ability to understand speech that includes consonant sounds (100%) with no background noise when the speech was at a very high level (70 dB HL). Thus, under ideal listening conditions and with her hearing aid, this individual could be expected to detect and understand speech well. If speech levels are reduced or in the presence of background noise, the ability to understand speech would be compromised.

In the left ear, a profound mixed loss is present due to congenital ossicular anomalies, active middle-ear disease, and significant damage to the cochlea. No form of amplification in the left ear can improve this individual's ability to use this ear effectively. She relies on the hearing in the right ear alone.

Further complicating the picture, this individual has active middle-ear disease in the right ear, and she is not able to wear her hearing aid all of the time. During these periods, she has a mild hearing loss that is not corrected. As a result, even though she ought to be depending totally on communication through the auditory channel, she relies on American Sign Language (ASL) in addition to spoken language.

This individual has another problem that is common to individuals who have significant conductive losses with normal cochlear hearing but is not often described. With her low-frequency conductive hearing loss, this person hears her own internal noises much louder than do those without this conductive loss. When she chews gum or food, the noise masks incoming sounds, and she is unable to understand a talker standing in front of her or sitting across from her at a dinner table. The audiometric results for this individual illustrate the complexities of the hearing problems that can be encountered with CHARGE syndrome.

Very Large Bilateral Ossicular Conductive Hearing Losses

The results shown in Figure 3–4 illustrate the largest conductive losses that the author has ever found with CHARGE syndrome or any other disorder. Bone-conduction thresholds for this 12-year-old male with CHARGE were measured for only the right ear and are assumed to be the same in the left ear. The average conductive loss measured with standard supra-aural earphones is 67 dB in the right ear and 78 dB in the left ear.

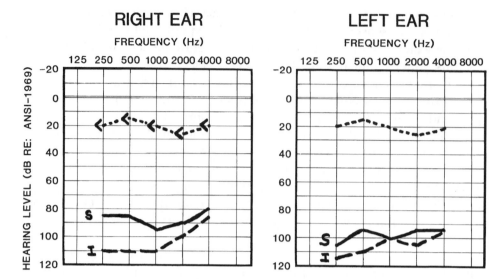

FIGURE 3–4. Audiograms for 12-year-old male with CHARGE syndrome. "S" and the solid line are for unmasked pure-tone, air-conduction thresholds obtained using supra-aural earphones. "I" and the dashed line are for unmasked pure-tone thresholds obtained using insert earphones. "Less than" symbol is for unmasked pure-tone, bone-conduction thresholds measured on the right mastoid; the dotted lines indicate these thresholds for both ears.

The thresholds then were remeasured using insert earphones that more closely approximated the signals that would be delivered by a behind-the-ear hearing aid: the thresholds worsened by 16 dB in the right ear and 7 dB in the left ear. These shifts occurred because the conductive losses are so large that the signals from the standard supra-aural earphones are so intense that the earphone acts as a bone vibrator. The thresholds obtained with insert earphones are closer to what would be expected with hearing aids. With standard supra-aural earphones, in this special case, the amount of the loss was underestimated, and the power requirements for the hearing aid were underestimated as well.

The measurement of hearing and the treatment of hearing loss with CHARGE syndrome can challenge even the most experienced pediatric audiologist. The unique anomalies, behaviors, and technical considerations for evaluating an individual with CHARGE syndrome require special professional attention. However, it is critical to note that the successful management of hearing loss has been shown to be highly-correlated with the development of symbolic communication that can enable an individual with CHARGE, who might otherwise be isolated, to communicate with the world at large (Thelin & Fussner, 2005).

AMPLIFICATION

A large majority of individuals with CHARGE have hearing loss and can benefit from some form of amplification. In most cases, the goal of amplification is to make speech audible so that communication can develop through the auditory channel and symbolic language can be learned. However, a significant percentage of those with CHARGE will not develop spoken language even with the optimal form of amplification. But for those individuals, often other benefits such as awareness of speech and environmental sounds may contribute greatly to the individual's sensory input and orientation in the environment. The criterion for successful amplification is that it is worn regularly and that it contributes to any aspect of perception that frees the individual from sensory isolation. If communication using some form of amplification is not possible, signed language can be used by itself or in combination with spoken language (total communication) as the means to establish symbolic language. Many individuals with CHARGE use both signed and spoken language.

The greatest chance for the acquisition of symbolic language occurs when hearing loss is treated successfully by six months of age (Yoshinaga-Itano, Sedey, Coulter, & Mehl, 1998). If amplification or other treatment is provided months or years later, the chances for the development of normal language decrease. However, if hearing loss is present or suspected, attempts need to be made to fit amplification *regardless of the age of the individual or the prognosis*. Children with CHARGE have the great ability to reach milestones of development and learning well beyond expected ages (see Chapter 24, "Life Cycle"). Delayed achievement, such as developing language abilities unexpectedly when amplification is used, is a great source of gratification for parents and a pleasant surprise for professionals.

Significantly, Thelin and Fussner (2005) found that acquisition of symbolic language is not related to the degree of hearing loss. Some individuals with moderate hearing losses have a great deal of difficulty hearing, understanding, and communicating—even with amplification. At the same time, some individuals with severe-to-profound hearing losses use amplification successfully and use spoken language. Thelin and Fussner (2005) also found that the acquisition of symbolic language *was* related to the initiation of communication therapy by three years of age; this included therapy using spoken language, signed language, or both. One young adult with CHARGE commented that her thought processes for spoken and signed language are different and that they reinforce each other when she wishes to express herself.

A number of options for amplification are used by children with CHARGE. The choice of a particular option depends on sensory, behavioral, anatomical, physiological, and medical factors. Parents who have discussed hearing with other parents often will become aware of a solution that has worked well for one child and will seek information about that particular instrument or device for their own child. Because the types and degrees of the hearing loss differ so greatly from child to child, the solution for one child with CHARGE may be inappropriate for another child. In the following sections, an overview is presented of several different forms of amplification that are used by individuals with CHARGE.

Air-Conduction Hearing Aids

Air-conduction hearing aids have microphones that sense incoming sound, amplify/process the sound, and deliver the sound to the eardrum. The most common form of these aids are behind-the-ear (BTE) aids that are situated on and behind the ear with a tube routing sound from the aid to an ear mold fitted in the ear canal. An important feature of these aids is that the microphones pick up sound in natural locations—near the ears. These are the most common types of hearing aids. Contemporary BTE aids are really computers that perform many transformations on incoming signals. The sound in specific frequency regions is adjusted to be maximally audible without being intolerably loud for a particular ear. BTE aids can be used for losses ranging from mild to profound. In most cases, the first attempts at amplification are made with BTE hearing aids. It is the form of amplification with which audiologists are most familiar. If BTE aids do not provide adequate benefit, other forms of amplification will be considered.

Before hearing aids can be fitted, the individual's hearing must have been determined separately for the two ears. This is especially true for those with CHARGE, because the type and degree of hearing loss often are very different in the two ears. Before amplification is fitted, ear-specific and frequency-specific hearing thresholds should be obtained or estimated using behavioral audiometry or auditory brainstem responses.

FM auditory trainers are special devices that are designed to minimize background noise (or improve the signal-to-noise ratio). With an FM system, a parent, therapist, or classroom teacher wears a microphone that picks up the voice with a minimum of background noise and transmits a radio-frequency signal to a receiver (boot) attached to the individual's hearing aid. The individual wearing the FM auditory trainer is able to hear that one person optimally, which can be a great advantage if the individual's best hearing is poor.

Frequency transposition hearing aids are BTE hearing aids that move sound energy from one frequency region to another. The purpose is to move information that is important for understanding speech from a frequency region of inaudibility to a region of audibility.

Although BTE hearing aids typically provide a great deal of benefit, a number of obstacles to their successful use are common for those with CHARGE. Some of these obstacles are as follows:

■ Misshapen pinnas with soft cartilage may not support BTE hearing aids well (Figure 3–5). The aids may fall off the ears and may need

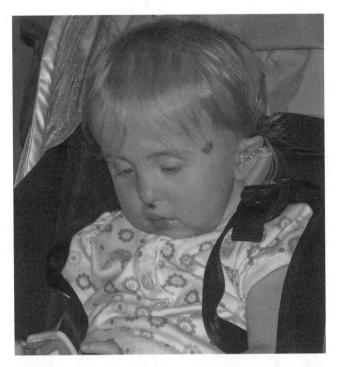

FIGURE 3–5. The floppy ear cartilage seen in CHARGE often makes it difficult to keep BTE aids on the ear.

to be held in place with toupé tape, a "*huggie*" which secures the aid to the ear, or other device.

■ Narrow ear canals may cause difficulties in making ear molds and keeping their sound channels clear.

■ Middle-ear effusion draining through a perforated eardrum may clog a hearing aid ear mold and prevent the sound from reaching the ear. If there is drainage in the ear canal, the use of an ear mold may be contraindicated medically.

■ With the large hearing losses that are common in CHARGE, very high levels of amplification may be required—especially with large conductive components. If the ear mold does not fit securely (and, in some cases, even when it does fit securely), squealing feedback may occur. Squealing feedback is can be very audible to the hearing aid user as well as to others who are nearby. The squealing masks audible signals. The squealing can be eliminated by reducing the gain of the hearing aid, which may greatly compromise or eliminate the benefit of the device. Manufacturers recently have developed hearing aids that utilize blue tooth technology to minimize feedback in cases in which large amounts of gain are required.

■ BTE aids (and all other types of amplification) need to be checked one or more times each day to determine that they are functioning properly.

Two other types of air-conduction aids deserve mention: in-the-ear (ITE) aids and body-worn aids. ITE aids fit completely inside the pinna. Typically, the ear canals of individuals with CHARGE are too small to house them, and they usually do not have enough gain to amplify properly. Also, when the pinna and ear canal grow, the replacement procedure involves mailing the hearing aid to the manufacturer for a week or so. (With BTE aids, the old ear mold is used while the new one is being fabricated.) Body-worn aids have a hearing aid "box" that fits into a pocket, a long cord, a receiver, and an ear mold. This was the style of hearing aids used 50 years ago. If the individual is not mobile or if very large amounts of gain are needed, a body-worn aid may be recommended.

Bone-Conduction Hearing Aids

This is hearing aid for a person with a large conductive hearing loss or conductive loss with not too much cochlear loss. With this type of aid, a bone-conduction oscillator or vibrator is placed on some part of the skull; and it stimulates both cochleas, which are embedded in the temporal bone of the skull. If the cochlea is functioning normally, the individual will be able to hear normally regardless of the conductive hearing loss. A small percentage of individuals with CHARGE have this type of loss. A majority have mixed loss with significant cochlear loss in the high frequencies. In these cases, a bone conduction aid will produce sound that is missing the high frequencies. Speech would be audible but unintelligible. Thus, bone-conduction aids are appropriate for only a small percentage of individuals with CHARGE. A standard bone-conduction hearing aid is held on the head with a cumbersome spring-steel head band. A preliminary trial for the aid can be conducted easily by putting the aid on and viewing the response of the person wearing it. A more extensive trial includes the measurement of hearing thresholds across the range of audible frequencies.

Standard bone-conduction hearing aids are uncomfortable to wear and have low fidelity. An implanted version of the bone-conduction aid, the Cochlear Corporation Baha [bone-anchored hearing aid], has a titanium screw embedded in the skull behind an ear (see Color Plate 4). The Baha attaches to the screw and forms a very firm coupling to the skull. With this coupling, amplification and fidelity are better than with a standard bone-conduction aid. The Baha can provide more amplification than the standard bone-conduction aid. As a result, individuals with mixed loss may be suitable candidates for implantation. Success with Baha is dependent upon the acceptance of the screw by the skull and by maintaining hygiene in the hole in the skin around the screw.

Anecdotally, some parents of children with CHARGE report great satisfaction with Baha implantation, and other parents were very disappointed. The reasons for these findings have not yet been described in the literature.

Hearing loss can be overcome with air- or bone-conduction amplification if the cochlea is capable of encoding a message that can be interpreted by the brain. If the cochlea cannot perform that function, then amplification is of little value, and cochlear implantation is considered as a means of delivering the neural signal to the brain (see Chapter 9, "Cochlear Implantation").

REFERENCES

Bamiou, D. E., Worth, S., Phelps, P., Sirimanna, T., & Rajput, K. (2001). Eighth nerve aplasia and hypoplasia in cochlear implant candidates: the clinical perspective. *Otology and Neurotology, 22*, 492-496.

Bauer, P. W., Wippold, F. J., 2nd, Goldin, J., & Lusk, R. P. (2002). Cochlear implantation in children with CHARGE syndrome. *Archives of Ototlaryngology Head and Neck Surgery, 128*, 1013-1017.

Dhooge, L., Lemmerling, M., Lagache, M., Standaert, L., Govaert, P., & Mortier, G. (1998). Otological manifestations of CHARGE association. *Annals of Otology, Rhinology, and Laryngology, 107*, 935-941.

Edwards, B. M., Van Riper, L. A., & Kileny, P. R. (1995). Clinical manifestations of CHARGE Association. *International Journal of Pediatric Otorhinolaryngology, 33*, 23-42.

Lanson, B. G., Green, J. E., Roland, J. T., Jr., Lalwani, A. K., & Waltzman, S. B. (2007). Cochlear implantation in children with CHARGE syndrome: Therapeutic decisions and outcomes. *Laryngoscope, 117*, 1260-1266.

MacArdle, B. M., Bailey, C., Phelps, P. D., Bradley , J., Brown, T., & Wheeler, A. (2002). Cochlear implants in children with craniofacial syndromes: assessment and outcomes. *International Journal of Audiology, 41*, 347-356.

Mitchell, J. A, Giangiacomo, J., Hefner, M. A., Thelin, J. W., & Pickens, J. M. (1985). Dominant CHARGE Association. *Ophthalmic Paediatric Genetics, 6*, 271-276.

Morimoto, A. K., Wiggins, R. H., 3rd, Hudgins, P. A., Hedlund, G. L., Hamilton, B., Mukherji, S. K., . . . Harnsberger, H. R. (2006). Absent semicircular canals in CHARGE syndrome: Radiologic spectrum of findings. *American Journal of Neuroradiology, 27*(8), 1663-1671.

Morita, T., Naito, Y., Tsuji, J., Nakamura, T., Yamaguchi, S., & Ito, J. (2004). Relationship between cochlear implant outcome and the diameter of the cochlear nerve depicted on MRI. *Acta Otolaryngologica, Supplement 551*, 56-59.

Nadol, J. B., Jr. (1997). Patterns of neural degeneration in the human cochlea and auditory nerve: implications for cochlear implantation. *Otolaryngology-Head and Neck Surgery, 117*(3 Pt 1), 220-228.

Nadol, J. B., Jr., & Xu, W. Z., (1992). Diameter of the cochlear nerve in deaf humans: implications for cochlear implantation. *Annals of Otology, Rhinology, and Laryngology, 101*, 988-993.

Satar, B., Mukherji, S. K., & Telian, S. A. (2003). Congenital aplasia of the semicircular canals. *Otology and Neurotology,24*, 437-446.

Shah, U. D., Ohlms, L. A., Neault, M. W., Willson, K. D., McGuirt, W. F., Hobbs, N., . . . Healy, G. B. (1998). Otologic management in children with CHARGE association. *International Journal of Pediatric Otorhinlaryngology, 44,* 139–147.

Shelton, C., Luxford, W. M., Tonokawa, L. L., Lo, W. W., & House, W. F. (1989). The narrow internal auditory canal in children: a contraindication to cochlear implants. *Otolaryngology-Head and Neck Surgery, 100,* 227–231.

Stremel-Thomas, K., & Bashinski, S. M. (2009, July). *Impact of cochlear implants in CHARGE syndrome: Preliminary findings.* Paper presented at the meeting of the 9th International CHARGE Syndrome Conference, Chicago, IL.

Thelin, J. W., & Fussner, J. C. (2005). Factors related to the development of communication in CHARGE syndrome. *American Journal of Medical Genetics, 133A,* 282–290.

Thelin, J. W., Mitchell, J. A., Hefner, M. A., & Davenport, S. L. H. (1986). CHARGE syndrome. Part II. Hearing loss. *International Journal of Pediatric Otorhinolaryngology, 12,* 145–163.

Yoshinaga-Itano, C., Sedey, A. L., Coulter, D. K., & Mehl, A. L. (1998). Language of early- and later-identified children with hearing loss. *Pediatrics, 102,* 1161–1171.

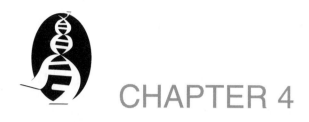

CHAPTER 4

Overview of Balance and the Vestibular System

CLAES MÖLLER, M.D., Ph.D.

*T*he ability to walk upright on two legs and keep equilibrium is dependent on the integrity of a complex system consisting of three major receptor organs: the vestibular, the visual, and the somatosensory systems (see Color Plate 6). The impulses from the vestibular (labyrinth) part of the inner ear, the eyes, and the stimuli from skin muscles, tendons, and joints (somatosensory) are so harmoniously balanced that, under normal conditions, they are well integrated. Afferent (incoming) signals from all three systems are conveyed into the brainstem and cerebellum where they are processed and then transmitted through efferent (outgoing) nerve fibers, mainly to muscles and eyes to maintain coordinated movements.

Assessment of these three systems and the central nervous processing in the brain is essential when evaluating children and adults with CHARGE syndrome because most persons with CHARGE have malformed vestibular organs, diminished or absent signals, and balance problems along with vision loss which will give severe balance problems especially at night. Ideally, the assessment of an individual always should include tests of the vestibular organs, the eyes, somato-sensation and tests of integration of these signals in the brain.

THE VESTIBULAR SYSTEM

The vestibular system is a sensory system that has access to the cerebral cortex with conscious perception and memory, but also a system regulating body posture and eye position. Five different parts of the vestibular organ are of special importance (Figure 4-1). The vestibular system is also called "the labyrinth" due to the complicated structure. Five different parts manage to monitor balance of the head by estimating movements in all directions, acceleration, deceleration and also the gravity. These five components are called the utriculus, sacculus and the three semicircular canals which are oriented perpendicular to one another in order to record all type of head movements (back-forward, side to side, turning, etc).

The vestibular part of the inner ear is filled with the same fluid as in the cochlea (peri and endolymph). The hair cells are joined together in a "swinging door," called the cupula, where they react with excitation (electrical impulses) in response to endolymph movements. When the head is turned, the flow of the endolymph in the semicircular canals will be clockwise in one ear and counter-clockwise in the other. This will result in an excitation in one

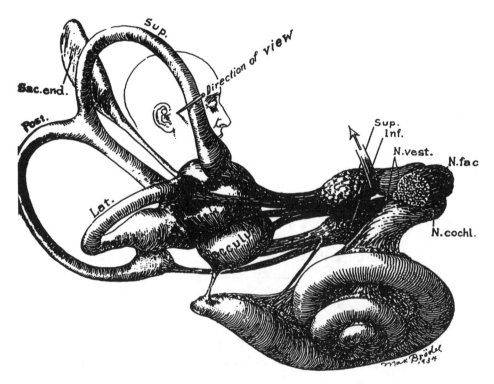

FIGURE 4–1. The inner ear. Courtesy of Claes Möller.

ear and an inhibition in the other, acting like a swing. The signals pass to the brainstem through the vestibular nerve (close to the auditory nerve) where they send their electrical impulses to the vestibular nuclei, which will pass the signal in two different directions. One direction is through cranial nerves to the muscles of the eyes in order to direct the eyes so that they can move in the opposite direction and speed as compared to the head. This reflex (vestibulo-ocular reflex, VOR, Figure 4–2) is in place to keep a steady image on the retina—the biological equivalent of a steady cam. The result is that the eyes move slowly in the opposite direction of the head, and when they reach their maximal position to the side, a quick-restoring eye movement moves the eye back to the central position. This eye movement is called *nystagmus*. If this reflex is not functioning, as in many individuals with CHARGE, performing quick head movements will not produce nystagmus, and the image will be blurry. The other pathway from the vestibular organ is through the cerebellum, which is the part of the brain that "organizes" movements to make them smooth.

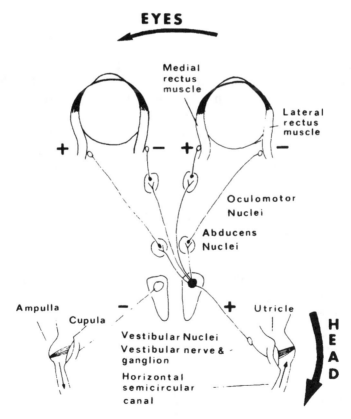

FIGURE 4–2. The Vestibular Ocular Reflex (VOR). Courtesy of Claes Möller.

THE VISUAL SYSTEM

The visual system can have fast eye movements (saccades) and slow ones (smooth pursuit). The aim of the saccades is to direct the gaze toward an object. Smooth pursuit refers to tracking: stabilizing a moving target on the fovea (retina) by producing eye velocities closely matching the target. Smooth pursuit works closely with the vestibular system. Smooth pursuit is most effective when tracking objects at low frequencies and speed, while the vestibular system is most effective at high frequencies.

In daily life activities, humans perform visual tracking by a combination of smooth pursuit, saccadic, vergence eye movements (the eyes converge on an object) together with the vestibulo-ocular reflex. A person with CHARGE who has large colobomas and vestibular areflexia (no vestibular signals) will have significant difficulties in spotting a target, tracking, and with balance since the eyes will not move correctly, and the picture will not be located steadily on the same place in the retina.

THE SOMATOSENSORY SYSTEM

The somatosensory system relates to multiple types of sensations in the body, including touch, pressure, pain, and muscle position. This system has a high degree of complexity, including contraction and relaxation in opposing muscle groups. Most of these reflexes work intimately with input from the vestibular and visual system. Many individuals with CHARGE have not only vestibular and visual dysfunction, but also cranial nerve pathologies that result in decreased function in some facial and neck muscles.

THE CEREBELLUM

The vestibular signals communicate with visual and somatosensory signals through the cerebellum in the back of the brain. The cerebellum often acts as an inhibitor on the vestibulo-ocular reflex. Other locations in the brainstem also will compare and moderate the signals from these three systems. Coordination of these systems is crucial for the development of normal motor milestones (see the following section) in a small child.

ASSESSMENT OF BALANCE AND VESTIBULAR FUNCTION

Identification and diagnosis of balance dysfunction is generally difficult. In adults, the case history and a thorough test battery is of utmost importance.

In children, it is more difficult to get a good case history, and some of the tests cannot be performed.

Children and adults with CHARGE have significant balance problems due to bilateral vestibular areflexia, deafness, decreased vision (deafblindness), and sometimes weak muscles, paralysis, etc. Most children with CHARGE that this author has examined (~30) have significantly delayed motor milestones in which a walking age of 4–5 years is common. When a child is suspected of having a balance disorder, it is wise to develop a strategy of down-to-earth questions, balance assessment, and most importantly, observation of the child.

One of the first symptoms in a young child with bilateral vestibular areflexia or severe vestibular dysfunction is delayed motor milestones. Before a correct diagnosis is made, many children with a bilateral vestibular areflexia are as "floppy infants," which leads to a suspicion of other CNS disorders. Questions concerning a child with late motor milestones should focus on certain events that parents might remember. Examples of questions directed toward a suspicion of bilateral vestibular hypofunction or areflexia are shown in Table 4–1. In a child with a complete bilateral vestibular loss, milestones will be delayed and all questions except motion sickness will be answered "yes." A person with bilateral vestibular areflexia cannot experience motion sickness.

ASSESSMENT

Balance assessment is, of course, dependent on the age of the child, but many tests can be performed from a very early age. A thorough ear, nose, and throat evaluation is mandatory along with assessment of cranial nerves, muscle, and

TABLE 4–1. Examples of Questions to Look for Decreased or Absent Vestibular Function

At what age did the child lift his head, roll around?

At what age did the child sit unsupported?

At what age did the child start to crawl, and in what way?

At what age did the child walk unsupported?

Did the child experience difficulties in learning to bicycle?

Does the child have problems when walking in darkness and on uneven surfaces?

Does the child experience motion sickness?

Does the child have problems in gymnastics and sport activities?

Is the child considered to be clumsy?

deep tendon evaluation. The performance in young children shows a large variation and depends on cooperation between the examiner, the child, and parent. This is, of course, even more so in a child with CHARGE. Standing on two legs closely together with closed eyes is very difficult to do if there is a bilateral vestibular loss, and standing on one leg with closed eyes is impossible.

Observation of the child during daily activities in different settings and light conditions with different visual vestibular and somatosensory stimuli can be time consuming but helpful. For instance, very young children with CHARGE prefer to scoot on their backs or crawl with their heads down on the ground. This is probably due to the bilateral vestibular loss combined with severely reduced vision. Older children have problems walking on uneven ground, performing certain tasks in the gymnasium like walking on a beam even if they can see if fairly well, or learning to ride a bicycle. In addition, since they do not get dizzy, they can twirl around or ride a merry-go-round for long periods of time.

Specialized laboratory procedures are listed in Table 4–2. Since imaging of the temporal bones usually shows malformed or even absent semicircular canals, further testing is indicated when it is important to know whether one or both sides are affected and whether the individual has some or no function.

SUMMARY

Objective testing of balance problems and vestibular function in children and adults with CHARGE is very helpful for a complete picture of the difficulties. Careful taking of a case history along with clinical tests and information from the visual examination will provide a medical and functional diagnosis of the balance problems. The vestibular test protocol produced by the *European work group on genetics of hearing impairment* (http://www.gendeaf.org) may be helpful in determining which test will be most useful in a particular case.

TABLE 4–2. Laboratory Tests of Vestibular Function

- *Video-oculography.* Videonystagmography, VNG, is a procedure in which infrared cameras are fitted in light-occluding goggles to record eye movements from voluntary control of the eyes and, more importantly, from stimulation of the vestibular system. With VNG, a rapid screening can be performed by rotating a patient in the office chair. If no nystagmus is observed during rotation, there is a strong indication of bilateral vestibular areflexia, which is very common in CHARGE.

- *Bithermal binaural caloric tests.* In the clinical vestibular evaluation, the caloric tests are often the most important because they are used to determine whether the semicircular canals can detect the motion of the head and direct the movement of the eyes to stabilize visual images when the head is in motion (VOR function). The tests are done by injecting warm and cool water into ear canals (with intact eardrums) and measuring changes in eye movement. The tests are challenging because the examinee must remain still while warm and cool water, which may cause vertigo, is injected into the ear canals.

- *Rotatory tests.* These are VNG tests in which the individual being evaluated is seated with goggles in a rotating chair in a completely darkened chamber. The VOR is tested by measuring eye movements in response to rotational stimulation. It is an excellent detector of a common anomaly in CHARGE—bilateral vestibular loss. It can be done with a baby seated on the lap of an adult.

- *Ocular tracking.* Several mechanisms that control ocular movement can be evaluated by recording eye movements while the eyes focus on targets. These tests are used primarily to evaluate neural vestibular and ocular pathways and the cerebellum.

- *Vestibular head impulse test.* This test is a fairly new test making it possible to discover a large unilateral vestibular lesion. The test can be performed from 4–5 years of age. The patient is asked to fixate on the examiner's nose while the head is rapidly turned approximately 50–60 degrees to one side. Abnormal eye movements may be detected if there is marked asymmetry in peripheral vestibular function.

- *Dynamic posturography* (*balance* and *stability* while in motion). This highly structured test challenges the balance of a person who is standing without assistance by denying vision, giving false visual information, and permitting the floor to tilt. It is used to assess the utilization of visual, vestibular, and sensory systems to maintain balance. This form of evaluation has great value in the assessment of individuals who are able to stand independently.

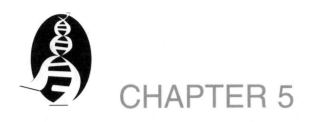

CHAPTER 5

Consequences of Vestibular Dysfunction

DAVID M. BROWN, M.A., D.SC. (HON)

*O*f all the many sensory impairments associated with CHARGE syndrome, absence of, or significant damage to, the vestibular sense is perhaps the most far-reaching in its implications, the least understood, and often the most overlooked. If people have any idea at all what the term "vestibular sense" means, they usually think that it relates to only the development of good balance, and so they might assume that vestibular issues will result in poor head control, delayed standing and walking, and a wobbly and insecure gait. Although all of these outcomes are likely, many others also need to be acknowledged and managed. Jean Ayres told us that "The vestibular system is the unifying system. . . . All other types of sensation are processed in reference to this basic vestibular information. The activity in the vestibular system provides a 'framework' for the other aspects of our experience. Vestibular input seems to 'prime' the entire nervous system to function effectively" (Ayres, 1979, p. 37).

Failure to acknowledge and deal with these issues probably will undermine any efforts that we make to help a child with CHARGE to develop skills in areas like vision, hearing, hand-eye coordination, receptive and expressive language, and so on. Most importantly, the vestibular sense plays a key role in helping us to develop effective self-regulation of our arousal level, the ability to maintain a calm but alert state. This is a sensory system that plays an extremely important role in enabling us to do almost everything that we do in our daily lives.

Postural issues, during both static and mobile activities, obviously will be a very noticeable outcome of an abnormal vestibular system in individuals with CHARGE. Very persistent low muscle tone might be associated with severe vestibular problems (Figure 5–1), and this is compounded by the lack of motivation to move and resist gravity, which results in a significant lack of "exercise" in every sense of the word. Protective reactions, standing, cruising, and independent walking all usually develop late. When children do move independently, they use unusual patterns like back scooting, rolling, or the five-point crawl (see Figure 1–3). After a child begins walking, he or she often develops a characteristic gait, some aspects of which may remain evident for many years (Figure 5–2). It is important to remember that these vestibular deficits never go away, although their presence may be masked by the adaptive skills and persistent concentration and hard work of the individual concerned.

Strong links exist between the vestibular sense and vision, and so the ability to maintain a stable visual field may be affected. It may be difficult for the eyes to follow objects smoothly as they move, and it may be hard to differentiate whether it is the object or oneself that is moving. Some children may appear to "go blind" if their postural security is too challenged, focusing all their attention and energy on getting into a secure position as an urgent priority. They may show some well-developed visual (and other) skills when they are flat on their backs or on their sides on a stable surface with their

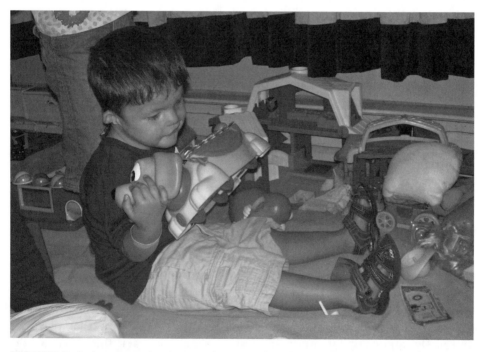

FIGURE 5–1. Low muscle tone can be associated with vestibular dysfunction. This slumping posture while sitting is typical for children with CHARGE.

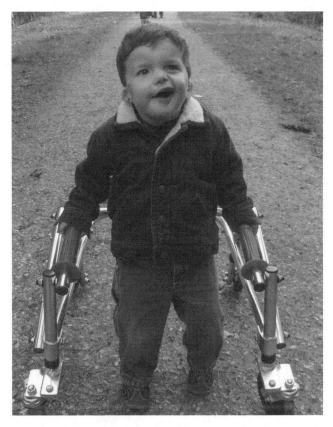

FIGURE 5–2. Walking may be delayed significantly in CHARGE, and gait may be unusual for life.

heads fully supported. As they get older, children may use residual vision to help them to stay upright, compensating for having a poor vestibular sense by using the strong visual impressions made by horizontal and, especially, vertical lines in a room (for example, corners, the edges of windows, doors, table tops, and wall-mounted pictures). They may have much less equilibrium outdoors, where these strong visual markers are largely absent or beyond their range of vision, or in dark environments. One result might be a reluctance to go outdoors, for example, during recess at school, and another might be an inability to perform certain tasks (kicking a ball, walking on an uneven surface, walking while carrying a large object) when they are outdoors that they can do well when they are indoors.

In the future, it is likely that we will discover close links between significant vestibular impairment and many of the currently "unexplained" CHARGE behavioral features such as difficulty with the self-regulation of arousal levels, sudden and apparently unpredictable mood changes, poor memory, and executive dysfunction. Significant difficulties with the vestibular sense cause disorientation, confusion, and fatigue in most aspects of daily living, particularly when other sensory impairments are present. Unless people involved with the child are prepared to understand these difficulties and adopt a supportive and nonjudgmental attitude, then the child is likely to develop a strong distrust and dislike of others, as well as a very poor self-image. This is especially regrettable when people repeatedly stop children from doing the very things that enable them to function—things like adopting specific postures or using self-regulation strategies that are interpreted negatively as "self-stimulating behaviors."

REFERENCE

Ayres, J. (1979). *Sensory integration and the child.* Los Angeles, CA: WPS.

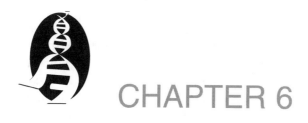

CHAPTER 6

Balance and Mobility

JAMES W. THELIN, Ph.D., SARAH E. CURTIS, Au.D.,
JILL FUSSNER MADDOX, Au.D., AND
LORI S. TRAVIS, Au.D.

*T*he anomalies that typically are present in children with CHARGE syndrome often result in the delay of the development of balance and mobility. The causes for these delays may include the following factors:

- Bilateral aplasia or dysplasia of the semicircular canals of the vestibular mechanism

- Visual impairment due to ocular colobomas or other anomalies

- Orthopedic disorders, including scoliosis

- Low muscle tone

- Neurological anomalies

Although delays in the development of balance and mobility likely have multiple causes, vestibular dysfunction is considered to be a major factor. The vast majority of individuals with CHARGE have substantial structural vestibular anomalies, most commonly of the semicircular canals that sense angular acceleration (Amiel et al., 2001; Collins & Buchman, 2002; Dhooge et al., 1998; Morgan et al., 1993; Morimoto et al., 2006; Murofushi et al., 1997; Satar, Mukherji, & Telian, 2003; Wiener-Vacher, Amanou, Denise, Narcy, & Manach, 1999; Wright, Brown, Meyerhoff, & Rutledge, 1986). Clinically, these anomalies are diagnosed with computerized tomography and magnetic resonance imaging.

Vestibular function in CHARGE has been measured by several investigators using physiologic tests (Abadie et al., 2000; Admiraal & Huygen, 1997; Tsuzuku & Kaga, 1992; Weiner-Vacher et al., 1999). All investigators found abnormal vestibular function, which included unresponsiveness to earth-vertical axis rotation, dampened responses in rotational chair tests, and reduced vestibulo-cular reflex (VOR) responses. (See Chapter 4 and Figure 4–2 for a diagram of the VOR.) In our experience, a majority of the individuals with CHARGE have not had radiographic imaging studies to document the integrity of the vestibular structures, and almost none have received an evaluation of vestibu-lar function using clinical physiologic measurement techniques. In many cases, the individuals are incapable of the cooperation necessary to make calibrated measurements. As a result, estimates of functional capability typically are not measured directly but are inferred from images of the vestibular structures.

At the University of Tennessee, three studies were conducted on individ-uals with CHARGE syndrome, which yielded information related to the devel-opment of balance and mobility. The first study (Thelin & Fussner, 2005) was an attempt to determine whether the acquisition of symbolic communication in 28 individuals with CHARGE syndrome was related significantly to any of 50 factors relating to physical status, sensory function, patterns of behavior, and communication therapy. Excepting a few individuals in the experimental group with severe neurological involvement and severe growth deficiency, the acquisition of symbolic communication was found to be related signifi-cantly to three factors: (1) successful management of hearing loss; (2) com-munication therapy initiated by 3 years of age; and (3) the ability to walk independently. The finding that the acquisition of symbolic communication was related to the ability to walk independently was unexpected.

The ability to walk or use symbolic communication may be due to the severity of medical involvement, but we were unable to find a significant rela-tionship between communication and any physical anomaly. Petroff (2001) reported a similar relationship between symbolic communication and the ability to walk independently for individuals with other forms of deafblind-ness (see Chapter 24 for a discussion of the CHARGE-related variables found associated with the age of walking). Davenport (2002) has proposed that an individual with vision and hearing impairment may be able to communicate effectively only if the talker is situated within a "communication bubble" that varies with background noise and lighting. It may be that an individual who walks independently has the ability to make critical adjustments in position to be able hear and see the surroundings; whereas those who cannot walk independently must accept the communication conditions without making adjustments. In summary, the combination of all factors that contribute to bal-ance and mobility are related in some manner to the development of sym-bolic communication.

In a second study, Travis and Thelin (2007) obtained information on the developmental milestones of nine individuals with CHARGE syndrome to determine whether any of the individuals were developing normally. Listed here are the age expectations for the development of the ability to walk independently and the results of the study:

Typically developing children:	Average = 12 months
Individuals with CHARGE syndrome:	Average = 42 months
	Range = 30 to 84 months

Another milestone that was examined was the ability to climb stairs with alternating feet. The age expectations and results are listed here:

Typically developing children:	Average = 30 months
Individuals with CHARGE syndrome:	Average = 108 months
	Range = 48 to 132 months

These data indicate that the development of mobility in CHARGE syndrome, which is very likely influenced by vestibular dysfunction, is grossly delayed, with a very broad range. The delays were very substantial for learning to walk independently and even greater for the more complex ability of walking up stairs with alternating feet. It is important to note that each of the individuals in this group eventually achieved the milestone of climbing stairs with alternating feet—despite being as much as 102 months beyond expectation for a typically developing child (Figure 6–1). This is important because it supports parents who almost universally maintain hope that their children will achieve certain levels of functioning even when others have lost hope.

In a third study, Krivenki and Thelin (2009) attempted to determine whether the VOR and/or cervico-ocular reflex (COR) was present in individuals with CHARGE syndrome. The VOR has sensors in the semicircular canals that route messages through the brainstem to the muscles of the eyes to control eye position. The properly functioning VOR stabilizes images while the head is in motion. The COR has the same action except that the sensors are located in the neck. These mechanisms are the "steady cameras" for the visual system. In CHARGE, VOR/COR function can be compromised or eliminated if neural signals to the eye muscles are abnormal or absent and if vision is compromised significantly by colobomas of the eye. If an individual with normal vestibular structures and function loses the VOR/COR, the horizon moves whenever the head moves, similar to a conventional, handheld camera. Therefore, the *loss* of the VOR/COR is very disorienting. Since the semicircular canals have been found to be malformed or missing in the vast majority of individuals with CHARGE syndrome, and since vision is disrupted by the presence of ocular colobomas, it was suspected that in many cases, the VOR and COR would not be present.

Because many individuals with CHARGE have a minimal ability to cooperate for long periods of time, a 60-second procedure was used in which the

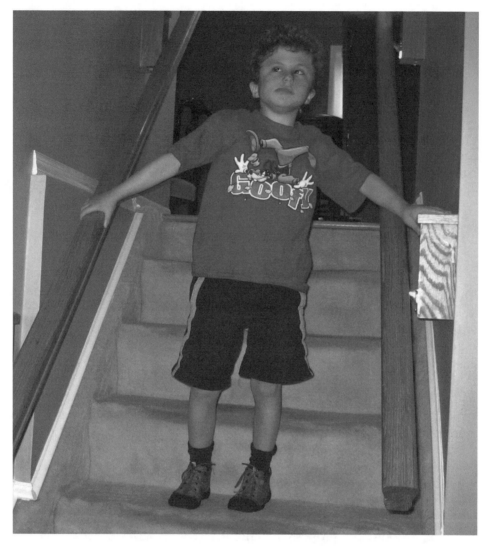

FIGURE 6–1. Older child finally able to go down stairs using alternate legs.

examiner sat behind a research participant who was seated in a swivel chair. The examiner reached over the participant and used handheld videonystagmography goggles over the participant's eyes, turning the chair from side-to-side to stimulate the VOR or turning the head side-to-side to stimulate the COR. The goggles measured the eye movements in darkness, and they were recorded on videotape and analyzed by visual inspection. The presence of horizontal nystagmus (a saw-tooth movement of the eyes) with head motion indicated the presence of a functioning VOR or COR mechanism. Congenital nystagmus is a constant oscillation of the eyes that intensifies with visual fixation. These individuals will have difficulty with mobility and reading because of constantly shifting visual images.

The 73 participants ranged in age from 1 to 31 years: 56 with CHARGE syndrome and 17 typically developing participants. Useful results were obtained on 87% of participants; valid results could not be obtained on a few participants who were too young or uncooperative. The VOR was absent for 29 of 29 individuals with CHARGE and present for 15 of 15 individuals who were developing typically. The COR was absent for 12 of 13 individuals with CHARGE and present for 13 of 13 individuals with typical development. Congenital nystagmus was present in 7 of 42 individuals with CHARGE and was not present in 15 of 15 individuals with typical development.

The vast majority of individuals with CHARGE syndrome in this study had no VOR or COR. If these individuals are able to stabilize images while the head is in motion, they must be using other mechanisms such as the saccule and utricle, the structures in the inner ear responsible for detecting horizontal and vertical acceleration, to achieve this function. Note that while individuals with CHARGE often have decreased ability to balance and ambulate, they do not complain of dizziness (Figure 6-2). Some parents have reported the opposite: children who wish to go on a roller coaster as many times as possible in succession. These findings provide evidence that individuals with CHARGE must use unique mechanisms for balance and mobility.

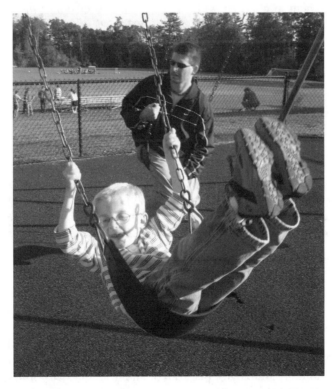

FIGURE 6–2. Children with CHARGE generally do not get dizzy and often crave experiences like swinging.

CONCLUSIONS

A substantial portion of the body of knowledge about the consequences of vestibular dysfunction in CHARGE has been obtained by perceptive observation and not with objective tests. However, objective tests often provide information about the dysfunction of specific structures that may be amenable to treatment. In the research conducted on individuals with CHARGE, clear evidence demonstrates relationships between vestibular function and the presence of the VOR, the ability to walk independently, motor development, and the acquisition of symbolic language.

REFERENCES

Abadie, V., Wiener-Vacher, S., Morisseau-Durand, M. P., Poree, C., Amiel, J., Amanou, L., . . . Manach, Y. (2000). Vestibular anomalies in CHARGE syndrome: Investigations on and consequences for postural development. *European Journal of Pediatrics*, *159*, 569-574.

Admiraal, R. J., & Huygen, P. L. (1997). Vestibular areflexia as a cause of delayed motor skill development in children with the CHARGE association. *International Journal of Pediatric Otorhinolaryngology*, *39*, 205-222.

Amiel, J., Attiee-Bitach, T., Marianowski, R., Cormier-Daire, V., Abadie, V., Bonnet, D., . . . Lyonnet, S. (2001). Temporal bone anomaly proposed as a major criteria for diagnosis of CHARGE syndrome. *American Journal of Medical Genetics*, *99*, 124-127.

Ayres, J. (1979). *Sensory integration and the child.* Los Angeles, CA: WPS.

Collins, W. O., & Buchman, C. A. (2002). Bilateral semicircular canal aplasia: a characteristic of the CHARGE association. *Otology & Neurotology*, *23*, 233-234.

Davenport, S. L. H. (2002). Influence of sensory loss on development: The communication bubble. In M. Hefner, & S. L. H. Davenport (Eds.), *CHARGE Syndrome: A Management Manual for Parents* (Version 2.1, Section IV-2B). Columbia, MO: CHARGE Syndrome Foundation.

Dhooge, I., Lemmerling, M., Lagache, M., Standaert, L., Govaert, P., & Mortier, G. (1998). Otological manifestations of CHARGE association. *Annals of Otology, Rhinology, and Laryngology*, *107*(11 Pt 1), 935-941.

Krivenki, S. E., & Thelin, J. W. (2009). *Vestibulo- and cervico-ocular reflexes in CHARGE syndrome.* Dallas, TX: American Academy of Audiology.

Morgan, D., Bailey, M., Phelps, P., Bellman, S., Grace, A., & Wyse, R. (1993). Ear-nose-throat abnormalities in the CHARGE association. *Archives of Otolaryngology— Head & Neck Surgery*, *119*, 49-54.

Morimoto, A. K., Wiggins, R. H., 3rd, Hudgins, P. A., Hedlund, G. L., Hamilton, B., Mukherji, S. K., . . . Harnsberger, H. R. (2006). Absent semicircular canals in CHARGE syndrome: radiologic spectrum of findings. *American Journal of Neuroradiology*, *27*, 1663-1671.

Murofushi, T., Ouvrier, R. A., Parker, G. D., Graham, R. I., da Silva, M., & Halmagyi, G. M. (1997). Vestibular abnormalities in CHARGE association. *Annals of Otology, Rhinology, and Laryngology, 106*, 129–134.

Petroff, J. G. (2001). *National transition follow-up study of youth identified as deaf-blind: parent perspectives.* Monmouth, OR: Teaching Research.

Satar, B., Mukherji, S. K., & Telian, S. A. (2003). Congenital aplasia of the semicircular canals. *Otology & Neurotology, 24*, 437–446.

Thelin, J. W., & Fussner, J. C. (2005). Factors related to the development of communication in CHARGE syndrome. *American Journal of Medical Genetics, 133A*, 282–290.

Travis, L. S., & Thelin, J. W. (2007). *Vestibular function, balance, and development in CHARGE syndrome.* 8th International CHARGE Syndrome Conference, Costa Mesa, CA.

Tsuzuku, T., & Kaga, K. (1992). Delayed motor function and results of vestibular function tests in children with inner ear anomalies. *International Journal of Pediatric Otorhinolaryngology, 23*, 261–268.

Wiener-Vacher, S. R., Amanou, L., Denise, P., Narcy, P., & Manach, Y. (1999). Vestibular function in children with the CHARGE association. *Archives of Otolaryngology—Head & Neck Surgery, 125*, 342–347.

Wright, C. G., Brown, O. E., Meyerhoff, W. L., & Rutledge, J. C. (1986). Auditory and temporal bone abnormalities in CHARGE association. *Annals of Otology, Rhinology, and Laryngology, 95*(5 Pt 1), 480–486.

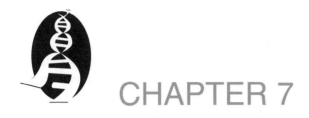

CHAPTER 7

Smell:
The Olfactory System

VÉRONIQUE ABADIE, M.D., PH.D.,
CHRISTEL CHALOUHI, M.D., PATRICK FAULCON, M.D.,
AND PIERRE BONFILS, M.D., PH.D.

ANATOMY AND EMBRYOLOGY

Development of the olfactory system begins very early in the human embryo. Olfactory bulbs have their definitive structure at day 56 (Bossy, 1980). Cells of the olfactory placode (thickening in the embryonic tissue) then differentiate to gonadotropinic cells and migrate to the hypothalamic region of the brain along the terminal nerve (also known as CN 0), the olfactory nerve (CN I), and the vomeronasal nerve. One section of the olfactory system projects into the anterior part of the hypothalamus, where it is responsible for odor perception and discrimination. The other section projects to the limbic system and the hippocampus, where the behavioral impact of olfaction and olfactory emotional memory reside. The olfactory epithelium (tissue composed of cells) is located high within the nasal vault and averages 1–2 cm^2 surface area on each side of the nose. In the fetus, the olfactory epithelium is a continuous sheet of cells, but in adults, it is a mixture of olfactory neuroepithelium and nonolfactory respiratory epithelium, a proportion that decreases with age. The olfactory mucosa contains several types of cells, especially the cell bodies of olfactory receptor neurons. Olfactory receptor neurons are bipolar neurons that project a single dendrite to the surface of the olfactory epithelium and a single axon to the olfactory bulb.

The nasal cavity of the typical human has 10 to 20 million olfactory receptor neurons. Unlike many neurons, they have the very special ability to renew themselves through life (Hadley, Orlandi, & Fong 2004). About 500 genes are known to encode for odorant receptors (proteins at the surface of these neurons), which is a significant proportion of the total number of genes in humans. Axons of these primary neurons expressing the same odorant receptor converge in the olfactory bulb on the same loci, termed *glomeruli*. Buck (2004) provided evidence that one odorant can activate multiple receptors, and a receptor can be activated by multiple odorants. Several primary olfactory neurons project on one glomerulus of the secondary neurons, which convey the information to the olfactory cortex (Buck & Axel, 1991; Buck, 2004). Olfaction occurs not only when molecules are carried in the inspired or sniffed air, but also up from the mouth during chewing and swallowing. Odorant molecules are transported across the olfactory mucus that blankets the surface of the olfactory epithelium. Regulation of this mucus may influence the degree of smell perception (Hadley, et al., 2004).

DEVELOPMENT OF OLFACTION: NORMAL AND DEFICIENT OLFACTION

Data suggest that olfaction is functional during prenatal life and leaves memories until after birth. At birth, newborns have highly efficient olfactory abilities, allowing them to discriminate the odor of their mothers' skin or milk from those of other mothers and to modify their feeding behavior according to the milk flavor. These very early experiences engrave food preference for a long time (Maier, Chabanet, Schaal, Leathwood, & Issanchou, 2008; Marlier & Schaal, 2005). Despite the difficulty of olfaction evaluation in infancy, all these data suggest that human neonatal and infantile olfaction plays a role both in mother-child bonding and infant feeding behavior. Nevertheless, it has been shown that reproducible behavioral modifications (breathing rhythm, mobility, and sight) indicate that healthy infants and toddlers (3 months to 3 years) have good olfaction abilities (Gordon-Pomares, Schirrer, & Abadie, 2002).

Several studies have shown that olfaction improves from the age when it becomes testable (7–8 years old) until about 40 years. These observations may be in part due to the methods of olfaction testing. After puberty, females have better olfaction abilities than males. From the age of about 40 years, olfaction abilities decrease, which partly may explain anorexia in the elderly (Doty et al. 1984; Richman, Sheehe, Wallace, Hyde, & Coplan, 1995). Olfaction in adults is likely involved in several areas, including appetite, emotional memory, and sexual bonding. Acute hyposmia or anosmia in adults may be responsible for depression and feeling of poor quality of life. Studies regarding congenital hyposmia are few, however; in particular, patients with Kallmann syndrome (congenital hyposmia and hypogonadism) seem to not demonstrate major effects of hyposmia, suggesting that hyposmic patients compensate for their deficit by other sensorial and cognitive means, especially if the defect exists before birth.

As is often the case in science or medicine, new ideas emerge at the same time from different origins and converge to the same hypothesis, leading to new knowledge. Thus, during the 1990s, four observations led to the hypothesis of an olfaction deficiency in children with CHARGE syndrome. First was the finding of anomalies of the forebrain, especially the rhinencephalon in autopsies of newborns or fetuses with suspicion of CHARGE syndrome (Pagon, Graham, Zonana, & Yong, 1981). Second was the observation of severe feeding disorders in children with CHARGE, lasting much longer than expected by the initial dysfunction of the brainstem and cranial nerves. Third was the improvement in the endocrinological understanding of the genital hypoplasia, delayed puberty, and growth retardation of these children. Several authors showed that pituitary function was mostly normal: the hormonal anomalies in individuals with CHARGE were due to hypothalamic hypogonadotropic hypogonadism (Pinto et al., 2005). That is, the hormones were not produced by the pituitary because they were not stimulated by the hypothalamus. The frequency of anomalies on the upper airways in CHARGE syndrome (e.g., choanal atresia, pharyngeo-laryngomalacia, tracheostomy, cleft palate) was an additional inducement to speculate about olfaction function in these patients. Finally, there was an interest in investigating how an additional sensory loss in children with multiple sensory deficiencies might contribute to our understanding of their behavior.

ASSESSMENT OF SMELL

Even if the ability of a young child to smell normally is obvious, quantitative measurement is difficult. Before it was possible to evaluate olfaction in children with CHARGE, it was first necessary to have suitable and standardized tests in other children. In 2004, when we initiated our study, there were no olfactory tests suitable for children younger than 12 years. We adapted the French Biolfa olfactory test that has been previously validated in healthy young adults (Bonfils, Faulcon, & Avan, 2004). This test is interesting because of its simplicity and because it is divided into a quantitative trial and a qualitative trial. The threshold test consists of nine aqueous dilutions of three components: eugenol, aldehyde C14, and PEA (smelling of cloves, peach, and rose, respectively). The lowest concentration at which one of these odors is detected is termed "detection threshold."

In each trial, we asked the child which of two stimuli (an odor or a blank), presented sequentially and in random order, smelled stronger (the forced-choice procedure). The first test began at the third level of difficulty. If a child failed to detect an odor, the next trial was performed at the next higher concentration level. The second part of the test is a qualitative evaluation in which the child is asked to recognize an odor presented at a concentration corresponding to his or her own olfactory detection threshold as previously measured.

From the eight odors available for adults, we chose the six most likely to be familiar to children, in order to be sure we were specifically testing olfaction and not the cognitive processes of the children: citronella (lemon), cis-3-hexenol (grass), L-carvone (mint), 1-Octene-3-ol (mushroom), vanillin (vanilla), and para-cresyl acetate (horse dung). Moreover, drawings representing 10 odors were presented systematically to the child in order to help with memory and oral expression. The test was scored by the number of olfactory items out of six correctly identified. The same investigator performed all the tests. For children with CHARGE, one parent was present during the test in order to avoid communication difficulties with the investigator.

We first showed that typical children have similar, or even better results than adults (vanilla: 84% of success by children versus 55% by adults; mint: 88% of success by children versus 51% by adults). We found that the test was understandable by children as young as 5 years old. Recently, a team from Australia and Germany published similar results screening olfactory function in school-age children (Laing, et al., 2008)

We then tested 14 children with CHARGE (8 girls, 6 boys, ages 7½ to 18 years). The results indicated olfaction deficiency in every one: half ($n = 7$) were anosmic, and the others were hyposmic (3 severely hyposmia, 3 moderately hyposmia and 1 mildly hyposmia). Six out of 14 (42%) had histories of choanal atresia, tracheostomy, or cleft palate. Of these six, half were anosmic and half were hyposmic, no different from the larger group.

In this preliminary study, we did not identify any statistical correlation between olfactory efficiency and the feeding disorders (duration of tube feeding, poor appetite, or difficulties with pieces chewing and swallowing). The olfactory deficiency was not correlated with the other sensory deficits. Regarding the level of developmental disability, we divided the group into two subgroups (high- and low-functioning level). We found that all the children of the low group were anosmic, but we also found anosmic children in the high group, suggesting that anosmia could be one of the factors that correlates with final developmental level. All nine children who underwent a brain MRI had anomalies of the olfactory bulbs and tracts, but without correlation between radiological and functional results (Chalouhi, et al., 2005).

Knowing that probably all (or at least a very large majority of) individuals with CHARGE have olfaction deficiency is important for several reasons: first, for recognizing the overlap between CHARGE and Kallmann syndrome; second, for a better understanding of feeding disorders of infants with CHARGE and to understand their unique feeding behaviors and preferences; and finally, to consider the possible influence of hyposmia on memory, behavioral, social bonding, and other attachment difficulties.

A Note on Kallmann Syndrome

The phenotype described by olfaction deficiency, hypogonadotropic hypogonadism (HH) characterized by delayed or absent puberty and abnormal anatomy of olfactory bulbs, is called Kallmann Syndrome (KS). KS is a heterogeneous situation with two distinct molecular loci identified: Kal-1 encodes anosmin-1 and is responsible for X-linked KS, and Kal-2 encodes a fibroblast growth factor receptor1 (FGFR-1) and is responsible for autosomal recessive KS (Cadman, Soo-Hyun, Youli, Gonzalez-Martinez, & Bouloux, 2007). Some patients with KS have additional features, such as renal anomalies, choanal atresia, hearing loss, and, of course, it is important to rule out CHARGE syndrome in the presence of these additional findings (Jongmans, et al., 2009; Klein, Friedman, Brookshire, Brown, & Edman, 1987).

Regarding CHARGE syndrome diagnosis, arhinencephaly, or congenital absence of the olfactory bulbs, tract, or nerves, could be considered a major diagnostic criterion of CHARGE, except that it is extremely difficult to confirm in infancy, the most common time period for a diagnostic evaluation to be performed. One mode of obtaining this information would to be focus an MRI on the olfactory tracts in addition to the inner ear and other portions of the brain. In our research, this rhinencephalon anomaly was present in all but one of the children investigated. In older individuals, the lack of a sense of smell might be helpful in confirming a diagnosis of CHARGE syndrome. Note that in individuals with CHARGE, except for rare cases, the pubertal hormonal deficiencies are not due to growth hormone deficiency, but rather hypogonaotropic hypogonadism.

Olfaction and Feeding

Many reasons exist for feeding problems in newborns and young children with CHARGE syndrome, most notably a lack of sucking and swallowing coordination due to brainstem and cranial nerve dysfunction, oral or esophageal malformations, upper airway obstructions, early surgery, early and long lasting hospitalization, along with mother-baby separation, etc. Our data regarding the importance of olfaction in the neonatal period strongly suggest that olfaction deficiency in babies with CHARGE further disturbs their feeding skills. Many toddlers with CHARGE are picky eaters, with strong preferences for specific textures, tastes, and consistencies. Given our new understanding of olfaction in CHARGE, it is quite likely that children would give more importance to textures than to "taste," which is really mostly smell. Some parents report that their children have a peculiar habit of stuffing their mouths with too quickly with too much food too quickly. One can now imagine that they need to feel in contact with the food in order to sense and appreciate it.

As an intervention, one might first try odor education, by surrounding the infant with a high level of fragrances and by using their trigeminal sensitivity for what seems normal. Trigeminal sensitivity facilitates the discrimination of taste (sweet, salt, sour, and bitter) and the perception of irritant odors. Thus, infants and children with CHARGE are more likely to enjoy food purees, which are clearly salty or sweet and even sour or spicy.

Older children may not be aware of odors that are unpleasant (e.g., body odor, foot odor) or have specific social meaning (e.g., perfumes, baking cookies) to others. They may not form odor memories, memories associated with a particular person, place, or food. We do not yet know how these different experiences change the world of an individual with CHARGE.

We do not know the impact of olfaction deficiency on the behavioral challenges of individuals with CHARGE. However, it is important to stimulate all of the senses for children with CHARGE to allow them better access to their world and perhaps along with that a better understanding of social interaction.

REFERENCES

Bonfils, P., Faulcon, P., & Avan, P. (2004). Screening of olfactory function using the Biolfa olfactory test: investigation in patients with dysosmia. *Acta Oto-laryngolocia, 124,* 1–9.

Bossy, J. (1980). Development of olfactory and related structures in staged human embryos. *Anatomy Embryology, 161,* 225–236.

Buck, L. B. (2004). The search or odorant receptors. *Cell, 116*(2), S117-9, 1 page following S119.

Buck, L., & Axel, R. (1991). A novel multigene family may encode odorant receptors: a molecular basis for odor recognition. *Cell, 65,* 175–187.

Cadman, S. M., Soo-Hyun, K., Youli, H., Gonzalez-Martinez, D., & Bouloux, P. M. (2007). Molecular pathogenesis of Kallmann's syndrome. *Hormone Research, 67,* 231–242.

Chalouhi, C., Faulcon, P., Le Bihan, C., Hertz-Pannier, L., Bonfils, P., & Abadie, V. (2005). Olfactory evaluation in children: Application to the CHARGE syndrome. *Pediatrics, 116,* 81–88.

Doty, R. L, Shaman, P., Applebaum, S. L., Giberson, R., Siksorski, L., & Rosenberg, L. (1984). Smell identification ability: Changes with age. *Science, 266,* 1441–1443.

Gordon-Pomares, C., Schirrer, J., & Abadie, V. (2002). Analysis of the olfactory capacity of healthy children before language acquisition. *Journal of Developmental and Behavioral Pediatrics, 23,* 1–5

Hadley, K., Orlandi, R. R., & Fong, K. J. (2004). Basic anatomy and physiology of olfaction and taste. *Otolaryngological Clinics of North America, 37,* 1115–1126.

Jongmans, M. C., Van Ravenswaaij-Arts, C. M., Pitteloud, N., Ogata, T., Sato, N., Claahsen-Van der Grinter, H. L., . . . Hoefsloot, L. H. (2009). CHD7 mutations in patients initially diagnosed with Kallmann syndrome-the clinical overlap with CHARGE syndrome. *Clinical Genetics, 75,* 65–71.

Klein, V. R., Friedman, J. M., Brookshire, G. S., Brown, O. E., & Edman, C. D. (1987). Kallmann syndrome associated with choanal atresia. *Clinical Genetics, 31,* 224–227.

Laing, D. G., Segovia, C., Fark, T., Laing, O.N., Jinks, A. L., Nikolaus, J., & Hummel, T. (2008). Tests for screening olfactory and gustatory function in school-age children. *Otolaryngology—Head and Neck Surgery, 139,* 74–82.

Maier, A. S., Chabanet, C., Schaal, B., Leathwood. P. D., & Issanchou, S. N. (2008). Breastfeeding and experience with variety early in weaning increase infants' acceptance of new foods for up to two months. *Clinical Nutrition, 27*, 849–857.

Marlier, L., & Schaal, B. (2005). Human newborns prefer human milk: Conspecific milk odor is attractive without postnatal exposure. *Child Development, 76*, 155–168.

Pagon, R. A., Graham, J. M., Zonana, J., & Yong, S. L. (1981). Coloboma, congenital heart disease and choanal atresia with multiple anomalies: CHARGE association. *Journal of Pediatrics, 99*, 223–227.

Pinto, G., Abadie, V., Mesnage, R., Blustajn, J., Cabrol, S., Amiel, J., . . . Netchine, I. (2005). CHARGE syndrome includes hypogonadotropic hypogonadism and abnormal olfactory bulb development. *Journal of Clinical Endocrinology and Metabolism, 90*, 5621–5626.

Richman, R. A., Sheehe, P. R., Wallace, K., Hyde, J. M., & Coplan J. (1995). Olfactory performance during childhood. II. Developing a discrimination task for children. *The Journal of Pediatrics, 127*, 421–426.

PART II

Medical Issues in CHARGE

*C*HARGE syndrome is medically complex. *CHD7*, the only gene currently recognized to cause CHARGE, is a regulatory gene that affects other genes. Multiple organ systems are affected, apparently due mostly to *CHD7* having its primary effect on the embryologic neural crest. Part II is organized around the major organs and organ systems involved. The most difficult thing to convey is how these conditions interact. In each chapter, we have made liberal reference to other chapters where additional information can be found, as a way of assisting the reader in making these connections.

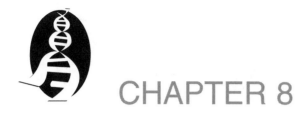

CHAPTER 8

Otologic Issues

SWAPNA K. CHANDRAN, M.D., AND
UDAYAN K. SHAH, M.D.

INTRODUCTION

External ear anomalies and hearing loss have long been recognized as cardinal features of CHARGE syndrome. Revised diagnostic criteria include the prevalence of anomalies in every area of the ear; external ear, hearing, balance, and facial nerve disorders are all seen as components of CHARGE syndrome.

ANATOMY OF A NORMAL EAR

The external ear is divided into the pinna, or auricle, and the external auditory canal. The pinna can be further divided into anatomical subparts, which are shown in Figure 8-1. Along with the middle ear, the external ear collects and funnels sound energy to the inner ear.

The middle ear consists of the tympanic membrane (TM) or "ear drum," the tympanic cavity, three ossicles ("bones of hearing"), two muscles, several tendons, and the Eustachian tube. The middle ear is connected to the mastoid bone via the *aditus ad antrum*, and the Eustachian tube connects the middle ear to the nasopharynx.

The three middle ear ossicles (malleus, incus, and stapes) convert the sound energy from the air medium of the middle ear to the fluid medium of the inner ear. The ossicles act as a lever system that conducts sound energy

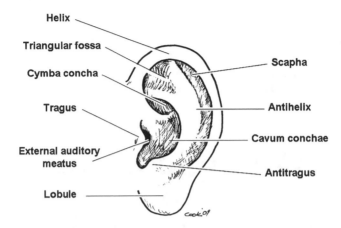

FIGURE 8–1. The pinna or outer ear with parts labeled. Courtesy of Steven Cook, M.D., used with permission.

from the tympanic membrane to the oval window on the cochlea. Also contained within the middle ear is the facial nerve (CN VII), the motor nerve allowing for muscle movement of the face and stapedial muscle. CN VII courses through the middle and inner ear and near the ossicles and the oval window, until it exits the skull via the stylomastoid foramen.

The inner ear system contains both the vestibular structures and the cochlea, which are organs for balance and hearing, respectively (Figure 8–2). The vestibular system consists of three semicircular canals, the utricle, and the saccule. The semicircular canals sit perpendicularly to one another and are paired bilaterally. They are responsible for maintaining balance in an angular plane. The utricle and the saccule sit between the semicircular canals and the cochlea and are responsible for balance in the linear plane.

The cochlea receives mechanical sound energy at the oval window via the ossicular chain. Within the cochlea is a fluid medium in which lie the sensory cells of hearing, the hair cells. Movement of the hair cells produces electrical stimulation and neural transmission of sound via the auditory nerve to the auditory cortex of the brain.

This simplified view of the function of the three parts of the ear allows for classification of conductive and sensorineural hearing loss (Color Plate 7). Conductive hearing loss is considered related to deficits in the function of the external or middle ear. Sensorineural hearing loss often is attributed to deficits in the function of structures in the cochlea and/or auditory nerve (CN VIII). Mixed hearing loss involves both the conductive and sensorineural systems.

EMBRYOLOGY

The outer and middle ear structures are developed from the first and second branchial structures, which each have an outer "groove" of ectoderm, a mid-

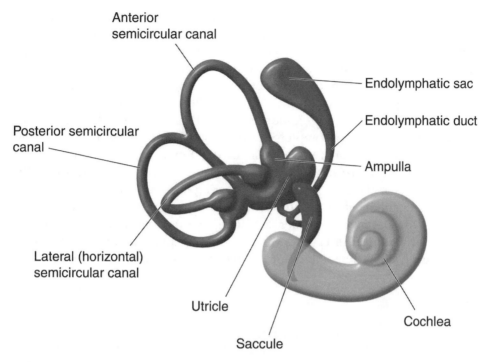

Anterior semicircular canal

Endolymphatic sac

Endolymphatic duct

Posterior semicircular canal

Ampulla

Lateral (horizontal) semicircular canal

Utricle

Cochlea

Saccule

FIGURE 8–2. The middle and inner ear with parts labeled. Photo from Shutter-stock®. All rights reserved.

dle "arch" of mesoderm, and an inner "pouch" of endoderm. By the sixth month of gestation, the ossicles have achieved adult size (Rodriguez, Shah, & Kenna, 2007).

The otic capsule, the bone that surrounds the organs of hearing and balance, forms the attachment of the footplate as well as the inner ear structures. The inner ear structures consist of a membranous labyrinth surrounded by a bony labyrinth. The membranous structures include the utricle, saccule, endolymphatic duct and sac, and the cochlear duct. These structures all contain endolymphatic fluid. The bony labyrinth is filled with perilymph.

The embryologies of the outer, middle, and inner ear structures, including the nerves and muscles, are related closely and all can be affected in individuals with CHARGE.

EXTERNAL EAR ANOMALIES

Bilateral and/or asymmetric external ear anomalies are seen in most children with CHARGE syndrome, with a reported incidence from 68% to 100%. Some authors mention that the external ear anomalies in CHARGE occasionally can be so distinctive that a presumptive diagnosis may be made on that basis alone (Davenport, Hefner, & Thelin, 1986; Dhooge, et al., 1998).

Typical CHARGE ears are short and wide, with a triangular concha with little or no lobe. They often are rotated posteriorly and may appear low set but usually are not (see Color Plate 8). Other frequent findings include discontinuity between the antihelix and antitragus, prominent or missing crura, and/or an unfolded or "snipped off" appearance of the helical fold. Weak cartilage leads to a floppy ear (Davenport, Hefner, & Mitchell, 1986).

Microtia, defined as an abnormally small ear, with stages ranging from minor abnormalities to complete absence of the external ear and external canal stenosis or atresia are rare in CHARGE (Dhooge, et al., 1998).

No definite correlation exists between the degree of deformity of the external ear and the type or degree of hearing loss. Patients with less severe external ear anomalies range from having no hearing loss to severe mixed hearing loss (Davenport, Hefner, & Thelin, 1986). Deformed or floppy ears may require surgical intervention to have adequate structure to accommodate hearing aids. The auditory canals may be narrow and/or tortuous.

MIDDLE EAR ANOMALIES

The frequency of ossicular abnormalities range from 54% to 86% in children with CHARGE (Morimoto, et al., 2006). Middle ear abnormalities range from absent or hypoplastic structures to dysmorphic ossicular masses. Fixation or fusion of the ossicular chain along any portion of the transducer system is common, with the malleus head often fixated to the anterior wall.

The muscular components of the middle ear also can be abnormal. The stapedius muscle and tendon, as well as its bony attachment to the temporal bone (the pyramidal eminence) was found to be absent in several series (Dhooge, et al., 1998). Furthermore, the oval window was found to absent in 23% to 100% of cases reported (Morgan, et al., 1993). The round window niche also has been reported to demonstrate abnormalities, namely obliteration. The cause of the obliteration is uncertain as it may result as a bony malformation of the ossicles or secondary to chronic otitis media or sinusitis.

Incidence of recurrent or persistent middle ear disease (middle ear effusion/otitis media [OM]) with or without tympanic membrane perforation in patients with CHARGE syndrome is reported as greater than 50% (Shah, et al., 1998). Otitis media in this population is thought to be secondary to Eustachian tube dysfunction resulting from the various craniofacial abnormalities including cleft lip and palate and perhaps even the anomalous middle-ear cleft. These findings include, but are not limited to, choanal atresia, cleft lip and palate, unilateral facial paralysis, and flattening of the malar eminences (Davenport, Hefner, & Mitchell, 1986; Thelin, Mitchell, Hefner, & Davenport, 1986).

The presentation of OM in children with CHARGE is unique because it is usually unrelenting or presents at an age when OM is uncommon (older children). Management of OM usually is surgical with either pressure equalization (PE) tubes and/or mastoidectomy (Shah, et al., 1998).

The constellation of malformations found within the middle ear demonstrate an embryologic defect in the second branchial arch system, which also contributes to the facial nerve deficits discussed later in this chapter.

INNER EAR ANOMALIES

Inner-ear anomalies can be subdivided into cochlear (hearing) and vestibular (balance) components. Both systems converge via their respective sensory nerves at the internal auditory canal (IAC).

The cochlear abnormalities found in CHARGE syndrome range from subtle modiolar deficiencies in which the bony core of the cochlea is malformed, to more severe partition defects such as the Mondini malformation, in which there are fewer than the normal 2.5 turns of the cochlea around the modiolus. Morimoto, et al. (2006) reported cochlear abnormalities in 81% of ears examined. The most common finding in patients with CHARGE undergoing cochlear implant placement for bilateral severe hearing loss is the Mondini malformation (Lanson, Green, Roland, Lalwani, & Waltzman, 2007). Additionally, a flattened cochlear promontory or basal turn of the cochlea has been reported (Bauer, Wippold, Goldin, & Lusk, 2002).

Cochlear (or auditory) nerve abnormalities arise both within the cochlea and at the level of the internal auditory canal where the nerve enters the brainstem. At the level of the cochlea, the cochlear nerve may have an abnormally thickened bony covering over the aperture, called a "trapped cochlea." Absent, hyopoplastic or dysplastic cochlear nerves have been identified in patients with CHARGE (Morimoto, et al., 2006).

The vestibular anomalies identified in those with CHARGE syndrome range from hypoplastic to absent structures. The most common finding is absence of the semicircular canals, seen in 26/26 cases studied by Morimoto, et al. (2006). However, almost half of dysplastic or absent semicircular canals are associated with normal vestibules (Morgan, et al., 1993). Additionally, the combination of a hypoplastic incus and an abnormal semicircular canal is thought to be characteristic of patients with CHARGE syndrome, as almost half may demonstrate this concomitant finding (Morgan, et al., 1993).

Other findings of the anomalous inner ear in CHARGE syndrome include a narrow internal auditory canal, which can be associated with an aplastic or absent cochlear nerve and an abnormal vestibular aqueduct (Morimoto, et al., 2006). The vestibular aqueduct may be absent or wide; some demonstrate an aberrant course with a reversed angle. The clinical implications of structural vestibular anomalies are detailed in this and subsequent sections.

THE FACIAL NERVE

The facial nerve (CN VII) exits the brain stem, enters the ear via the internal auditory canal, and traverses the middle ear prior to exiting at the stylomastoid foramen. It is the associated nerve of the second branchial arch; therefore, embryonic derangements that occur in the middle ear may affect the course of the seventh cranial nerve.

An aberrant facial nerve is extremely common in patients with CHARGE syndrome and may make surgery such as cochlear implantation difficult. In vitro studies have demonstrated that both the labyrinthine and tympanic segments in CHARGE syndrome can be more anterior or posterior than normal or directly overlay the oval window niche (Morgan, et al., 1993; Morimoto, et al., 2006).

Facial nerve palsy is a common finding in CHARGE syndrome, occurring in more than 50% of patients and is considered a major diagnostic criterion (Blake, et al., 1998; Verloes, 2005). The palsy can be unilateral, which is more common, or bilateral. Cases in which the bony facial canal is dehiscent (ruptured), thereby exposing bare nerve, are susceptible to recurrent (intermittent) facial palsy occurring in the setting of OM.

Facial nerve problems can result in dry eyes that require lubrication with "artificial tear" solutions and can impair oral continence (maintaining saliva), therefore further complicating oral feeding and speech. Bilateral facial palsy significantly can impair social interactions.

HEARING LOSS AND HABILITATION

For more information on hearing loss and habilitation, see also Chapter 3.

Hearing loss is the most common finding in CHARGE syndrome, with a reported frequency of 85% to 100%. Early studies classified the degree of hearing loss as ranging from mild to profound. As more investigations into the hearing-loss patterns in patients with CHARGE have been done, a spectrum of hearing-loss patterns have been identified. Conductive (CHL), sensorineural (SNHL), and mixed hearing losses have been identified in patients with CHARGE. Some reports of progressive hearing loss have been noted (Dhooge, et al., 1998; Thelin, et al., 1986).

The high prevalence of hearing loss warrants early detection, classification, and habilitation. Audiologic intervention is especially important in children with CHARGE as hearing and vision impairment coexist. In cases in which the CHL is secondary to Eustachian tube dysfunction or middle-ear effusion, pressure equalization tubes, and in some cases adenoidectomy, should be utilized. These tubes may be necessary well past early childhood. Ossicular abnormalities also may be amenable to surgical repair. Risk to the potentially aberrant (ectopic) facial nerve and oval window should be considered prior to surgery.

Many individuals with CHARGE benefit from amplification via hearing aids. Dilemmas may arise with poor or difficult fitting of the hearing aid secondary to pinna abnormalities (both shape and rigidity). Bone conduction aids and surgical correction of ossicular malformation may or may not be an option, depending on the cochlear hearing loss.

Cochlear implantation is a more recent method of auditory habilitation for individuals with CHARGE (see Chapter 9). Again, as with any surgical intervention in an embryologically deranged ear, care must be taken with facial nerve anatomy.

VESTIBULAR FUNCTION AND REHABILITATION (SEE ALSO CHAPTER 4)

For more information on vestibular function and rehabilitation, see also Chapter 4.

The manifestations of a hypoplastic or dysplastic vestibular system can be found in Table 8-1. The degree and location of the anomalies along with concomitant ear or other sensory deficits contribute to the severity and quality of the impairment. The delays in achieving motor milestones experienced by children with CHARGE are multifactorial and secondary to combinations of semicircular canal anomalies; visual impairment; neurological impairment; prolonged hospital stays, and multiple surgical procedures (Blake, Kirk, & Ur, 1993).

TABLE 8–1. Vestibular Manifestation of CHARGE Syndrome

Hypotonia during the first years of life

Poor head support

Slower placing responses of the upper extremities

Delay in sitting without support (never before 1 year)

Delay in walking (not before 2 years)

Difficulties in transitioning from one position to another

Problems with walking in the dark

Problems with walking on uneven ground

CONCLUSION

The otologic manifestations and functional deficits of CHARGE syndrome are derived from embryologic derangements of first and second branchial arches, the otic capsule, and neurologic impairment. Since all parts of the ear can be affected, early identification of the extent of malformation of each is critical to the choice of therapies, both medical and surgical. For instance, pinna reconstruction may be needed so hearing aids stay on or, in older children, for cosmetic improvement that can have an effect on self esteem. Tympanostomy tube insertion is common, but reconstruction of middle-ear structures is not. The issues with cochlear implantation are discussed in Chapter 9, and detailed discussions of the complexities encountered in the assessment and management of hearing loss are in Chapter 3. The identification of vestibular loss, the effect on development, and the approaches to therapy are covered in Chapter 4.

REFERENCES

Bauer, P. W., Wippold, F. J., Goldin, J., & Lusk, R. P. (2002) Cochlear implantation in children with CHARGE Association. *Archives of Otolaryngology—Head and Neck Surgery, 28*, 1013-1017.

Blake, K. D., Davenport, S. L., Hall, B. D., Hefner, M. A., Pagon, R. A., Williams, M. S., et al., (1998). CHARGE association: an update and review for the primary pediatrician. *Clinical Pediatrics, 37*, 159-173.

Blake, K., Kirk, J. M., & Ur, E. (1993). Growth in CHARGE association. *Archives of Diseases in Childhood, 68*, 508-509.

Davenport, S. L., Hefner, M. A., & Mitchell, J. A. (1986). The spectrum of clinical features in CHARGE syndrome. *Clinical Genetics, 29*, 298-310.

Davenport, S. L., Hefner, M. A., & Thelin, J. W. (1986). CHARGE syndrome: Part I. External ear anomalies. *International Journal of Pediatric Otorhinolaryngology, 12*, 137-143.

Dhooge, I., Lemmerling, M., Lagache, M., Standaert, L., Govaert, P., & Mortier, G. (1998). Otological manifestations of CHARGE association. *Annals of Otology, Rhinology and Laryngology, 107*, 935-941.

Lanson, B. G., Green, J. E., Roland, J. T., Jr., Lalwani, A. K., & Waltzman, S. B. (2007). Cochlear implantation in children with CHARGE syndrome: therapeutic decisions and outcomes. *Laryngoscope, 117*, 1260-1266.

Morgan, D., Bailey, M., Phelps, P., Bellman, S., Grace, A., & Wyse, R. (1993). Ear-nose-throat abnormalities in the CHARGE association. *Archives of Otology—Head & Neck Surgery, 119*, 49-54.

Morimoto, A. K., Wiggins, R. H., Hudgins, P. A., Hedlund, G. L., Hamilton, B., Mukherj, S. K., . . . Harnsberger, H. R. (2006). Absent semicircular canals in CHARGE syndrome: radiologic spectrum of findings. *American Journal of Neuroradiology, 27*, 1663-1671.

Rodriguez, K., Shah, R., & Kenna, M. (2007). Anomalies of the middle and inner ear. *Otology Clinics of North America, 40*, 81–96.

Shah, U. K., Ohlms, L. A., Neault, M. W., Willson, K. D., McGuirt, W. F., Jr., Hobbs, N., Healy, G. B. (1998). Otologic management in children with the CHARGE association. *International Journal of Pediatric Otorhinolaryngology, 44*(2),139–147.

Thelin, J. W., Mitchell, J. A., Hefner, M. A., & Davenport, S. L. (1986). CHARGE syndrome. Part II. Hearing loss. *International Journal of Pediatric Otorhinolaryngology, 12*, 145–163.

Verloes, A. (2005). Updated diagnostic criteria for CHARGE syndrome: A proposal. *American Journal of Medical Genetics, 133A*, 306–308.

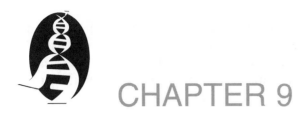

CHAPTER 9

Cochlear Implantation

N. WENDELL TODD, M.D., M.P.H.

INTRODUCTION

As the hearing impairment in CHARGE is often at least partially sensorineural, cochlear implantation (CI) is a consideration for many children with CHARGE, but each patient is to be especially regarded. The comparatively small external ear canals restrict visualization of the tympanic membrane, cause difficulties in performing physiologic audiologic tests, and create problems in fitting hearing aid ear molds. Moreover, the narrow canal contributes to poor clearing of cerumen (wax), which can occlude hearing aid ear molds and prevent proper amplification.

The middle-ear problems seen in children with CHARGE include otitis media ("ear infection") and congenital abnormalities of the ossicles such that sound is not effectively transmitted to the inner ear. Middle-ear disease that usually resolves in typically developing children in later childhood may persist into adulthood for individuals with CHARGE.

In the inner ear, any or all of the structures (semicircular canals, saccule, utricle, cochlea, and auditory nerve) can be affected. At least as shown in imaging studies (computed tomography, CT, and magnetic resonance imaging, MRI), the more phylogenetically and ontogenetically ancient pars superior is [surprisingly] more affected: hypoplastic semicircular canals and [presumably] utricle. In contrast, the more recent (in both phylogeny and ontogeny) pars inferior is comparatively less affected: dysplastic cochlea and [presumably] saccule. For hearing impairment attributable to cochlear and/or cochlear nerve problems, acoustic amplification with hearing aids is attempted first. If the benefit with hearing aids is not enough to enable acceptable hearing, then cochlear implantation may be considered. Each of the preceding factors is taken into account before the decision to implant is made.

INDICATIONS FOR COCHLEAR IMPLANTATION

For the child with CHARGE syndrome in whom acoustic amplification does not provide a boost into the range of audible frequencies required to understand speech (often called the "speech banana"), cochlear implantation may be a consideration. Implantation also may help individuals with "auditory neuropathy/dys-synchrony," in which the cochlear nerve does not transmit in a sufficiently organized manner for human listening. Cochlear implantation may afford "electric hearing"—that is, electrical stimulation of the cochlear (auditory) nerve fibers such that the individual can "hear." For auditory neuropathy/dys-synchrony patients, electric stimulation by cochlear implant seems to demand or regiment organized information transmission into the cochlear nerve. For the surgeon, the simplistic mantra is, "Getting the electrons to the neurons." Unfortunately, especially for individuals with CHARGE, the likelihood of enabling listening-speaking communication is less than 100%, and the risks are high of a disappointing result, infection, and facial paralysis. Therefore, candidates for cochlear implantation should meet the criteria that follow. It is important to note that the decision to implant depends on as many nonhearing related factors as hearing-related factors.

Appropriately Motivated Family

A motivated family is required, with realistic expectations for the outcomes of implantation and a willingness to provide the time, support, access to therapy, and work to help the individual with CHARGE to benefit from the device.

Audiologic Criteria

Essentially, the most important criterion is either such poor hearing that hearing aids do not boost sounds in the speech frequencies into the audible range or to use the cochlear implant to overcome the effects of auditory neuropathy/ or dys-synchrony, a form of hearing impairment in which typically there is normal function of the outer hair cells of the cochlea, but neural transmission in the auditory pathway is disordered.

Otologic Criteria

MRI and CT imaging must demonstrate the presence of a cochlea into which an electrode array can be inserted, the presence of an adequate cochlear nerve (Shelton, et al., 1989), and a facial nerve positioned such that it is unlikely to be damaged in the implantation surgery. Otitis media must be controllable.

General Health Criteria

The child must be deemed able to withstand general anesthesia, and there should be the expectation for adequate wound healing. Immunizations should be up-to-date and are more extensive than for other children. Information on the extra risks of bacterial meningitis with CI can be obtained from the Centers for Disease Control guidelines (http://www.cdc.gov/vaccines and then search "cochlear").

A schematic drawing of the auditory system and the CI device is shown in Color Plate 9 (Rauschecker & Shannon, 2002). Running down the left side of the figure is a depiction of the components of a CI device. The microphone picks up incoming sound, converts it to an electrical signal, and delivers it to the sound processor whose output is directed to a transmitter that is "coupling" to a receiver implanted in the skull under the skin. The coupling between the transmitter and receiver is magnetic so that signals can be delivered through the skin. The receiver is connected to the electrode array that is inserted into the cochlea by wires. In CHARGE syndrome, the success of the implantation surgery is related to the ability of the surgeon to implant the receiver–stimulator package in the skull and CI electrode array into a cochlear labyrinth that may be very abnormal in terms of the location, shape, and size of critical landmarks and structures.

Running up the right side of Color Plate 9 is a depiction of the pathway for CI stimulation. The electrode array in the cochlea (green) sends signals that activate auditory nerve fibers (brown), which travel through the brainstem to the auditory cortex where neural activity becomes hearing. The success of the implant depends on the precise placement of the CI electrode array, programming it to deliver useful signals, the ability of the auditory nerve to be stimulated, and the integrity of the pathways to the cortex.

In Figure 9–1, pictures of a young boy are shown of the surgical wound from CI surgery and a post-surgical dressing. In Figure 9–2, the CI transmitter that is coupled magnetically to the side of the head is shown on a young adult.

When it has been determined that a child might benefit from cochlear implantation, the issues arise as to whether unilateral, bilateral sequential, or same day implantation is optimal. In children whose only disorder is deafness, there is a mounting body of evidence of the benefits of bilateral implantation (Balkany, et al., 2008; Eapen & Buchman, 2009). For children with CHARGE,

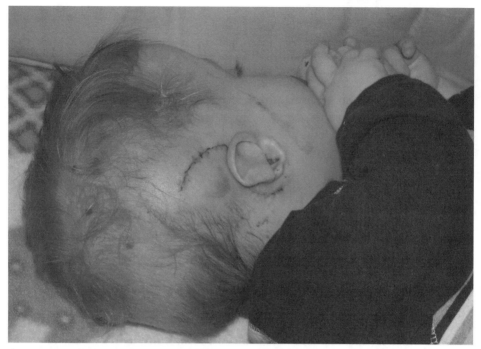

A

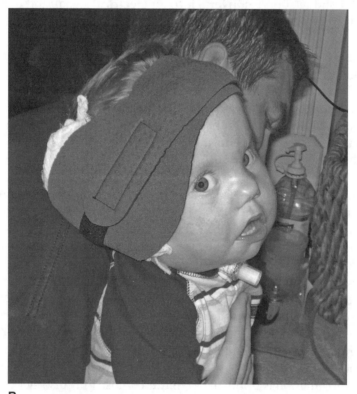

B

FIGURE 9–1. A. A young child immediately after cochlear surgery. **B.** Recovery from cochlear surgery.

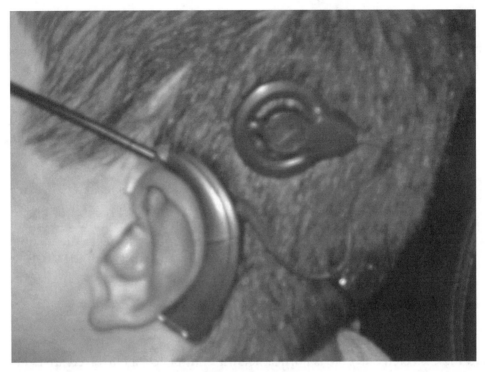

FIGURE 9–2. A boy who has CHARGE with an implant. Notice the CHARGE outer ear (see Chapter 8).

who often have differences between the cochleas and auditory nerves for the two ears, very little information is available at this time about the benefits of bilateral implantation.

COMPLICATIONS AND PROBLEMS WITH COCHLEAR IMPLANTATION

In the case of CHARGE, the likelihood of an outcome enabling listening-speaking communication is relatively low, and the risks are many, including poor outcome, infection, inadvertent stimulation of the facial nerve, and facial paralysis. Many relatively poor outcomes are attributable to anatomical and surgical challenges: fewer cochlear neurons that can be accessed for electrical stimulation, the high occurrence of ear infections, and often unusual location of the facial nerve that may be stimulated inappropriately by the implant or damaged by the surgery (MacArdle, et al., 2002). The surgeon must address these concerns during preoperative assessment before the decision to implant is considered seriously. This is in addition to the technical feat of the implantation itself in anomalous structures.

A common problem with CI in CHARGE syndrome is the parents' disappointment related to unrealistic expectations for the behavioral outcome of the surgery. For the majority of children with CHARGE syndrome, vision is sufficient for signed communication. But the family often wants the child to have at least some listening-speaking communication. Realistic family expectations, often a challenge to assess and achieve in implant candidates without CHARGE, are far more challenging in patients with CHARGE syndrome and their families. For the surgeon, implant team, and parents, there is always the question of whether the benefits of CI are likely to outweigh the risks, effort, and costs.

Many children with CHARGE have significant problems related to balance and mobility (see Chapter 6). Another factor to consider is that recent evidence indicates that cochlear implantation may affect adversely vestibular function (Jacot, Van Den Abbeele, Debre, & Wiener-Vacher, 2009). However, the vestibular effects from CI have not yet been studied in individuals with CHARGE.

OUTCOMES

If the expected outcome is normal hearing and speech, all involved are likely to be disappointed. However, when the expected/desired outcome is improved hearing and sound awareness and improved oral communication, CI may be considered successful in many instances. Lanson et al. (2007) report the course of the largest published series of CI in patients with CHARGE to date: results on 10 patients, three months to seven years after implantation. Two manifested infections were so severe as to prompt implant removal (and subsequent replacement in each child). Disappointingly, the most optimistically summarized communication outcomes were as follows: one child with no communication; five using manual communication; and four using total communication. However, all 10 demonstrated improved audiometric results and enhanced connectivity to their environments. Given the multisensory deprivation that occurs in CHARGE, improvements in audition that would be considered unacceptable for a typically developing individual may have major positive consequences on many aspects of communication and development for individuals with CHARGE.

REPORTS OF TWO PATIENTS IMPLANTED BY THE AUTHOR

Reports of two cases are presented here to illustrate the complexity of the issues in cochlear implantation from the perspective of the ear surgeon.

CASE 1

A now 14-year old girl, known to the author since infancy, had multiple surgeries for bilateral choanal atresia, patent ductus arteriosus, tracheo-esophageal fistula, and cleft lip and palate. She began walking independently at four years of age. Hearing aids were introduced at age four months in conjunction with auditory-verbal therapy (from which she graduated at age seven). Her hearing impairment was severe mixed loss in each ear, left ear slightly worse than right.

Computed tomography at age five showed quite small pneumatization of each mastoid, severely hypoplastic semicircular canals, and abnormal ossicles. Her fifth set of tympanostomy tubes was placed at age five.

With acoustic amplification no longer benefitting her left ear, she received a left cochlear implant at age six (Cochlear Corporation Nucleus 24). The procedure included radical mastoidectomy with fat obliteration and closure of the external ear canal.

At age 14, the right tympanic membrane had been clinically normal for about five years, and she continues to use a hearing aid on that side. The implanted left ear is doing well, and she communicates by listening and speaking. Sometimes she effectively can use a speaker telephone with a familiar person. She attends regular 7th grade, receiving extra help in one subject. She writes her own poetry (see Sidebar 9–1).

Sidebar 9–1

Case 1 is a 14-year-old girl who loves to write poetry and shares (with her parents' permission) the following verse, which she presented at the retirement of her beloved auditory-verbal therapist:

To Maryann:
Running feet, like the pistons on a train
people of all genders, disabilities, color, size, and shapes
They're running with the stream,
Their loyalty, faith, and love continue through the years
Many leave the race as they die
The light and wind leave their faces
I lift my face to the wind as I run
That's life in the running of the people's hearts and minds
The small pools are forgotten
I can now run with the mainstream and that is my life

CASE 2

A now 11-year-old boy first presented to the author at age six with the question of whether another attempt at cochlear implantation could be considered. At age five, he had undergone an unsuccessful attempt at implanting the left cochlea. During surgery, the facial nerve was found to be splayed over the deformed stapes and promontory and anterior to both the oval and round windows. No cochlear lumen was found during cochleostomy attempts. The tympanic membrane defect was addressed by tympanoplasty at that time.

This child's features of CHARGE include having bilateral colobomas, choanal atresia, characteristic outer ears, hearing impairment, dysphagia, and gastro-esophageal reflux. He began walking independently at age 18 months. Despite all the problems, he was assessed as having above average intelligence.

Lifelong otitis media had required five sets of tympanostomy tubes and adenoidectomy. He first received hearing aids at age 4½ years. On the left, amplification with hearing aids never provided meaningful benefit. At age 6, aided hearing in his right ear had decreased to such an extent that he was not able to continue as a listening-speaking communicator. He continued to suffer from near-monthly purulent drainage in both ears through the open tympanic membranes (the tympanoplasty at age five was not successful). Despite attending an auditory-oral school, his speech skills degraded. Behavior was becoming problematic.

Imaging studies at age 6 showed each ear to have only one turn (the basilar) of the cochlea, a slightly enlarged vestibule, and no identifiable semicircular canals. In addition, there was concern about a possibly isolated left cochlea (also termed absent cochlear fossette, meaning congenital absence of bony canal for the cochlear nerve; this observation is consistent with absent cochlear nerve, or at least severely deficient number of cochlear neurons). Diagnostic measurements made at the University of Michigan found that electrical stimulation onto the promontory yielded satisfactory brainstem responses from the left cochlea; that is, the "promontory stimulation" test elicited satisfactory waveforms generated in his brainstem. With this concern put to rest, the remaining problems were devising a technique for electrode insertion and reducing the risk of infection from the recurrently active otitis media (which can increase the risk of infecting the cochlear implant that may lead to meningitis).

Cochlear implantation (MED-EL model PULSARci100) was accomplished at age 6, inserting via the vestibule, i.e., inserting the electrode array posterior-superior to the facial nerve, feeding the array into the cochlea, and wedging the hub in the labyrinth. Concomitant radical mastoidectomy with obliteration (fat graft) was done. Twenty months after implantation, using the cochlear implant in his left ear and the hearing aid in his right ear, he was able to use the speaker telephone, including talking with nonfamiliar persons. Now, at age 11, he attends regular 5th grade, with extra help in a couple of subjects. Inflammation at the implanted ear has not occurred to date.

COCHLEAR IMPLANTATION SURGERY IN THE FUTURE

Cochlear implantation has been beneficial for some individuals with CHARGE. However, it also has not been beneficial for a significant number of individuals. This is in part due to the wide range of anatomical and physiological anomalies with this disorder (Bauer, et al., 2002). In the future, ear surgeons will have a greater understanding of the issues associated with implantation when temporal bone information becomes available (Haginomori, Sando, Miura, & Casselbrant, 2002). New physiologic methods for the measurement of auditory nerve function also will assist the surgeon in predicting success, and special surgical approaches, such as the middle cranial fossa approach when there is facial nerve involvement (Todd, 2007), may enable better outcomes.

REFERENCES

Balkany, T., Hodges, A., Telischi, F., Hoffman, R., Madell, J., Parisier, S., . . . Litovsky, R. (2008). William House Cochlear Implant Study Group: Position statement on bilateral cochlear implantation. *Otology and Neurotology*, *29*(2), 107–108.

Bauer, P. W., Wippold, F. J., 2nd, Goldin, J., & Lusk, R. P. (2002). Cochlear implantation in children with CHARGE syndrome. *Archives of Ototlaryngology Head and Neck Surgery*, *128*, 1013–1017.

Curr, O. (2009). *Otolaryngol Head Neck Surgery*, 17(5), 351–355.

Eapen, R. J., & Buchman, C. A. (2009). Bilateral cochlear implantation: Current concepts. *Current Opinion in Otolaryngology & Head and Neck Surgery*, Advanced online publication.

Haginomori, S., Sando, I., Miura, M., & Casselbrant, M. L. (2002). Temporal bone histopathology in CHARGE association. *Annals of Otology, Rhinology, & Laryngology*, *111*(5 Pt 1), 397–401.

Jacot, E., Van Den Abbeele, T., Debre, H. R., & Wiener-Vacher, S. R. (2009). Vestibular impairments pre- and post-cochlear implant in children. *International Journal of Pediatric Otorhinolaryngology*, *73*, 209–217.

Lanson, B. G., Green, J. E., Roland, J. T., Jr., Lalwani, A. K., & Waltzman, S. B. (2007). Cochlear implantation in children with CHARGE syndrome: Therapeutic decisions and outcomes. *Laryngoscope*, *117*, 1260–1266.

MacArdle, B. M., Bailey, C., Phelps, P. D., Bradley, J., Brown, T., & Wheeler, A. (2002). Cochlear implants in children with craniofacial syndromes: assessment and outcomes. *International Journal of Audiology*, *41*, 347–356.

Rauschecker, J. P., & Shannon, R. V. (2002). Sending sound to the brain. *Science*, *295*, 1025–1029.

Shelton, C., Luxford, W. M., Tonokawa, L. L., Lo, W. W., & House, W. F. (1989). The narrow internal auditory canal in children: a contraindication to cochlear implants. *Otolaryngology Head & Neck Surgery*, *100*, 227–231.

Todd, N. W. (2007). Cochlear implantation via the middle fossa: Surgical and electrode array considerations. *Cochlear Implants International*, *1*, 12–28.

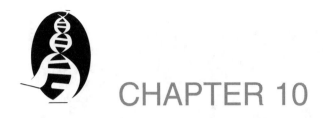

CHAPTER 10

Rhinologic (Nasal) Issues

CHRISTOPHER R. GRINDLE, M.D., AND
UDAYAN K. SHAH, M.D.

INTRODUCTION

CHARGE syndrome includes a predisposition to a variety of rhinologic issues. Patients with CHARGE have altered nasal, skull base, and oral anatomy that may contribute significantly to rhinologic disease. Examples of this include choanal atresia/choanal stenosis, cleft palate, adenoid hypertrophy, upper airway obstruction, and sinusitis (Coniglio, Manzione, & Hengerer, 1988).

CASE 1

Case 1 was born via an uncomplicated term vaginal delivery to a healthy mother. Prenatal ultrasound had indicated a cardiac defect (ventricular septal defect) and bilateral choanal atresia. Initial respiratory distress and cyanosis (blue skin and lips) were treated successfully by suctioning of the mouth and oral airway placement with bag-mask ventilation. Neither nasal cavity could be suctioned fully as catheters could not be passed posteriorly into the nasopharynx (area of throat behind the nose), consistent with the prenatal ultrasonography indicating probable choanal atresia. Computed tomography (CT) confirmed bilateral choanal atresia (Figure 10-1). Genetics evaluation prompted a diagnosis of CHARGE syndrome based on the clinical findings of

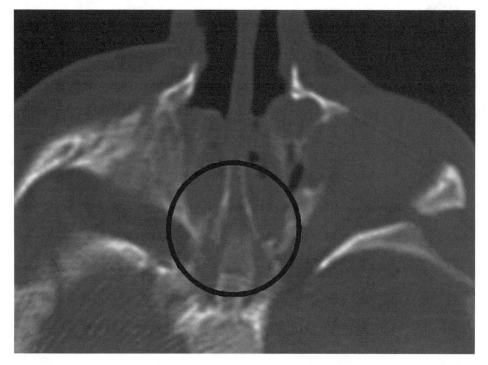

FIGURE 10–1. Axial computed tomography scan. Choanal atresia is circled. Blockage is indicated by the white bony obstruction within the circle. Nose oriented to top of photo. Figure courtesy of Dr. Riccardo D'Eredita.

ocular colobomas, cardiac defect, choanal atresia, genitourinary anomalies, and sensorineural hearing loss. Surgery to correct the heart defect was completed first. After the baby was stable from this repair, the choanal atresia was treated with five procedures: one trans-nasal repair that opened both nasal vaults and four subsequent trans-nasal revisions over the next 14 months. At age four years, the child is doing well with respect to his nasal airway.

CHOANAL ATRESIA/CHOANAL STENOSIS

Choanal atresia (CA) refers to a blockage of the posterior nasal cavity. Choanal atresia or stenosis (narrowing of the passageway, CS, Figure 10-2) is seen in 35% to 60% of patients with CHARGE syndrome (Blake, et al., 1998; Jongmans, et al., 2006). CHARGE syndrome is the most common syndrome observed in patients with CA (Hengerer, Brickman, & Jeyakumar, 2008; Tellier et al., 1998).

Choanal atresia may be unilateral or bilateral. CA is a rare cause of upper airway obstruction, occurring in 1 in 5000 to 7000 live births. It may be seen

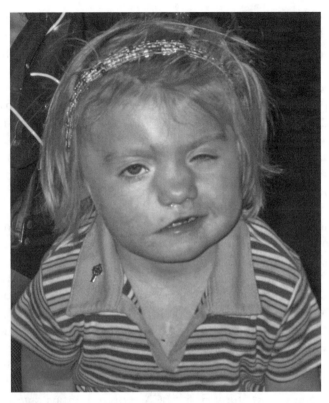

FIGURE 10–2. Persistent nasal drainage occurs with choanal stenosis. Note the typical CHARGE face and unilateral facial palsy.

more often in girls than boys (commonly a 2:1 ratio of female to male is cited, e.g., Samadi, Shah, & Handler, 2003), and unilateral choanal atresia (UCA) is more common than bilateral choanal atresia (BCA) (Hengerer, et al., 2008). Various theories exist regarding the etiology of CA or CS, including failure of the posterior nasal membrane to rupture, persistence of the buccopharyngeal membrane, or incomplete opening of the embryologic nasal cavity (Hengerer, et al., 2008; Morgan et al., 1993). The presence of CA warrants evaluation for other findings that may be seen in infants with CHARGE syndrome.

Bilateral choanal atresia is immediately life threatening, as newborns are obligate nose breathers (they cannot breathe orally). Neonates born with BCA present in respiratory distress and have stridor (noisy breathing) and cyclic cyanosis (blue skin due to lack of oxygen) that are relieved temporally with crying (Tellier, et al., 1998). Rapid intervention is required in the form of an oral airway, using a McGovern nipple, intubation (a breathing tube), or, rarely, tracheotomy. These methods bypass the area of obstruction and allow for delivery of air to the lungs until correction of the BCA can be achieved. Unilateral choanal atresia typically presents as unilateral nasal congestion with mucoid nasal discharge (Jongmans, et al., 2006). It may be mistaken for chronic unilateral rhinosinusitis. It may be diagnosed at birth or may go undiagnosed for years since the child can breathe through the other side of the nose.

Historically, it was taught that 90% of atresia is bony and 10% membranous, but recent reports have shown that most children have a combination of bony and membranous atresia (Hengerer, et al., 2008). Diagnosis of CA/CS is suspected by history and presentation. Inability to pass a small suction catheter through the nare soon after birth is highly suggestive of CA/CS, and confirmation may be made by flexible fiberoptic nasopharyngoscopy (NPL) and/or by fine-cut CT. These studies are complementary in trying to determine preoperatively the type of CA/CS to aid in surgical planning and to assess for concomitant aerodigestive and nasopharyngeal anomalies such as laryngomalacia (floppy epiglottis and larynx) seen by NPL, or an excessively narrow nasopharynx seen by both CT and NPL (Hengerer, et al., 2008).

Various treatment methods exist for the surgical treatment of CA (Hengerer, et al., 2008; Park, Brockenbrough, & Stankiewicz, 2000). The first step is to maintain the airway. This can be done with an oral airway or with a McGovern nipple, which is simply a large nipple with the end cut off and secured in the baby's mouth to keep an open airway. Surgery generally is safe and effective, allowing for the creation of a nasal airway. This can be done by working through either the nose or the mouth and palate. Most children undergo surgery via the trans-nasal route. The need for multiple surgeries is common. In one report, surgery for BCA required an average of 4.9 procedures, while children with UCA required an average of 2.7 procedures (Tellier, et al., 1998).

Families should be prepared for multiple procedures and/or the need for definitive airway management via tracheotomy. The medical, surgical, and anesthesia team should be aware of the potential cardiac and airway anomalies that exist in patients with CHARGE syndrome that may require special operative anesthetic techniques and result in a prolonged recovery (Blake, et al., 2009).

Speech and language issues associated with CA/CS may include both hyponasality (a stuffy-nose sound) as well as hypernasality (too much air escaping from the nose) in children with CHARGE. Hypernasality is usually due to palatal problems (inadequate closure by the palate at the back of the throat during speech). Hyponasality can be due to a continued blockage of the nasal airway, and although not in itself an indication for surgery, increasing hyponasality may portend airway obstruction, accompanied by feeding problems. Along with airway concerns, speech and feeding issues impact development, and the care required for nasal obstruction can add tasks onto an often already overwhelmed family. Often, hyponasality can be managed with the use of nasal saline and gentle suctioning using an anterior bulb or small nonlatex catheters to wash out the mucus and promote the clearance of secretions. Nasal steroid sprays often are not helpful because the problem is structural, with bony or membranous obstruction rather than mucus membrane swelling. Decongestant nasal sprays are not recommended for long-term use. Surgery may be useful to further open the airway with nasal turbinate (interior sides of the nose) reduction or revision of the choanal atresia repair. Accurate surgical diagnosis with preoperative CT scanning as well as intraoperative endoscopy guide surgical decision making. This, coupled with family discussions balancing expected improvements against surgical and anesthetic risk, guide in achieving the best possible patient outcomes in regards to rhinologic issues in CHARGE.

ADENOID PROBLEMS IN CHARGE

Anatomic studies utilizing high-resolution CT have shown that patients with CHARGE syndrome have a narrowed nasopharynx (Coniglio, et al., 1988). It is in this area that adenoid tissue is found. As a result, even minimal enlargement of adenoid tissue may obstruct the choanae. Symptoms of adenoid hypertrophy include mouth breathing, hyponasal speech, sleep apnea, and persistent or recurrent rhinosinusitis, otitis media, or both. Management is by adenoidectomy (removal of the adenoid tissue). Children with CHARGE who may have a complete or submucus cleft palate may require only partial adenoidectomy to prevent velopharyngeal insufficiency (escape of air and food through the nose when speaking or eating). Additionally, adenoidectomy must be approached with caution in patients with known velopharyngeal insufficiency because removal of adenoid tissue can make this worse.

Adenoidectomy does not always reverse the symptoms. Often in children with CHARGE syndrome, even with small tonsils, removal of the tonsils is considered and performed via a variety of techniques. The rationale for concurrent tonsillectomy when tonsils are small is that each incremental improvement in the airway will benefit the child's airway and eating status. Discussion of concurrent tonsillectomy must consider the additional bleeding risk. Around 1% to 2% of children experience bleeding after tonsillectomy, which may necessitate a return trip to the operating room. On very rare occasions, this bleeding may be life-threatening. On occasion, adenotonsillar size may contribute to obstructive sleep apnea, which may be difficult to distinguish from seizure disorder or attention deficit hyperactivity disorder. A polysomnogram (sleep study) with a pH probe study (to evaluate the contribution of gastroesophageal reflux) with electroencephalography may help to clarify the various contributing factors to sleep, reflux, and seizure disorders in CHARGE.

SINUSITIS

Chronic or recurrent rhinosinusitis is frequently encountered in patients with CHARGE syndrome. Nasal discharge that is purulent, usually with fever but sometimes without, in addition to irritability (including sudden changes in behavior) and headache are seen. Usually the maxillary (under the eyes) and ethmoid (between the nose and eye) sinuses are most affected until teen years, when the frontal sinuses (above the eyes) develop and can be the source of sinusitis. The contracted nasopharynx and limited nasal airways of people with CHARGE contribute to altered airflow though the nose, predisposing to drying of the nasal membranes with subsequently decreased clearance of mucus. In addition, gastroesophageal reflux disease (GERD) promotes the development of rhinosinusitis in individuals with CHARGE. Diagnosis of sinusitis can be difficult in individuals with limited communication skills. In some cases, imaging of the sinuses is necessary to confirm the diagnosis.

Medical management begins with nasal saline sprays, directed "back" toward the ear rather than "up" toward the eyes. Nasal decongestants such as oxymetazoline (Afrin) are not to be used for more than three days to avoid the development of "rebound" congestion and worsening of nasal obstruction and rhinosinusitis (Asher, McGill, Kaplan, Friedman, & Healy, 1990). Antibiotics often are helpful to treat sinusitis in CHARGE, and surgery other than adenoidectomy is not needed often.

When necessary, surgery may help to open the sinuses and assist drainage in patients who fail medical therapy. Many children with CHARGE have had multiple surgeries for chronic sinusitis. These surgeries may include adenoidectomy to remove obstructing and/or infected lymphoid tissue or sinus surgery to improve the ventilation and/or drainage of the paranasal sinus. Management of sinusitis needs to include a detailed discussion with individuals presenting with sinusitis about the symptoms which cause concern. As stated, the diagnosis of sinusitis may be difficult especially in children who are deafblind without formal language. Sinusitis may present as irritability, fatigue, or disinterest in whatever is asked of them at school or at home or with a sudden change in behavior, including apparently aggressive behavior. Because persons with CHARGE may be under-reactive for pain (see Chapter 30), pain associated with sinusitis may go unnoticed until it is above the threshold and is suddenly unbearable.

CONCLUSION

Children with CHARGE syndrome are predisposed by their anatomy to problems with nasal airflow and infections. An informed proactive interdisciplinary approach allows for expedient and long-term management of these often difficult problems. Families and other providers benefit from candid discussion on the pace and duration of treatment, including consideration of a realistic time frame and office visit schedule, when managing these often chronic rhinologic concerns.

Nasal problems can have a major effect on the child, family, and caregivers. At birth, choanal atresia can be life-threatening. Enlarged adenoids can obstruct the airway, block the eustachian tubes, aggravate otitis media, affect speech, and even mimic seizures. Sinusitis can occur occasionally or become a chronic debilitating problem. Lack of smell (see Chapter 7) has a profound impact on the child's understanding of the world about him or her, especially if deafblindness is also present.

REFERENCES

Asher, B. F., McGill, T. J., Kaplan, L., Friedman, E. M., & Healy, G. (1990). Airway complications in CHARGE association. *Archives of Otolaryngology—Head and Neck Surgery*, *116*, 594-595.

Blake, K. D., Davenport, S. L., Hall, B. D., Hefner, M. A., Pagon, R. A., Williams, M. S., . . . Graham, J. M., Jr. (1998). CHARGE association: an update and review for the primary pediatrician. *Clinical Pediatrics*, *37*, 159-173.

Blake, K. D., MacCuspie, J., Hartshorne, T. S., Roy, M., Davenport, S. L., & Corsten, G. (2009). Postoperative airway events of individuals with CHARGE syndrome. *International Journal of Pediatric Otorhinolaryngology*, *73*(2), 219-226.

Coniglio, J. U., Manzione, J. V., & Hengerer, A. S. (1988). Anatomic findings and management of choanal atresia and the CHARGE association. *Annals of Otology Rhinology and Laryngology*, *97*, 448-453.

Hengerer, A. S., Brickman, T. M., & Jeyakumar, A. (2008). Choanal atresia: embryologic analysis and evolution of treatment, a 30-year experience. *Laryngoscope*, *118*, 862-866.

Jongmans, M. C., Admiraal, R. J., van der Donk, K. P., Vissers, L. E., Baas, A. F., Kapusta, L., . . . van Ravenswaaij, C. M. (2006). CHARGE syndrome: the phenotypic spectrum of mutations in the CHD7 gene. *Journal of Medical Genetics*, *43*, 306-314.

Morgan, D., Bailey, M., Phelps, P., Bellman, S., Grace, A., & Wyse, R. (1993). Ear-nose-throat abnormalities in the CHARGE association. *Archives of Otology—Head & Neck Surgery*, *119*, 49-54.

Park, A. H., Brockenbrough, J., & Stankiewicz, J. (2000). Endoscopic versus traditional approaches to choanal atresia. *Otolaryngology Clinics of North America*, *33*, 77-90.

Samadi, D. S., Shah, U. K., & Handler, S. D. (2003). Choanal atresia: A twenty-year review of medical comorbidities and surgical outcomes. *Laryngoscope*, *113*, 254-258.

Tellier, A. L., Cormier-Daire, V., Abadie, V., Amiel, J., Sigaudy, S., Bonnet, D., . . . Lyonnet, S. (1998). CHARGE syndrome: Report of 47 cases and a review. *American Journal of Medical Genetics*, *76*, 402-409.

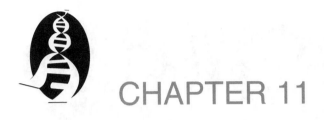

CHAPTER 11

Airway

MICHAEL J. RUTTER, M.D., FRACS, JEREMY D. PRAGER, M.D., AND EVAN J. PROPST, M.D.

*A*lthough the CHARGE acronym and the diagnostic criteria specifically identify choanal atresia as the only airway anomaly, clinicians with experience in managing patients with CHARGE almost always identify at least one other airway anomaly. This chapter begins with an overview of these anomalies and briefly describes pertinent airway issues, relevant diagnostic investigations, and the clinical management of this complex patient population. Airway anomalies are presented in anatomical sequence from the oral cavity to the lungs (Color Plate 10).

PHYSICAL ANOMALIES

Oral Malformations

Oral malformations commonly are seen in children with CHARGE syndrome. When micrognathia (abnormally small lower jaw) is present, glossoptosis (posterior displacement of the tongue) is universal. Moreover, even in patients with mild micrognathia, glossoptosis may be significant. Cleft lip and palate are present in up to 20% of patients (Blake, et al., 1998; Jongmans, et al., 2006) (Figure 11-1). Dental anomalies such as oligodontia (congenital lack of more than six teeth) and delayed eruption of teeth have also been reported (Al, Cottrell, & Hughes, 2002).

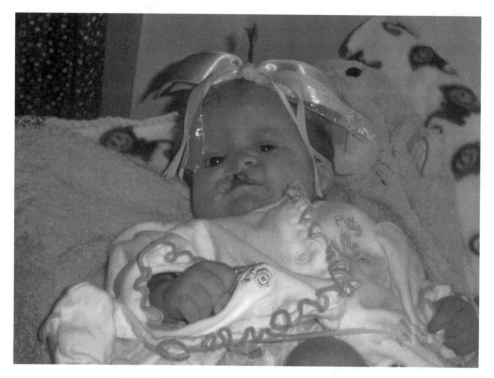

FIGURE 11–1. Infant with cleft lip and palate.

Posterior Choanae

Choanal atresia refers to the congenital failure of one or both of these nasal passages to open. See Chapter 10 for a discussion of choanal atresia and stenosis in CHARGE syndrome.

Larynx

The larynx in patients with CHARGE is characterized by prominent anterior-lying arytenoid cartilages (see Color Plate 10) that often are diagnosed incorrectly as laryngomalacia (floppy, immature cartilage of upper larynx). Adding to this confusion, children with CHARGE syndrome often have respiratory distress, feeding difficulties, and aspiration—all of which are also seen in patients with severe laryngomalacia. It is significant to note that, whereas supraglottoplasty is an extremely effective surgical intervention for patients with laryngomalacia, this procedure tends to worsen aspiration in patients with CHARGE (White, Giambra, Hopkin, Daines & Rutter, 2005).

Subglottic stenosis (narrowing of region just below the vocal cords) is generally considered to be either congenital or acquired. In many patients with CHARGE, however, congenital and acquired stenoses often are combined. Children with even mild stenosis at birth (congenital stenosis) may require prolonged or repeated periods of intubation. This, in turn, may lead to the development of an additional acquired stenosis. Interestingly, although congenital subglottic stenosis has a tendency to improve spontaneously, acquired subglottic stenosis is unlikely to do so without surgical intervention (Morgan, et al., 1993). The reported incidence of subglottic stenosis in patients with CHARGE varies from 8% to 22% (Morgan, et al., 1993; White, et al., 2005), perhaps reflecting differences in referral patterns and the disproportionate percentage of patients with airway problems in the latter institution. Other rarely seen laryngeal anomalies are laryngeal cleft and laryngeal web.

Although the anatomic characteristics of the larynx may be superficially the most impressive feature, laryngeal physiology is of greater clinical significance. In essence, it is the abnormal neuromuscular input of the CHARGE larynx that dominates the clinical picture. Abnormal sensation and muscular control result in vocal cord dysfunction and a strong tendency toward aspiration. These same disorders of sensation and muscular control also afflict the pharynx of most children with CHARGE syndrome.

Many children with CHARGE have an underlying cardiac defect that ultimately requires repair. This repair has the inherent risk of damage to the recurrent laryngeal nerves, particularly the left recurrent laryngeal nerve, which passes by and under the aorta. A resultant left vocal cord paralysis makes an already bad airway situation worse in terms of airway compromise and aspiration.

Pharynx

Upper airway obstruction and swallowing difficulties are common in children with CHARGE syndrome. These difficulties result from many factors, including neuropathies of cranial nerves V (trigeminal), VII (facial), IX (glossopharyngeal), and X (vagus) (see also Chapters 12 and 13). These nerves are responsible for oral cavity, pharyngeal, and laryngeal sensation, tone, and reflexive and voluntary motor function. Pharyngeal and laryngeal sensory deficits, hypotonia, and lack of coordination play a role in the predisposition to upper airway obstruction and swallowing difficulties seen in these patients (Naito, et al., 2007).

Trachea

Patients with CHARGE often have a tracheoesophageal fistula (TEF, abnormal connection between the trachea and the esophagus) with or without esophageal atresia (EA). Although all children with a tracheoesophageal fistula have tracheomalacia (abnormal collapse of tracheal walls), the actual incidence of tracheomalacia in patients with CHARGE is somewhat higher than can be explained by TEF alone. In addition, some children who do not have a TEF have tracheomalacia or tracheobronchomalacia (collapsible trachea and bronchi). A tracheostomy often is required (Figure 11–2).

Cranial Neuropathies

Most patients with CHARGE have involvement of the cranial nerves known as neuropathies (Blake, Hartshorne, Lawland, Dailor, & Thelin, 2008). Color Plate 11 illustrates the normal sensory and motor innervation of the oral cavity, pharynx, and larynx. Dysfunction of cranial nerves IX and X is considered the likely etiology of swallowing difficulties and aspiration, both of which are very common in children with CHARGE syndrome. These nerves are involved in laryngeal and pharyngeal sensation and movement, including the swallowing reflex. The glossopharyngeal nerve (CN IX) generally provides taste sensation from the posterior tongue as well as sensation from the oral cavity,

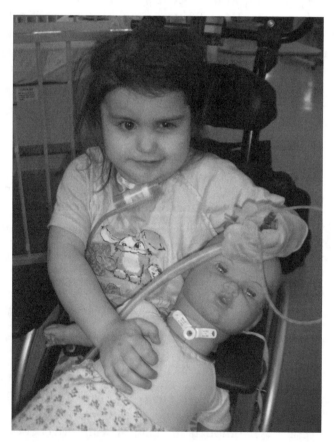

FIGURE 11–2. Child with a tracheostomy and her doll with a tracheostomy.

oropharynx, and hypopharynx. The vagus nerve (CN X) provides sensation from the epiglottis and larynx and innervates the muscles of the soft palate, pharynx, and larynx. Other neuropathies involving cranial nerves V, VII, and VIII (vestibulocochlear nerve) also have been reported in patients with CHARGE (Morgan, et al., 1993; Byerly & Pauli, 1993).

EVALUATION AND MANAGEMENT

Most infants with CHARGE present with airway distress or aspiration shortly after birth. This warrants airway evaluation and management by an interdisciplinary team comprising pediatric subspecialists in otolaryngology, pulmonology, and gastroenterology as well as experienced speech and language pathologists. The most common early presentation is infants with bilateral choanal atresia. These infants commonly present with apneic spells (stop breathing). Initial evaluation generally is performed by the pediatric service. This evaluation involves the placement of a 6-French suction catheter in the nose to determine whether it can be passed into the nasopharynx (MacDonald, Mullett, & Seshia, 2005). When this cannot be done, consultation with an otolaryngologist is the next step. A more comprehensive evaluation is provided by flexible nasopharyngoscopy, which permits direct visualization of the posterior choanae. If choanal atresia is confirmed or even suspected, a computed tomography (CT) scan of the nose and nasopharynx is indicated. It is advisable to decongest and suction the nose just prior to the CT scan. The CT scan also should include specific images of the inner ear (both cochlea and vestibule), as this information is helpful both in confirming a diagnosis of CHARGE syndrome and in determining the extent of hearing loss and balance abnormalities in these children.

Transnasal flexible laryngoscopy is also desirable, as this provides information regarding the pharynx, tongue base, and larynx, including vocal cord mobility. This is not possible in a setting of bilateral choanal atresia; in these patients, transoral flexible laryngoscopy may be performed.

Although transnasal or transoral evaluations with flexible telescopes ideally are performed with the child awake, formal evaluation of the larynx, trachea, and bronchi with the child under general anesthesia is desirable. Laryngoscopy and bronchoscopy allow a more detailed examination of the airway. The tongue base should be evaluated for glossoptosis (posterior displacement of tongue). The larynx should be examined for laryngomalacia, tall, anterior-lying arytenoids, short vocal cords, laryngeal cleft, or glottic web. The subglottis should be evaluated for stenosis and the posterior tracheal wall for evidence of a tracheoesophageal fistula. Tracheobronchomalacia also may be noted. Coordination with other specialists who need to examine the child under anesthesia (e.g., ophthalmology) is advisable, to limit the number of anesthesias necessary.

Aspiration and Swallowing

For more information on aspiration and swallowing, see also Chapter 12.

Chronic pulmonary disease resulting from aspiration is a common cause of death in patients with CHARGE syndrome. As shown in Table 11-1, three substances can be aspirated—food and drink, saliva, and refluxate. Investigation and management depend on what substance or substances are being aspirated. Aspiration of food and drink can be evaluated with multiple tools. Flexible bronchoscopy and bronchoalveolar lavage (BAL) can provide supportive evidence of aspiration if lipid-laden macrophages are present (Boesch, et al., 2006).

Fiber-optic endoscopic evaluation of swallowing (FEES) involves placement of a flexible nasopharyngoscope through the nose and choana to allow visualization of the glottis from above. Patients are asked to swallow food and

TABLE 11–1. Evaluation and Management of Aspiration in CHARGE Syndrome

Aspirated Substance	Evaluation	Management
Food and drink	Flexible bronchoscopy with bronchoalveolar lavage (BAL)	Selective oral feeding
	Functional endoscopic evaluation of swallowing (FEES)	Nasogastric tube feeding
		Gastrostomy tube feeding
	FEES with sensory testing (FEEST)	
	Video swallow study (VSS)	
	Dye study (in patients who have a tracheotomy)	
Saliva	Radionuclide salivagram	Anticholinergic (glycopyrrolate)
	Computed tomography (CT) chest scan	Botulinum toxin injection
	Dye study (in patients who have a tracheotomy)	Salivary gland excision or duct ligation
		Tympanic neurectomy
		CPAP
		Laryngeal separation
Reflux	Multichannel intraluminal impedance with Ph monitoring (MII-pH)	Changing food consistency
	Radionuclide scans	Promotility agents
	Dye study (in patients who have a tracheotomy)	Proton pump inhibitor
		Fundoplication
		Gastrojejunal feeding

liquid of different consistencies. FEES is used to evaluate vocal fold mobility, management of secretions, spontaneous clearing swallows, and hypopharyngeal sensation. FEES with sensory testing (FEEST) allows quantification of laryngeal sensation and accurately predicts aspiration. The ability to achieve and sustain airway protection during swallowing is assessed using trials of liquid and semisolids to investigate spillage, penetration, aspiration, response to aspiration and residue (a problem resulting from poor pharyngeal contraction). A speech and language pathologist is present and may recommend modifications in swallowing techniques and food consistencies.

A video swallow study (VSS) also can be used to evaluate aspiration of food and drink. In VSS, fluoroscopy is used to provide a real-time look at all phases of swallowing. Particular attention should be paid to premature spillage, laryngeal penetration, aspiration, residue, patient reaction/sensitivity, and clearing responses to these abnormalities. As in FEES, a speech and language pathologist is present to offer recommendations regarding swallowing and oral intake.

In patients with CHARGE who have a tracheotomy tube, a dye study may be performed. Food coloring is added to various consistencies of food, and the presence of aspiration is confirmed when colored secretions are present in the tracheotomy tube.

Management of aspiration of food and drink depends on the severity of the aspiration. Aspiration of certain consistencies can be alleviated by modifications of swallowing technique or avoidance. Temporary feeding can be achieved through a nasogastric tube. For longer rehabilitation or for aspiration that is unlikely to resolve, a gastrostomy tube can be placed. Many individuals with CHARGE require gastrostomy tubes for many years.

Saliva

Aspiration of saliva can be evaluated using a number of techniques. Radionuclide salivagrams are performed by placing a small quantity of radiotracer in the buccal pouch (cheek) and recording serial images until clearance from the mouth occurs. The presence of radioactivity in the trachea or bronchi indicates aspiration. It is important to note, however, that salivagrams have shown poor agreement with other tests for salivary aspiration, and further evaluation regarding the accuracy of this technique is needed (Boesch, et al., 2006).

FEES can demonstrate aspiration of oral secretions directly or imply impending aspiration by the presence of pooled secretions in the larynx and diminished laryngeal sensitivity. Pooled secretions and sensory deficits predict aspiration without challenging the patient with an oral bolus (Perlman, et al., 2004; Thompson, 2003).

High-resolution CT of the chest can demonstrate pulmonary changes consistent with chronic salivary aspiration. Although these changes are suggestive of salivary aspiration, they are not diagnostic. Because these patients often are kept on a nothing by mouth status or have significant oral aversions, VSS generally is not performed. In addition, flexible bronchoscopy with BAL is not useful because saliva does not contain lipid and, thus, does not contain lipid-laden macrophages.

Management of salivary aspiration should be individualized. Medical therapy with the anticholinergic agent glycopyrrolate can reduce the amount of saliva produced and aspirated. Botulinum toxin injection into salivary glands also has been used to reduce the amount of saliva produced (Blake & Mac-Cuspie, 2009), as has surgical removal of salivary gland tissue or duct ligation. Tympanic neurectomy can be used to decrease salivary gland activity. In patients who have a tracheotomy, continuous positive airway pressure (CPAP) can decrease the amount of aspiration by moving secretions back into the hypopharynx. Laryngotracheal separation offers a definitive and potentially reversible surgical method of preventing aspiration.

Refluxate

Although the 24-hour pH probe historically has been used to diagnose gastroesophageal reflux, this study is limited, as it can detect acidic reflux only and not nonacidic reflux. Multichannel intraluminal impedance with pH monitoring (MII–pH) allows for the diagnosis of both acid and nonacidic reflux events. This technique involves the diagnosis of refluxate by detecting changes in intraluminal resistance.

Radionuclide studies, also known as gastroesophageal scintigraphy or "milk scans," have been used as physiologic tests for aspiration of refluxate. Technetium-99-sulphur colloid is mixed in formula, and the child is fed. Serial images then are taken to detect tracer activity in the lung parenchyma. Although this finding may indicate aspiration, the technique is unable to differentiate between direct aspiration and reflux aspiration (Boesch, et al., 2006).

In the presence of confirmed gastroesophageal reflux, a positive dye study in a patient with a tracheotomy supports a diagnosis of aspiration of refluxate. When gastrostomy tube feeds are colored with green food dye and green-tinged secretions are subsequently suctioned from the tracheotomy tube, the diagnosis of refluxate aspiration is confirmed.

Mild aspiration may be treated by changing the consistency of food, using promotility agents such as erythromycin and administering proton pump inhibitors to reduce the acid content of reflux; however, fundoplication is the surgical antireflux procedure of choice for persistent or severe aspiration of reflux. Because less reflux exists if the stomach is empty, an alternative is gastrojejunal feeding.

Upper Airway Obstruction

Recurrent cyanosis and respiratory distress secondary to bilateral choanal atresia may be the first presentation of CHARGE. Respiratory distress also may present secondary to micrognathia, glossoptosis, and pharyngeal and laryngeal sensory and motor dysfunction. Severe life-threatening airway obstruction, stridor, and recurrent cyanosis all require immediate management. Temporizing measures such as the placement of an oral airway device, a McGovern nipple, or intubation should be used to establish a definitive airway. Because of micrognathia, glossoptosis, pharyngeal and laryngeal abnormalities, intubation may be challenging, and a tracheotomy may be required. Most patients with CHARGE syndrome present with symptoms related to stable chronic upper airway obstruction, which may be addressed in a nonemergent fashion.

Pharyngeal sensory and motor dysfunction plays a role in swallowing difficulties and aspiration and in upper airway obstruction. If these deficits are severe, they will manifest while the patient is awake and require urgent evaluation and management. Milder deficits may manifest as an obstruction during sleep. Approximately 50% of patients with CHARGE have symptoms ranging from hypopnea (decreased breathing) to desaturations and bradycardia during sleep (Roger, et al. 1999). Repeated episodes of hypopnea can lead to abnormal cerebral development and pulmonary hypertension.

In older children with CHARGE who are not tracheotomy dependent, several methods are available to evaluate airway obstruction. Nocturnal obstructive apnea usually is seen in conjunction with severe snoring and may be a consequence of enlarged tonsils and adenoid tissue. These patients are less likely to tolerate crowding of the nasopharynx or oropharynx and benefit from tonsillectomy and adenoidectomy. Polysomnography is considered the gold standard for diagnosis and allows for titration of CPAP; however, it does not allow determination of the site of obstruction. Cine magnetic resonance imaging (MRI) and fluoroscopy and flexible bronchoscopy with the child under light anesthesia usually can isolate the dominant source of obstruction, thus helping to direct appropriate surgical intervention (Figure 11-3).

A detailed discussion of the management of upper airway obstruction during sleep is beyond the scope of this chapter. Briefly, therapy ranges from CPAP to less invasive procedures such as tonsillectomy and adenoidectomy to more invasive procedures such as base of tongue reduction and tracheotomy. Therapy is tailored to the individual patient and often is conducted in a stepwise fashion.

As mentioned previously, the arytenoids in patients with CHARGE lie anteriorly and can contribute to airway obstruction. This often is misdiagnosed as laryngomalacia and managed with supraglottoplasty. Supraglottoplasty involves releasing shortened aryepiglottic folds responsible for prolapse of the arytenoids into the laryngeal inlet. Reduction of redundant mucosa overlying the arytenoid cartilages also may be performed as part of this procedure. However, in the majority of patients with CHARGE syndrome, supraglottoplasty is relatively contraindicated. Several studies have shown limited success in airway improvement as well as potential exacerbation of aspiration with this intervention (Roger, et al 1999; White, et al., 2005).

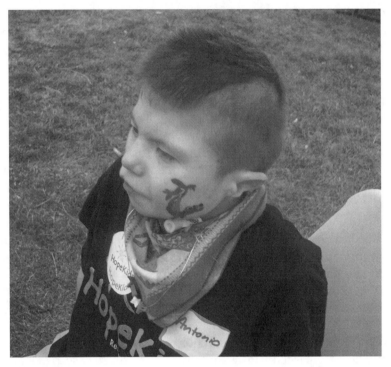

FIGURE 11–3. Older child with trach. Note typical CHARGE ears and scarf to catch saliva.

Role of Tracheotomy

Placement of a tracheotomy may be necessary in close to 30% of patients with CHARGE (Roger, et al., 1999). Several indications exist for tracheotomy, and regardless of the indication, early tracheotomy is thought to benefit the airway management of these complicated patients. The most frequent reason for tracheotomy placement is airway obstruction, the etiology of which often is multifactorial. In children with an unstable airway and in whom intubation is challenging, a tracheotomy may be required to secure a safe airway.

Although most children with bilateral choanal atresia do not require tracheotomy placement, this is not the case for children with CHARGE. Even when choanal atresia is addressed during the neonatal period, the likelihood of requiring a tracheotomy remains surprisingly high.

The pharyngeal and laryngeal sensory and motor dysfunction that leads to aspiration is also a common criterion for performing a tracheotomy. The addition of left recurrent laryngeal nerve palsy following cardiac surgery increases the likelihood of requiring a tracheotomy (Roger, et al., 1999).

Tracheotomy can aid in the diagnosis of aspiration via a dye study, although this is not a sufficient indication for surgery. After a tracheotomy is in place, it allows for improved pulmonary toilet through direct suctioning.

In addition, CPAP given though the tracheotomy can decrease the amount of aspiration by moving secretions superiorly back into the hypopharynx. This also can be used to treat tracheomalacia.

SUMMARY

Airway abnormalities are common in patients with CHARGE syndrome. These abnormalities are diverse and can involve multiple anatomic sites extending from the oral cavity to the lungs. Evaluation depends on the particular presentation and may range from urgent airway intervention to a more systematic aerodigestive examination. Most patients should undergo nasopharyngoscopy, laryngoscopy, bronchoscopy, and evaluation of swallowing, reflux, and airway obstruction during sleep. Treatment ranges from immediate measures to stabilize the airway to more complex medical and surgical management of specific issues. Complicated patients with multiple or severe abnormalities are likely to benefit from early tracheotomy. Patients with CHARGE syndrome are best managed by an interdisciplinary team comprising pediatric subspecialists in otolaryngology, pulmonology, gastroenterology, and speech and language pathology.

Acknowledgments. We would like to thank Aliza Cohen for assistance in writing, and Claire Miller, Program Director, Aerodigestive Center and Division of Speech Pathology, Cincinnati Children's Hospital Medical Center, for content contributions.

REFERENCES

Al, S. T, Cottrell, D. A., & Hughes, C. V. (2002). Dental findings associated with the malformations of CHARGE. *Pediatric Dentistry, 24*, 43–46.

Blake, K. D., Davenport, S. L., Hall, B. D., Hefner, M. A., Pagon, R. A., Williams, M. S., . . . Graham, J. M., Jr. (1998). CHARGE association: an update and review for the primary pediatrician. *Clinical Pediatrics, 37*, 159–173.

Blake, K. D., Hartshorne, T. S., Lawand, C., Dailor, A. N., & Thelin, J. W. (2008). Cranial nerve manifestations in CHARGE syndrome. *American Journal of Medical Genetics, 146A*, 585–592.

Blake, K., & MacCuspie, J. (2009, July). *Botox for dysphagia in CHARGE syndrome: A case study.* Poster presented at meeting of the CHARGE Syndrome Conference for Professionals, Chicago, IL.

Boesch, R. P., Daines, C., Willging, J. P., Kaul, A., Cohen, A. P., Wood, R. E., & Amin, R. S. (2006). Advances in the diagnosis and management of chronic pulmonary aspiration in children. *European Respiratory Journal, 28*, 847–861.

Byerly, K. A., & Pauli, R. M. (1993). Cranial nerve abnormalities in CHARGE association. *American Journal of Medical Genetics, 45*, 751–757.

Jongmans, M. C., Admiraal, R. J., van der Donk, K. P., Vissers, L. E., Baas, A. F., Kapusta, L., . . . van Ravenswaaij, C. M. (2006). CHARGE syndrome: the phenotypic spectrum of mutations in the CHD7 gene. *Journal of Medical Genetics, 43,* 306-314.

MacDonald, M. G., Mullett, M. D., & Seshia, M. M. (2005). *Avery's neonatology: Pathophysiology and management of the newborn* (6th ed.). Philadelphia: Lippincott Williams & Wilkins.

Morgan, D., Bailey, M., Phelps, P., Bellman, S., Grace, A., & Wyse, R. (1993). Ear-nose-throat abnormalities in the CHARGE association. *Archives of Otology—Head & Neck Surgery, 119,* 49-54.

Naito, Y., Higuchi, M., Koinuma, G., Aramaki, M., Takahashi, T., & Kosaki, K. (2007). Upper airway obstruction in neonates and infants with CHARGE syndrome. *American Journal of Medical Genetics, 143A,* 1815-1820.

Perlman, P. W., Cohen, M. A., Setzen, M., Belafsky, P. C., Guss, J., Mattucci, K. F., & Ditkoff, M. (2004). The risk of aspiration of pureed food as determined by flexible endoscopic evaluation of swallowing with sensory testing. *Otolaryngology-Head and Neck Surgery, 130,* 80-83.

Roger, G., Morisseau-Durand, M. P., Van Den Abbeele, T., Nicollas, R., Triglia, J. M., Narcy, P., . . . Garabedian EN. (1999). The CHARGE association: the role of tracheotomy. *Archives of Otolaryngology—Head & Neck Surgery, 125,* 33-38.

Thompson, D. M. (2003). Laryngopharyngeal sensory testing and assessment of airway protection in pediatric patients. *American Journal of Medicine, 115,* 166S-168S.

White, D. R., Giambra, B. K., Hopkin, R. J., Daines, C. L., & Rutter, M. J. (2005). Aspiration in children with CHARGE syndrome. *International Journal of Pediatric Otorhinolaryngology, 69,* 1205-1209.

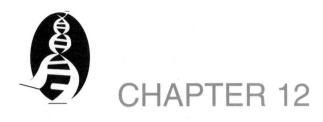

CHAPTER 12

Feeding Issues

JOAN ARVEDSON, Ph.D.

*F*eeding and swallowing difficulties are common in infants and children with CHARGE syndrome. These difficulties vary considerably in type and severity as expected given the wide range of combinations of signs and symptoms in individuals with CHARGE syndrome (Blake, Hartshorne, Lawand, Dailor, & Thelin, 2008; Blake & Prasad, 2006; Stromland et al., 2005). Multiple cranial nerve deficits are fundamental to the swallowing problems in infancy and may persist as children get older (Blake, Salem-Hartshorne, Daoud, & Gradstein, 2005; Lin, Siebert, & Graham, 1990). Some children progress to become total oral feeders in childhood, while others require a gastrostomy tube for supplemental feeding through adolescence and into adulthood (Issekutz, Graham, Prasad, Smith, & Blake, 2005). A description of "normal" feeding is included in the evaluation sections that follow.

Difficulties are associated with congenital structural anomalies (e.g., choanal atresia, clefting) and oral sensorimotor impairment. In some children, the problems may be primarily motor or primarily sensory based. Most children have some degree of involvement with both sensory and motor deficits. One would expect sensory and motor-based deficits as most cranial nerves involved in swallowing have both sensory and motor inputs (see Chapter 13). It is also quite common to find feeding difficulties that appear more behavioral based. Children learn to respond to difficult situations by food refusals and other behavioral "acting out" to escape situations that they may find scary or beyond their skill levels. Since infants and young children have limited communication skills, parents and other caregivers try to interpret fussing, arching, head turning, "shutting down," and other negative behaviors on the basis of cues that are not always clear. When cues are misinterpreted or over-ridden, problems become exacerbated.

This chapter includes a brief discussion of criteria for oral feeding in infancy, primary "red flags" as screening for feeding/swallowing problems, neural control of swallowing, evaluation of feeding/swallowing in infants and children to include clinical and instrumental examinations, and management approaches in individualized ways on the basis of the neurodevelopmental status and safety for swallowing.

CRITERIA FOR ORAL FEEDING IN INFANCY

A primary need for all infants, including those with CHARGE syndrome, is adequate nutrition for appropriate weight gain and growth (Blake, Kirk, & Ur, 1992). In order to meet those needs via oral nipple feeding, infants must be able to breathe through the nose. Infants are obligate nose breathers in order to suck, swallow, and coordinate breathing via breast or bottle feeding. A stable airway is a critical underpinning for oral feeding. Infants born with choanal atresia cannot feed orally in a typical way. Removal of a nipple every time an infant needs to breathe is far too disruptive to provide a sufficient volume of breast milk or formula to meet nutrition needs for appropriate growth. In those infants, supplemental tube feeding is needed for whatever duration is required for management to stabilize the airway. Even without choanal atresia, many infants with CHARGE are either not able to take in sufficient volume or have tracheal aspiration during oral feedings and need supplemental tube feedings. Aspiration of acidic reflux contents may have greater negative consequences on pulmonary function than aspiration with oral feedings.

Supplemental Tube Feeding

Supplemental tube feeding can be accomplished in several ways. An orogastric (OG) tube is logical initially as a temporary tube. OG tubes typically are used only for a short term given that they rest on the tongue and may interfere with suckling as well as posterior propulsion of the tongue in preparation for swallowing. They are dislodged easily. Choanal atresia, and in some instances choanal stenosis (even unilateral), will prevent the passage of a nasogastric (NG) tube. NG tubes (Figure 12–1) have a number of advantages over OG tubes; for instance, they do not interfere with tongue function. Disadvantages of NG tubes include stress on the infant when the tube is placed, the need for replacement when an infant pulls the tube out, some level of risk for placement into the airway instead of into the esophagus, tape on the face to keep the tube in place, upper esophageal sphincter kept open slightly by the tube,

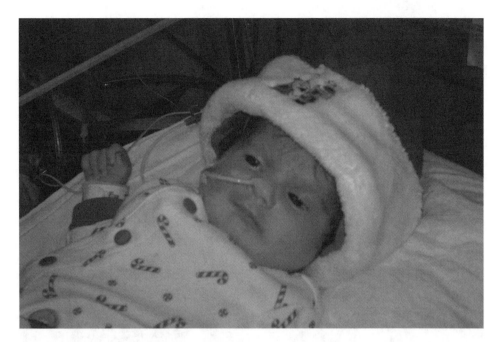

FIGURE 12–1. Infant with nasogastric (NG) tube for meeting nutrition and hydration needs, usually used for a fairly short time, at most several months.

and reduced nasal airflow with a tube blocking one nare. If the other nare is stenotic, nasal breathing can be reduced significantly, which will continue to have a negative impact on the potential for oral nipple feeding. When nonoral supplemental feeding is anticipated for more than just a few months, a gastrostomy tube (GT) or percutaneous endoscopic gastrostomy (PEG) tube usually is a more viable option (Figure 12-2). It is important for all professionals and parents to understand that tubes can be removed and that the presence of any type of tube does not preclude oral feeding experiences. A tube can be a facilitator for advancing oral feeding while ensuring that the infant/child's nutrition and growth needs are being met.

Aspiration and Gastrointestinal (GI) Tract (Gastroesophageal Reflux [GER], Gastroesophageal Reflux Disease [GERD], Eosinophilic Esophagitis [EE or EoE], and Constipation)

Aspiration and GER

Presence of aspiration and GER are primary factors associated with tube feeding at one year of age in children with CHARGE syndrome (Dobbelsteyn, Peacocke, Blake, Crist, & Rashid, 2008). GI tract issues that include GER are known to contribute to aversive responses to advancing textures and are reported to

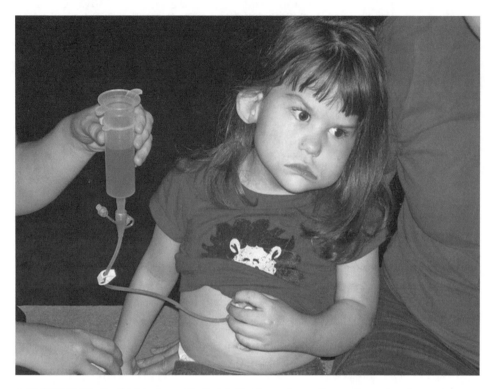

FIGURE 12–2. Child given Pedialyte™ via syringe through gastrostomy tube.

lead to long-term difficulty in feeding development in some instances (e.g., Dobbelsteyn, Marche, Blake, & Rashid, 2005; Strudwick, 2003). In their survey of parents of 39 children with CHARGE syndrome, Dobbelsteyn et al. (2008) reported that only GER (experienced by 89%) was associated significantly with tube feeding beyond 3 years of age. Fundoplication procedure for severe GER/GERD was used in 17 of 39 children (44%) with GER. Some children with fundoplication experienced side effects including gagging, retching, dumping syndrome, and gas bloat syndrome. On the other hand, fundoplications can fail with a reoperation rate of up to 19% (Rudolph et al., 2001), particularly in children with neurologic impairment as can be the case with CHARGE syndrome (Kimber, Kiely, & Spitz, 1998; Srivastava et al., 2009). The primary cause of fundoplication failure is herniation into the posterior mediastinum in the series reported by Kimber et al. (1998).

Although fundoplication was the mainstay of surgical management of GERD in past years, currently it is performed with less frequency (Lasser, Liao, & Burd, 2006). Fundoplication is a viable therapy when performed exclusively for management of GERD, especially for life-threatening GERD. It should be used only for effortless regurgitation seen with GERD, and not for children with frank vomiting as they will likely suffer complications and ultimately fail the procedure (Richards, Milla, Andrews, & Spitz, 2001). Srivastara et al.

(2009) stressed the need for prospective, multicenter, randomized control trials to evaluate management options to compare fundoplication and gastro-jejunal (GJ) feeding tube. Children with severe GERD or recurrent vomiting may require slow tube feedings over many hours each day. Prior to fundoplication, endoscopy should be performed to rule out nonreflux etiologies of vomiting that require other treatments, particularly eosinophilic esophagitis (Liacouras, 1997).

Eosinophilic Esophagitis

EE or EoE is an inflammatory disease of the esophagus that often mimics the signs of GERD (Noel & Tipnis, 2006). Although EE is less common than reflux esophagitis, it has become recognized and diagnosed with greater frequency in the past several years. EE is often associated with food allergy and atopy (Noel, Putnam, & Rothenberg, 2004). The inflammation process is unrelated to acid exposure, but possibly related to dietary antigen sensitivities (e.g., Markowitz, Spergel, Ruchelli, & Liacouras, 2003). This inflammation is associated with dysphagia, irritability, and in older children and adults food impaction (Noel & Tipnis, 2006) with muscosal changes (e.g., Lim et al., 2004). Diagnosis is made via histologic confirmation of a biopsy obtained during endoscopy. Treatment is specific and involves dietary changes and medications (Konikoff et al., 2006; Markowitz et al., 2003).

Constipation

In addition to GI tract issues focused on GER and EE, constipation is a common and aggravating problem for children with CHARGE syndrome and other neurologically based swallowing and feeding problems. The multiple causes for constipation include, but are not limited to, faulty innervations of the entire GI tract, inadequate fluid and/or fiber in the diet that also may place a child at risk for dehydration, lack of physical activity, lack of toilet training, side effects of medications, and inappropriate feeding regimens (e.g., Del Giudice et al., 1999; Sullivan, 1997). Cow's milk allergy can be related to constipation in some children (El-Hodhod, Younis, Zaitoun, & Daoud, 2010). Children who are constipated typically do not show interest in eating and drinking, and so they reduce their intake especially for fluid, which in turn aggravates the constipation, resulting in a vicious cycle. The importance of optimal nutrition and hydration cannot be overstated for all children. Dietitians and physicians are the primary professionals who make decisions with parents to minimize constipation issues. The availability of long-term outcome data contributes to increased understanding of the natural history of the problem of constipation (Walia, Mahajan, & Steffen, 2009). Newer pharmacological approaches provide optimism for treatment (Coccorullo, Quitadamo, Martinelli, & Staiano, 2009). Parents are encouraged to seek medical and nutrition advice whenever their infants and children do not have regular bowel movements, strain to have bowel movements, produce stools of exceptional size, or demonstrate any other out-of-the-ordinary circumstance. It is beyond the scope of this chapter to cover these GI topics in depth.

PRIMARY "RED FLAGS" WHEN SCREENING FOR FEEDING/SWALLOW PROBLEMS

The following questions should be helpful to all professionals, parents, and other caregivers in determining whether a child, regardless of underlying etiology, should be evaluated in depth by a feeding/swallowing specialist (adapted from Arvedson, 2008; Arvedson & Rogers, 1993, 1997). Professionals also need to keep in mind and to respect cultural differences around feeding.

How long does it take to feed the child? Feeding times greater than about 25–30 minutes on a regular basis may be a sign of a serious feeding problem and point to the need for further investigation.

Are there signs of respiratory distress? The infant or child who becomes increasingly congested as the feeding progresses, has a gurgly voice quality, and/or shows rapid or catch-up breathing (panting) may be having aspiration events or other pharyngeal phase swallowing problems.

Does the infant or child become irritable or lethargic during feedings? Irritability may relate to gastrointestinal discomfort, airway problems, neurologic issues, or behavioral issues. Lethargy or sleepiness may result from fatigue, sedating medications (e.g., anticonvulsants, muscle relaxants), or recurrent seizures.

Are mealtimes stressful? Regardless of the reasons for stress in child or parent, follow-up investigations are needed. Parents become very concerned when children do not eat easily and well. They may be force feeding without realizing it. Additional complications that can result from forced feeding may include inadequate weight gain, increased food refusals and, in severe cases, global behavior maladaptations.

Has the child slowed or stopped gaining weight in the previous two to three months? During the first two years of life in particular, appropriate steady weight gain is expected and critical for overall growth and for brain development. Lack of weight gain in a young child is equivalent to weight loss in an older child or adult.

NEURAL CONTROL OF SWALLOWING

Three distinct anatomic regions make up the swallow mechanism: oral cavity, pharynx, and esophagus. These regions can function separately, but they integrate their functions effectively through a neuronal network for swallowing.

The complexities of this system are beyond the scope of this chapter. Readers are encouraged to seek out other references (e.g., Dodds, 1989; Dodds, Stewart, & Logemann, 1990; Miller, 1999).

The neural control of swallowing involves four major components:

■ Afferent (incoming) sensory fibers contained in cranial nerves (Table 12–1)

■ Cerebral, midbrain, and cerebellar fibers that synapse (connect) with brain-stem swallowing centers

■ Paired swallowing centers in the brain stem

■ Efferent (outgoing) motor fibers contained in cranial nerves (Table 12–2)

Cranial nerve manifestations in CHARGE syndrome have been reported from evidence recorded by clinical presentations and specialized testing (e.g., Blake et al., 2008; Blustajn, Kirsch, Panigrahy, & Netchine, 2008; Chalouhi, Faulcon, Le Bihan, et al., 2005; Pinto, et al., 2005).

Sensory Aspects of Flavor Learning (Taste and Smell)

Disruptions in the sense of smell demonstrated in children with CHARGE syndrome include anosmia and mild to severe hyposmia (Chalouhi et al., 2005, and Chapter 7). Abnormal olfactory bulbs have been reported (Blustajn et al., 2008; Pinto et al., 2005). However, Chalouhi and colleagues found no correlation between the olfactory deficits and the severity of feeding problems.

TABLE 12–1. Sensory (Afferent) Cranial Nerves Involved in Swallowing

Cranial Nerve	Function
Trigeminal (V): mandibular division	Anterior 2/3 tongue; mucosa of cheek, floor of mouth, gums, temporomandibular joint; lower teeth; skin of lower lip and jaw
Trigeminal (V): maxillary division	Mucosa of nasopharynx, soft palate, hard palate, gums; upper teeth
Facial (VII)	Taste anterior 2/3 tongue
Glossopharyngeal (IX)	Taste and sensation posterior 2/3 tongue; sensation in mucosa of oropharynx, palatine tonsils, fauces
Vagus (X)	Sensation to mucosa of pharynx, larynx, viscera, epiglottis, esophagus

TABLE 12–2. Motor (Efferent) Innervation for Phases of Swallowing

Phase of Swallow	Innervation (cranial nerves + ansa cervicalis)
Oral	
Buccinator muscles of mastication (chewing)	CN V—mandibular branch, VII—inferior buccal branch
Orbicularis oris (lip closure)	CN VII—inferior and superior buccal branch
Facial muscles	CN VII
Tongue	
Intrinsic muscles (within tongue)	CN XII
Extrinsic muscles (move the tongue)	Ansa cervicalis (C1–C2)
Palatoglossus (initiation of swallowing)	CN XI (through pharyngeal plexus)
Pharyngeal	
Stylopharyngeus (bolus)	CN IX—muscular branch
Pharyngeal constrictors	CN X & XI—through pharyngeal plexus
Soft palate	
Tensor veli palatini muscle	CN V—mandibular branch
Levator veli palatini and uvular m.	CN X & XI—through pharyngeal plexus
Muscles of larynx	CN X—recurrent branch
Esophageal	
Suprahyoid muscles	CN V, VII, XII
Cricopharyngeus	CN X—recurrent and superior laryngeal external branches
Esophagus	CN X

It is well known that smell (odor) is involved intimately in taste of food and liquid. Newborn infants clearly distinguish odors among sweet, sour, and bitter (Hudson & Distel, 1999). The following tastes with preferences that have a strong innate component are commonly described: (1) sweet usually indicates energy-rich nutrients; (2) sour typically reflects the taste of acids; (3) salty allows modulating of diets for electrolyte balance; (4) bitter contributes to complexity and the enjoyment of beverages and foods, although it is not a dominant taste sensation (varied compounds do not share similar chemical structures and may include peptides, salts, plant-derived phenols and polyphenols, flavonoids, catechins, and caffeine (Drewnowski, 2001); (5) umami (or savory) is a term used to reflect the taste of amino acids (e.g., meat broth or aged cheese) (Bowen, 2006). Sweet, umami, and salty substances are innately preferred; whereas bitter and many sour substances are innately rejected (Beauchamp & Mennella, 2009).

The determinants of infant flavor preferences involve multiple sensory systems with taste receptors throughout the tongue. The sense of smell must be considered along with the development of taste preferences as found in studies of typically developing children (e.g., Liem & Mennella, 2003; Mennella & Beauchamp, 2005, 2008; Mennella, Pepino, & Reed, 2005). Research is needed in children with neurologic deficits, especially cranial nerve deficits. Based on anecdotal observations of children and parent reports, it is not uncommon for children who have had supplemental tube feedings over extensive time frames and, for whatever reason, have not been able to take regular diets from infancy, to show strong preferences for sour and salty foods. They lick salt off pretzels and crackers long before they feel safe enough to put the food into their mouths. They accept a couple drops of water flavored with lemon or pickle juice more readily than a sweet flavor.

Motor Aspects (Deficits Related to Cranial Nerve Damage)

Children with CHARGE syndrome having primarily motor deficits may show signs of oral and pharyngeal phase swallowing problems. Cranial nerves V, VII, IX, X, and XII provide innervations to muscles involved in the swallowing process (see Tables 12–1 and 12–2). Facial nerve (CN VII) damage may become evident by limited facial expression with the forehead usually involved, which leads one to suspect CN VII. If sensation to the anterior two thirds of the tongue, lips, and face is reduced, along with reduced motor strength and coordination, a child may have difficulty holding the lips together to contain food within the mouth. In addition, there may be difficulty using the tongue to form a bolus in order to propel food and liquid posteriorly into the pharynx. Damage to the glossopharyngeal (CN IX) and vagus (CN X) cranial nerves has a direct effect on the pharyngeal phase of swallowing and places children at risk for aspiration. Children with CHARGE syndrome appear less likely to have significant motor deficits related to cranial nerves V (trigeminal) and XII (hypoglossal), although specific studies of all aspects of tongue movement have not been reported in this population.

In every published survey since 1981, the majority of children with CHARGE have demonstrated coordination problems for swallowing attributed primarily to the dysfunction of cranial nerves IX and X (e.g., Blake et al., 1998; Tellier et al., 1998), placing them at risk for aspiration, usually silent (e.g., Arvedson, Rogers, Buck, Smart, & Msall, 1994; Asher, McGill, Kaplan, Friedman, & Healy, 1990; Roger et al., 1999; Giambra, Hopkin, Daines, & Rutter, et al., 2005). White and colleagues (2005) estimated the prevalence of aspiration in CHARGE syndrome at around 60% with more general swallowing problems seen even more frequently. Some children show signs of inefficiency in preparing a bolus or in timing of swallowing, but others do not. This author has seen children who feed eagerly with no obvious coordination problems by clinical observation but who then aspirate a significant volume as demonstrated during videofluoroscopic swallow study (VFSS). The vagus nerve (CN X) provides primary innervation to the esophagus, which also may be affected in children with CHARGE.

Malformations in CHARGE Syndrome Affecting Feeding

Substantial variability of all clinical characteristics can be expected in children with CHARGE syndrome. Anatomic and structural defects that vary in frequency and degree of severity may require medical and surgical management in order for a child to be able to meet nutrition and hydration needs (Table 12–3). Many of these conditions are discussed in detail in other chapters in this book.

EVALUATION OF SWALLOWING AND FEEDING

Evaluation of infants and children with swallowing and feeding concerns involves multiple considerations beyond a simple clinical observation of a feeding regardless of the underlying diagnosis. A comprehensive evaluation

TABLE 12–3. Anatomic/Structural Defects: Location, Phase of Swallow Impairment Likely, and Indications for VFSS

Anatomic or Structural Defect	Location	Oral Phase	Pharyngeal Phase	Esophageal Phase	Indications for VFSS
Choanal atresia/ stenosis	Nose/ nasopharynx	+	+		Sometimes
Cleft palate +/– cleft lip	Oral cavity	+			No
Laryngomalacia or laryngotracheo-malacia	Airway		+	+/–	Sometimes (GER common)
Laryngotracheal cleft	Airway		+	+	
Tracheoesophageal fistula (TEF)	Airway/ esophagus		+	+	Sometimes
Tracheoesophageal atresia	Airway/ esophagus		+	+	No, unless spit fistula is present s/p surgery

for infants and children with CHARGE syndrome must consider health status, broad environment, parent-child interactions, and parental concerns (Arvedson, 2008; Rogers & Arvedson, 2005).

Infants in NICU

In the newborn period, most infants with CHARGE syndrome are in a Neonatal Intensive Care Unit (NICU) where the primary physicians are neonatologists. In addition, other specialists usually include otolaryngologists and pulmonologists for airway concerns and gastroenterologists for GI tract issues (Table 12–4). Appropriate nonnutritive oral experiences are encouraged with

TABLE 12–4. Core Team Members and Primary Functions

Team Member	Function
Parents	Advocate for child; follow through depends on parental "buy in"
Physician (e.g., gastroenterologist, developmental pediatrician)	Medical director for team (coleader); medical evaluation and management; evaluation and management of GI tract issues; endoscopy, manometry, impedance, etc., of GI tract; pediatric and neurodevelopmental diagnosis
Dietitian	Nutrition needs assessment and ongoing guidance
Speech-language pathologist	Team coleader; clinic/bedside feeding and swallowing evaluation; videofluoroscopic swallow study (VFSS) with radiologist; flexible endoscopic evaluation of swallowing (FEES) with otolaryngologist; oral sensorimotor habilitation/rehabilitation
Psychologist	Evaluation of psychological and behavioral factors; evaluation of parent/child interactions; treatment/ intervention of behavioral feeding problems
Occupational therapist	Evaluation and treatment focused on posture, tone, self-feeding skills, and sensory issues
Nurse	Coordinator and primary contact for parents and other members of the team
Social worker	Assists families with community resources; respite needs; variety of support services
Physician specialists (otolaryngologist, pulmonologist, surgeon, radiologist, cardiologist, neurologist, etc.)	Evaluate and manage specific needs within the specialty; meet with core team members as needed for decision making/planning

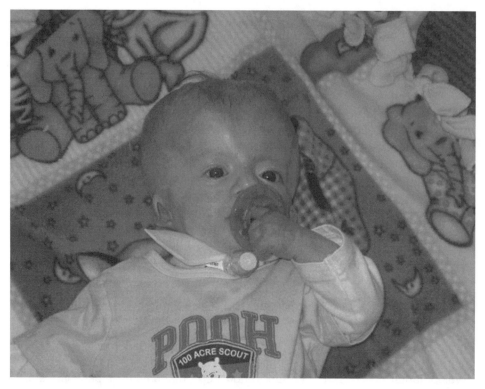

FIGURE 12–3. Infant doing non-nutritive sucking on a pacifier that helps facilitate readiness for nipple feeding, whether by breast or bottle.

pacifier as tolerated (Figure 12–3). Although an infant does not have to coordinate sucking, swallowing, and breathing with a pacifier, the infant does have to be able to breathe through the nose in order to keep the pacifier in the mouth. Nipple feeding at the breast or by bottle cannot be expected (or even assessed) until any upper airway obstruction is alleviated to a degree that nasal breathing can be achieved for at least short periods of time. The in-patient team members vary depending on the status and needs of the infant. Speech-language pathologists, occupational therapists, and physical therapists work closely with nurses and parents to facilitate readiness for oral feeding through on-going assessment and intervention that may include positioning, handling, monitoring state changes, readiness for oral feeding trials (e.g., McCain, 2003), advancing oral feeding, and discharge planning.

Assessment Process beyond NICU for Infants and Children with Feeding and Swallowing Disorders

The assessment process typically encompasses multiple dimensions that include, but may not be limited to: (1) review of family, medical, developmental, and feeding history; (2) physical examination (prefeeding assessment); (3) clinical feeding and swallowing evaluation; (4) other considerations (e.g., somatic growth patterns, neurodevelopmental status, orofacial structures, cardiopulmonary, GI function) (Arvedson, 2008). Many children with CHARGE are at risk for pharyngeal phase swallowing problems with aspiration (Sporik, Dinwiddie, & Wallis, 1997; White, et al., 2005). An instrumental swallow evaluation is recommended for those children because the pharyngeal and upper esophageal phases of swallowing cannot be delineated strictly by clinical observation. Other diagnostic tests may be ordered by physicians (these are beyond the scope of this chapter).

Oral Feeding Observation

Oral feeding observation is an integral part of a comprehensive evaluation. It is vital for professionals to understand and appreciate "normal" development of oral skills and the supporting systems that underlie successful oral feeding (Table 12–5). Observation of children's oral feeding requires a broad knowledge base, in order to contribute to comprehensive management decisions, even though the focus appears to be on what happens in the mouth and throat. Observation of oral feeding yields information related to bolus formation for liquid by bottle/nipple or cup, smooth or lumpy food by spoon or fork, and solid food with fingers or utensils (lip, jaw, and some aspects of tongue function), along with some reasonable inferences about bolus transit through the oral cavity over the tongue and timing for initiation of a pharyngeal swallow. Particular attention is paid to findings that may relate to cranial nerve (CN) function during every feeding assessment of transitional feeders or older chil-

TABLE 12–5. Developmental Feeding: Age Range of Introduction to Advance Textures

Age (months)	Type of Food
Term birth Preterm infants (about 34–37 weeks gestation)*	Liquid by nipple (breast or bottle)
5–6	Smooth puree (SP)
6–9	SP; textured puree; easily dissolvable solids
9–12	Soft, mashed, and diced solids; cup drinking
12–18	Chopped table food

*Feeding advances in preterm infants relate to adjusted age, not chronologic age for the first 2 years of life.

dren with CHARGE syndrome (Table 12-6). The range of possible findings is extensive and multifactorial. Multiple scales and checklists provide detailed guidance for interpreting these clinical observations, but standardization is lacking (e.g., Arvedson & Brodsky, 2002, pp. 324–330; Coster, Deeney, Halti-wanger, & Haley, 1998; Jelm, 1990; Kenny et al., 1989; Koontz-Lowman & Lane, 1999; Reilly, Skuse, & Wolke, 2000). It is not possible to define the pharyngeal physiology or upper esophageal function by a clinical feeding observation.

It is helpful for all professionals, each with a different focus, to observe parents feeding an infant or overseeing a meal with an older child. Parents simulate a "typical" meal environment when they come to a clinic or hospital, although everyone knows that it is impossible to make the situation like home. Findings are interpreted both on the basis of what is observed and on differences or similarities reported by caregivers. Most children show considerable variability in their oral feeding skills: They may feed better for a babysitter or nanny than for a parent; they may feed with less stress with one parent compared to another parent; they may feed better at one time of day compared to another (e.g., breakfast is better than dinner or the other way around, especially for tube feeders who get overnight feeds and are not hungry early in the day). Some of these children experience nausea for an hour or two after tube feeding is turned off. The factors surrounding meals, presence or absence of hunger, tolerance or intolerance of tube feeds, vomiting, constipation, and medications can have effects on oral feeding situations.

TABLE 12–6. Observations of Oral Feeding in Transition Feeders or Older Children That May Relate to Cranial Nerve (CN) Function

CN	Action	Expected Response	Response with CN Deficits
V	Food on tongue	Chewing	Lack of chewing, bolus not formed
VII	Sucking	Lips form seal on nipple or around straw	Lip seal not formed
	Food on lower lip	Upper lip and teeth pull food into mouth; lip closure	Lack of lip closure; limited lip action
	Smile	Lip retraction symmetrical	Asymmetric lip retraction or limited to no retraction
IX, X	Food in oral cavity, posterior	Pharyngeal swallow initiated less than 2 seconds	Delay longer than 2 seconds to initiate pharyngeal swallow
XII	Food on tongue	Shaping of tongue to include grooving, pointing, or protruding	Tongue flat, lacking elevation and thinning, atrophy, drooling

Global Aspects of Oral Feeding/Swallowing Evaluation

Observation of oral feeding starts with the environment and interactions between child and caregivers. Signs of stress are noted in child and in caregivers. Posture, position, and tone are important underlying factors that aid in determining global levels of functioning. Professionals make estimates of cognitive, receptive, and expressive language levels, as well as gross and fine motor skills. They need to know the status of hearing and vision. During the first two to three years of life, expectations of feeding-related skills are linked closely to the global neurodevelopmental levels of function. In addition, children who were born prematurely deserve to be considered on the basis of their adjusted age at least up to 24 months of chronologic age as well as the level of functioning for gross and fine motor skills. The child who is not sitting independently, not crawling, is producing only vowel-like cooing sounds, and is not babbling, is estimated to be functioning overall at about a six-month level, with some emerging skills a month or two higher. Such a child might not be expected to do finger feeding or to use a spoon or fork. If the child has been an oral feeder since infancy and is safe for oral feeding (i.e., not at risk for aspiration), one would expect primarily nipple feeding and spoon feeding of smooth purees by parent (Figure 12–4). Perhaps limited cup

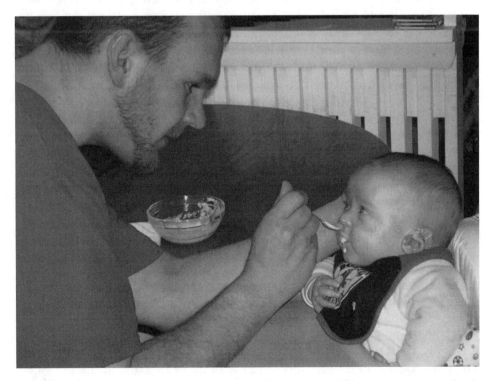

FIGURE 12–4. Child at about 6-month developmental skill level given spoon feeding experience by his father.

drinking practice and finger food exposure could be appropriate if the child shows interest. Critical and sensitive periods of development must be considered in introduction of textured food to children before the end of the first year of life or greater resistance may be displayed when introduction of lumpy textures is delayed (Illingworth & Lister, 1964).

Primary Question To Be Answered during a Clinical Feeding/Swallowing Evaluation

The primary question at the end of a feeding observation is: Can this child meet nutrition and hydration needs safely by total oral feeding? If the answer is "no" or questions remain regarding swallowing safety or possible risks for aspiration, follow-up instrumental examination(s) of swallowing likely will be needed. Other diagnostic tests may be requested by physicians. A nutrition panel may be requested by dietitians. There may be additional follow-up, as optimal management decisions can be made only when the etiology of the swallowing and feeding problems is established. Treatment based on signs and symptoms alone is not likely to be effective.

Children with CHARGE syndrome change over time with maturation and skill development in all areas of learning. Caregivers and professionals must keep in mind that these children, like all children, can experience acute events that may or may not be related to CHARGE. For example, one child with CHARGE, who had a tracheostomy tube until two years of age and feeding difficulties in infancy and early childhood, became stable on a combination of gastrostomy tube (GT) and oral feeding. She showed increased difficulties at age 4 with multiple pneumonias and increased aspiration with oral feeding. Neurologic work-up revealed hydrocephalus with Chiari malformation. A ventriculoperitoneal (VP) shunt was placed, followed by Chiari decompression. Swallowing improved, and she was decannulated within a few more months. By age 5½, she increased oral feeding with GT for hydration only. The tube was removed a few months later after she maintained oral feeding through a respiratory illness that included adequate liquid intake. This example reminds all readers that any change in feeding and swallowing patterns needs to be investigated.

Instrumental Swallowing Procedures

The choice of an instrumental swallowing procedure is made on the basis of specific questions and the ability of the procedure to answer the questions (Table 12–7). Ultrasonography (US) uses reflected sound as an imaging tool to visualize temporal relationships between movement patterns of oral and pharyngeal structures. Currently, US is used more for research purposes than for clinical purposes. The two examinations used most often with pediatric patients are (1) videofluoroscopic swallow study (VFSS) and (2) flexible endoscopic evaluation of swallowing (FEES). Advantages and disadvantages of each study are listed in Table 12–7.

TABLE 12–7. Instrumental Swallow Evaluations: Advantages and Disadvantages

Imaging Study	Swallow Phases	Advantages	Disadvantages
Ultrasonography	Oral primarily	Soft tissue delineation.	Limited primarily to oral function.
		Captures structures at rest and during function	Cannot detect laryngeal penetration or aspiration directly.
		No contrast material required.	Structural landmarks are difficult to identify—training is needed.
		No radiation exposure.	
		Extended time possible.	Availability of trained personnel may be limited
		Body positioning no problem—infant/child can be held by mother.	Laryngeal structures cast shadow obscuring view of airway.
		Equipment available at most major medical centers.	
Flexible endoscopic evaluation of swallowing (FEES), + sensory testing (ST)	Pharyngeal (laryngeal function can be assessed)	Readily available, can to taken to patient.	Incomplete examination of swallowing—no oral or upper esophageal visualization possible.
		Position of patient can be flexible.	If aspiration, not always clear when it occurred.
		Observation of structure and function of pharynx and larynx	
		May be repeated frequently.	Cannot evaluate coordination of pharyngeal function with tongue action, laryngeal excursion, and UES opening.
		Duration of study can be as long as desired.	
		Can test sensory component.	Minimally invasive, but some children become stressed with endoscope passage (usually settle readily).

continues

TABLE 12–7. *continued*

Imaging Study	Swallow Phases	Advantages	Disadvantages
Videofluoroscopic Swallow Study (VFSS)	Bolus formation, oral transit, pharyngeal, and upper esophageal phases	Dynamic visualization of phases of swallow through UES. Coordination of pharyngeal motility with tongue function can be seen in real time and reviewed frame-by-frame and in slow motion. If aspiration, can determine before, during, or after swallows and on what texture. Transit times can be measured. Available in most institutions.	Uses ionizing radiation, so studies should be of short duration. Positioning equipment can be cumbersome. Patient has to be taken to radiology suite. Requires trained personnel. Requires use of barium contrast that alters taste and texture, or preprepared barium products. Brief window in time that does not simulate a real mealtime.

Readers interested in details regarding criteria for referral for VFSS, preparation of infants and children, procedures, reading and interpreting X-ray findings, and management considerations are directed to several resources including, but not limited to, Arvedson (2007), Arvedson & Brodsky (2002, pp. 341–388), and Arvedson & Lefton-Greif (1998).

VFSS is the primary instrumental evaluation used to provide dynamic imaging of oral, pharyngeal, and upper esophageal phases of swallowing in lateral view (as standard) and anteroposterior (PA) view (when asymmetry is noted or suspected). The PA view can be helpful to delineate mass effect of palatine tonsils when they are seen on lateral view. The esophagus is scanned for transit of a bolus. An esophagram or upper gastrointestinal (UGI) study is needed for in-depth examination of the esophagus.

MANAGEMENT OF FEEDING/SWALLOWING DISORDERS IN CHILDREN WITH CHARGE SYNDROME

Basic principles of management for children with CHARGE syndrome are the same as those for all children with neurologic-based feeding and swallowing problems. Oral feeding goals are determined in light of adequate nutrition and gastrointestinal function, stable pulmonary function, and safety of swallowing (see Chapter 11). Caregivers and professionals must establish developmentally appropriate goals to advance oral sensorimotor and feeding skills for safe swallowing. These goals are determined within the context of maximal participation in the social and communication activities associated with mealtimes for each child and the rest of the family.

Because the underlying nutrition and hydration status is paramount for all children, supplemental nutrition routes are needed when it is not possible to meet those needs strictly orally. Decisions to accept feeding tubes usually are very difficult for parents, who often see a tube as a sign of failure with oral feeding. Professionals have an obligation to help parents understand that a feeding tube is not a last resort nor does a feeding tube need to be permanent. Instead, a feeding tube should be seen as a facilitator, not only for nutrition, but for advancing oral skills as well. Undernourished children typically display reduced energy as they may burn up a lot of calories during their prolonged meal times. They also may have more frequent upper respiratory illnesses if they are aspirating even intermittently with their oral feedings. Anecdotal reports from parents often are similar to this: "I wish I would have accepted the tube sooner. Now my child has more energy and stays healthy. She is making developmental gains and doing things she would never even try in the past. For example, she is now pulling to stand."

Although not all children can become total oral feeders, it would be highly unusual for a child to be strictly nonoral to a degree that no tastes would be allowed. Children have saliva that needs to be swallowed regularly.

In most instances, drooling results from less frequent swallowing of saliva and not to excessive saliva production. Stimulation of swallowing by presenting liquid and food in very small quantities should be possible so that the child can have pleasurable experiences. The best practice for swallowing is swallowing. Oral stimulation apart from tastes cannot be guaranteed to get a child to feed orally. Some children resist stimulation with vibrators, stroking to the face and mouth, or intraoral stimulation when a parent or therapist moves a Nuk brush or similar object around in a child's mouth. Only when these kinds of activities are pleasurable and nonstressful to a child as well as leading to a functional outcome of nonstressful oral manipulation of food and/or liquid followed by swallowing in a timely way, should they be included in a therapeutic regimen.

Examples of Specific Therapeutic Intervention Procedures

Interventions include, but are not limited to, varied approaches to oral sensorimotor stimulation and neuromuscular electrical stimulation (NMES). Direct oral sensorimotor treatment frequently is recommended for children with feeding and swallowing deficits, although evidence is limited regarding efficacy for specific strategies. Such treatment focuses on improving jaw, lip, cheek, tongue, and palate function, as those structures are under voluntary neural control and are accessible to a clinician for stimulation (Arvedson & Brodsky, 2002). Changes will affect bolus formation (oral preparatory phase of swallowing), oral transit, and in some instances, initiation of the pharyngeal swallow. Given that completion of the pharyngeal phase and the entire esophageal phase of swallowing are under involuntary neural control, oral sensorimotor intervention is not expected to affect those aspects of swallowing directly. In contrast, neuromuscular electrical stimulation (NMES) involves application of surface electrodes to the neck with a goal of stimulation to pharyngeal swallowing muscles. The goal is to make pharyngeal muscle swallowing action faster and stronger that should improve efficiency and safety of swallowing. However, little is known about the effects of transcutaneous stimulation on swallowing physiology. Electrical stimulation applied to skin or oral mucosa at low current levels activates sensory nerve endings in the surface layers providing sensory feedback to the central nervous system (Ludlow, et al., 2007). As current amplitude is increased, the electric field may depolarize nerve endings in muscles lying beneath the skin surface and may spread with diminishing density to produce muscle contraction. Ludlow and colleagues (2007) found that NMES applied at rest in adults with chronic pharyngeal dysphagia lowered the hyoid rather than elevating it as understood to be the expected movement in functional swallowing. They recommended that before surface electrical stimulation is used patients should be screened to determine whether there would be an increased risk of aspiration with a procedure that lowers the hyoid. That guideline was made for adults. Findings are needed for children of all ages.

A commonly used device for clinical intervention and for research with children and adults is VitalStim®, which was approved by the U.S. Food and Drug Administration in 2002, although that is not the only product available. The therapy usually is carried out by speech-language pathologists. In many instances, a VFSS is completed as a baseline measure before therapy is initiated and again after therapy is completed, often following 2–3 weeks of therapy with 3–5 sessions per week. No standard of practice exists to date, nor do data-based reports with children. Anecdotal reports suggest it has been successful in some cases, but not in others. Parents and professionals are encouraged to keep abreast of advances in all areas of potential management while they also seek best evidence for physiologic bases that support outcomes.

Sensory Based Issues in Intervention

Questions arise as to whether children with CHARGE syndrome have a primary sensory-based feeding/swallowing disorder or whether the behavioral responses may be a result of externally driven forces. That is, aversiveness actually can be imposed upon the child when caregivers and therapists do not "read" the child's cues appropriately. A fundamental principle for therapeutic intervention is to build in very small steps starting from what a child is doing at the time. An example follows: a child of 18 months of age (developmentally at about 10–12 month level) on PEG tube feeds for primary nutrition, no aspiration or obvious signs for risks for aspiration, presented at the feeding clinic with concerns that nutrition was borderline acceptable. The child was still vomiting on a combination of small bolus feeds during the day and continuous slow feeds over night, which indicated some level of volume sensitivity. He took small volume nipple feeding three times per day with variable efficiency. He had had no colds recently. He had been refusing spoon feeding of pureed baby food since it was first introduced at about 6 months of age. At this session, he turned his head away and fussed as the spoon was brought toward his mouth. When asked whether the child was ever presented with a dry spoon or a spoon dipped into his formula, parents stated "no." During the initial clinical session, the child was given a spoon, which he promptly put into his mouth, albeit upside down. He then allowed the clinician to place a spoon into his mouth. Then he accepted the spoon dipped into formula multiple times. The next step was rice cereal added to the formula (an even smaller amount than on the previous presentation). He accepted that spoon with no gag or cough. Later in the session, a wide-lipped open cup was presented containing the thin rice cereal. He accepted the first sip willingly and appeared to swallow with no delay. The next time, he reached for the cup and put his hands on it "to help." The parents were surprised and impressed.

The underlying principles in this scenario include the following: build on what the child does well, make the changes in *very* small steps, and make sure that every task request is developmentally appropriate. Although evidence-based guidance for intervention is limited, the clinician's evidence comes from a strong knowledge base of normal development for swallowing and feeding, along with all other aspects of neurodevelopment; neurologic-based swallowing and feeding deficits; neurosensory and neuromotor deficits; and behavior aspects. Professionals and parents are reminded that behavioral responses are the child's way to communicate, especially for those children who do not have functional verbal communication. Dobbelsteyn et al. (2005) described early oral sensory experiences and feeding development in five children with CHARGE syndrome. They found considerable variability in early oral sensory experiences, with all five children having some difficulty in feeding.

Variability is the key descriptor that must be kept in mind during all interactions for evaluation and management of feeding and swallowing disorders in children with CHARGE syndrome. Change over time is expected. Early identification and appropriate facilitation of skills are urged for all children with CHARGE. Facilitation of oral feeding skills should be pleasurable and non-stressful for child and parents with advances in oral feeding never interfering with nutrition and pulmonary status. In summary, children with CHARGE syndrome show considerable variability in their feeding and swallowing problems and in the ways they make gains over time. The unique individual differences are to be appreciated and celebrated.

REFERENCES

Arvedson, J. C. (2007). *Interpretation of videofluoroscopic swallow studies of infants and children. A study guide to improve diagnostic skills and treatment planning.* Gaylord, MI: Northern Speech Services.

Arvedson, J. C. (2008). Assessment of pediatric dysphagia and feeding disorders: clinical and instrumental approaches. *Developmental Disabilities and Research Reviews, 14,* 118–127.

Arvedson, J. C., & Brodsky, L. (2002). *Pediatric swallowing and feeding: Assessment and management.* (2nd ed.). Albany, NY: Singular Publishing Group, a division of Thomson Learning.

Arvedson, J. C., & Lefton-Greif, M. A. (1998). *Pediatric videofluoroscopic swallow studies: A professional manual with caregiver guidelines.* San Antonio, TX: Communication Skill Builders.

Arvedson, J., & Rogers, B. (1993). Pediatric swallowing and feeding disorders. *Journal of Medical Speech-Language pathology, 1,* 203–221.

Arvedson, J. C., & Rogers, B. T. (1997). Swallowing and feeding in the pediatric patient. In A. L. Perlman, & K. S. Schulze-Delrieu (Eds.), *Deglutition and its disorders* (pp. 419–448). San Diego, CA: Singular Publishing Group.

Arvedson, J., Rogers, B., Buck, G., Smart, P., & Msall, M. (1994). Silent aspiration prominent in children with dysphagia. *International Journal of Pediatric Otorhinolaryngology, 28,* 173–181.

Asher, B. F., McGill, T. J., Kaplan, L., Friedman, E. M., & Healy, G. B. (1990). Airway complications in CHARGE association. *Archives of Otolaryngology-Head and Neck Surgery, 116,* 594–595.

Beauchamp, G. K., & Mennella, J. A. (2009). Early flavor learning and its impact on later feeding behavior. *Journal of Pediatric Gastroenterology and Nutrition, 48*(Suppl. 1), S25–S30.

Blake, K. D., Davenport, S. L., Hall, B. D., Hefner, M. A., Pagon, R. A., Williams, M. S., . . . Graham, J. M., Jr. (1998). CHARGE association: An update and review for the primary pediatrician. *Clinical Pediatrics, 37,* 159–173.

Blake, K. D., Hartshorne, T. S., Lawand C., Dailor, A. N., & Thelin, J. W. (2008). Cranial nerve manifestations in CHARGE syndrome. *American Journal of Medical Genetics A, 146A*(5), 585–592.

Blake, K., Kirk, J. M. W., & Ur, E. (1992). Growth in CHARGE association. *Archives of Diseases in Childhood, 68,* 508–509.

Blake, K. D., & Prasad, C. (2006). CHARGE syndrome [Review]. *Orphanet Journal of Rare Diseases* 1:34. Retrieved April 12, 2009, from http://www.ojrd.com/content/pdf/1750-1172-1-34.pdf.

Blake, K. D., Salem-Hartshorne, N., Daoud, M. A., & Gradstein, J. (2005). Adolescent and adult issues in CHARGE syndrome. *Clinical Pediatrics, 44,* 151–159.

Blustajn, J., Kirsch, C. F., Panigrahy, A., & Netchine, I. (2008). Olfactory anomalies in CHARGE syndrome: Imaging findings of a potential major diagnostic criterion. *American Journal of Neuroradiology, 29,* 1266–1269.

Bowen, R.A. (2006). Physiology of taste. In *Pathophysiology of the digestive system.* Retrieved May 10, 2010, from http://www.vivo.colostate.edu/hbooks/pathphys/digestion/pregastric/taste.html.

Chalouhi, C., Faulcon, P., Le Bihan, C., Hertz-Pannier, L., Bonfils, P., & Abadie, V. (2005). Olfactory evaluation in children: application to the CHARGE syndrome. *Pediatrics, 116,* 81–88.

Coccorullo, P., Quitadamo, P., Martinelli, M., & Staiano, A. (2009). Novel and alternative therapies for childhood constipation. *Journal of Pediatric Gastroenterology and Nutrition, 48*(Suppl. 2), S104–S106.

Coster W, Deeney T, Haltiwanger J, & Haley S. (1998). *School Function Assessment (SFA).* San Antonio, TX: Therapy Skill Builders.

Del Giudice, E., Staiano, A., Capano, G., Romano, A., Florimonte, L., Miele, E., . . . Crisanti, A. F. (1999). Gastrointestinal manifestations in children with cerebral palsy. *Brain and Development, 21,* 307–311.

Dobbelsteyn, C., Marche, D. M., Blake, K., & Rashid, M. (2005). Early oral sensory experiences and feeding development in children with CHARGE syndrome: A report of five cases. *Dysphagia, 20,* 89–100.

Dobbelsteyn, C., Peacocke, S. D., Blake, K., Crist, W., & Rashid, M. (2008). Feeding difficulties in children with CHARGE syndrome: Prevalence, risk factors, and prognosis. *Dysphagia, 23,* 127–135.

Dodds, W. (1989). The physiology of swallowing. *Dysphagia, 3,* 171–178.

Dodds, W., Stewart, E. T., & Logemann, J. A. (1990). Physiology and radiology of the normal oral and pharyngeal phases of swallowing *American Journal of Radiology, 154,* 953–963.

Drewnowski, A., (2001). The science and complexity of bitter taste. *Nutrition Review, 59*(6), 163–169.

El-Hodhod, M. A., Younis, N. T., Zaitoun, Y. A., & Daoud, S. D. (2010). Cow's milk allergy related pediatric constipation: Appropriate time of milk tolerance. *Pediatric Allergy and Immunology, 21*(2, Pt. 2), e407–e412. [Epub 2009 June 25].

Hudson, R., & Distel, H. (1999). The flavor of life: perinatal development of odor and taste preferences. *Schweizer Medizinische Wochenschrift, 129*(5), 176-181.

Illingworth, R. S., & Lister, J. (1964). The critical or sensitive period, with special reference to certain feeding problems in infants and children. *Journal of Pediatrics, 65*, 840-848.

Issekutz, K. A., Graham, J. M. Jr., Prasad, C., Smith, I. M., & Blake, K. D. (2005). An epidemiological analysis of CHARGE syndrome: Preliminary results from a Canadian study. *American Journal of Medical Genetics, 133A*, 309-317.

Jelm, J. M. 1990. *Oral sensori-motor/feeding rating scale.* Tucson, AZ: Therapy Skill Builders.

Kenny, D., Koheil, R., Greenberg, J., Reid, D., Milner, M., Roman, R., & Judd, P. (1989). Development of a multidisciplinary feeding profile for children who are dependent feeders. *Dysphagia, 4*, 16-28.

Kimber, C., Kiely, E. M., & Spitz, L. (1998). The failure rate of surgery for gastro-oesophageal reflux. *Journal of Pediatric Surgery, 33*, 65-67.

Konikoff, M. R., Noel, R. J., Blanchard, C., Kircy, C., Jameson, S. C., Buckmeier, B. K., . . . Rothenberg, M. E. (2006). A randomized, double-blind, placebo-controlled trial of fluticasone propionate for pediatric eosinophilic esophagitis. *Gastroenterology, 131*(5), 1381-1391.

Koontz-Lowman, D., & Lane, S. J. (1999). Children with feeding and nutritional problems. In S. M. Porr, & E. B. Rainville (Eds.), *Pediatric therapy: A systems approach* (pp. 379-423). Philadelphia, PA: FA Davis.

Lasser, M. S., Liao, J. G., & Burd, R. S. (2006). National trends in the use of antireflux procedures for children. *Pediatrics, 118*(5), 1828-1835.

Liacouras, C.A. (1997). Failed Nissen fundoplication in two patients who had persistent vomiting and eosinophilic esophagitis. *Journal of Pediatric Surgery, 32*(10), 1504-1506.

Liem, D. G., & Mennella, J. A. (2003). Heightened sour preferences during childhood. *Chemical Senses, 28*, 173-180.

Lim, J. R., Gupta, S. K., Croffie, J. M., Pfefferkorn, M. D., Molleston, J. P., Corkins, M. R., . . . Fitzgerald, J. F. (2004). White specks in the esophageal mucosa: An endoscopic manifestation of non-reflux eosinophilic esophagitis in children. *Gastrointestinal Endoscopy, 59*(7), 835-838.

Lin, A. E., Siebert, J. R., & Graham, J. M., Jr. (1990). Central nervous system malformations in the CHARGE association. *American Journal of Medical Genetics, 37*, 304-310.

Ludlow, C. L., Humbert, I., Saxon, K., Poletto, C., Sonies, B., & Crujido, L. (2007). Effects of surface electrical stimulation both at rest and during swallowing in chronic pharyngeal dysphagia. *Dysphagia, 22*, 1-10.

Markowitz, J. E., Spergel, J. M., Ruchelli, E., & Liacouras, C. A. (2003). Elemental diet is an effective treatment for eosinophilic esophagitis in children and adolescents. *American Journal of Gastroenterology, 98*(4), 777-782.

McCain, G. C. (2003). An evidence-based guideline for introducing oral feeding to healthy preterm infants. *Neonatal Network, 22*(5), 45-50.

Mennella, J. A., & Beauchamp, G. K. (2005). Understanding the origin of flavor preferences. *Chemical Senses, 30*(Suppl. 1), i242-i243.

Mennella, J. A., & Beauchamp, G. K. (2008). Optimizing oral medications for children. *Chemical Senses, 30*, 2120-2132.

Mennella, J. A., Pepino, M. Y., & Reed, D. R. (2005). Genetic and environmental determinants of bitter perception and sweet preferences. *Pediatrics, 115*(2), e216-e222.

Miller, A. J. (1999). *The neuroscientific principles of swallowing and dysphagia*. San Diego, CA: Singular Publishing Group.

Noel, R. J., Putnam, P. E., & Rothenberg, M. E. (2004). Eosinophilic esophagitis. *New England Journal of Medicine, 351*(9), 940-941.

Noel, R. J., & Tipnis, N. A. (2006). Eosinophilic esophagitis—a mimic of GERD. *International Journal of Pediatric Otorhinolaryngology, 70*(7), 1147-1153.

Pinto, G., Abadie, V., Mesnage, R., Blustajn, J., Cabrol, S., Amiel, J., . . . Netchine, I. (2005). CHARGE syndrome includes hypogonadotropic hypogonadism and abnormal olfactory bulb development. *Journal of Clinical Endocrinology and Metabolism, 20*, 5621-5626.

Reilly, S., Skuse, D., & Wolke, D. (2000). *SOMA: Schedule for Oral Motor Assessment*. Eastgardens, New South Wales, Australia: Whurr.

Richards, C. A., Milla, P. J., Andrews, P. L., & Spitz, L. (2001). Retching and vomiting in neurologically impaired children after fundoplication: Predictive preoperative factors. *Journal of Pediatric Surgery, 36*(9), 1401-1404.

Roger, G., Morisseau-Durand, M. P., Van Den Abbeeloe, T., Nicollas, R., Triglia, J. M., Narcy, P., . . . Garabedian, E. N. (1999). The CHARGE association: the role of tracheotomy. *Archives of Otolaryngology-Head and Neck Surgery, 125*, 33-38.

Rogers, B., & Arvedson, J. (2005). Assessment of infant oral sensorimotor and swallowing function. *Mental Retardation and Developmental Disabilities Research Reviews, 11*, 74-82.

Rudolph, C. D., Mazur, L. J., Liptak, G. S., Baker, R. D., Boyle, J. T., Colletti, R. B., . . . Werlin, S. L. (2001). Guidelines for evaluation and treatment of gastroesophageal reflux in infants and children: Recommendations of the North American Society for Pediatric Gastroenterology and Nutrition. *Journal of Pediatric Gastroenterology and Nutrition, 32*(Suppl. 2), S1-S31.

Sporik, R., Dinwiddie, R., & Wallis, C. (1997). Lung involvement in the multisystem syndrome CHARGE association. *European Respiratory Journal, 10*, 1354-1355.

Srivastava, R., Downey, E. C., O'Gorman, M., Feola, P., Samore, M., Holubkov, R., . . . Dean, J. M. (2009). Impact of fundoplication versus gastrojejunal feeding tubes on mortality and in preventing aspiration pneumonia in young children with neurologic impairment who have gastroesophageal reflux disease. *Pediatrics, 123*(1), 338-345.

Stromland, K., Sjogreen, L., Johansson, M., Ekman Joelsson, B. M., Miller, M., Danielsson, S., . . . Granstrom, G. (2005). CHARGE association in Sweden: malformations and functional deficits. *American Journal of Medical Genetics, 133A*, 331-339.

Strudwick, S. (2003). Gastro-oesophageal reflux and feeding: the speech and language therapist's perspective. *International Journal of Otorhinolaryngology, 7*(Suppl.1), S101-S102.

Sullivan, P. B. (1997). Gastrointestinal problems in the neurologically impaired child. *Bailliere's Clinical Gastroenterology, 11*, 529-546.

Tellier, A., Cormier-Daire, V., Abadie, V., Amiel, J., Sigaudy, S., Bonnet, D., . . . Lyonnet, S. (1998). CHARGE syndrome: report of 47 cases and review. *American Journal of Medical Genetics, 76*(5), 402-409.

Walia, R., Mahajan, L., & Steffen, R. (2009). Recent advances in chronic constipation. *Current Opinions in Pediatrics, 21*(5), 661-666.

White, D. R., Giambra, B. K., Hopkin, R. J., Daines, C. L., & Rutter, M. J. (2005). Aspiration in children with CHARGE syndrome. *International Journal of Pediatric Otorhinolaryngology, 69*, 1205–1209.

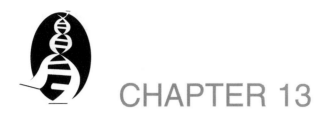

CHAPTER 13

Neurodevelopment

ELIZABETH GILLES, M.D.

NEUROLOGIC ISSUES

Neurologic findings in CHARGE syndrome run the gamut from developmental delay, cranial nerve dysfunction, epilepsy, sleep disorders, and behavioral problems to cognitive/executive function deficits.

Seizures and Epilepsy

Seizures occur in some children with CHARGE, and some develop epilepsy (recurrent unprovoked seizures). A seizure essentially is a transient event caused by abnormal brain electrical activity resulting in involuntary muscle activity, sensory symptoms, or altered responsiveness. The prevalence and incidence of seizures and epilepsy in CHARGE are unknown. Onset of seizures has been seen from infancy to adulthood. Although seizures can be a significant problem in CHARGE, no unique patterns exist. Treatment is based, as in other conditions, on seizure type.

Many nonepileptic events in children mimic seizures in that they are also paroxysmal and may have features suggestive of a seizure. Among the most common such events are breath-holding spells, fainting (syncope), gastroesophageal reflux with secondary esophagitis (Sandifer syndrome), and night terrors. A number of children with CHARGE have had airway obstruction and airway issues with resultant spells that looked like seizures. Therefore, evaluation of the airway is a critical part of the assessment of paroxysmal events.

Development

Intellectual Outcome

The degree of impairment and ultimate functioning depends on many factors including severity of visual, hearing and vestibular impairments, severity of cerebral dysgenesis, age at which intensive interventions begin, and quality of social stimulation (Raqbi, et al., 2003; Souriau, et al., 2005). Presumably, the more severe the cerebral dysgenesis, the worse intellectual/functional outcome compared with children without discernable structural abnormality. However, as in other conditions, imaging may show no abnormality, but functioning can be low, and vice versa. (See also Chapter 20.)

Motor Development

For more information on motor development, see also the "Introduction," section of Chapter 1 and Chapter 24.

Gross motor delay is almost universal in children with CHARGE. Most walk between 35-57 months, with 80% by 6-7 years, compared to typically developing children who walk independently at 9.4 months (range 8.2-17.6) (Hartshorne, Nicholas, Grialou, & Russ, 2007). Congenitally blind or severely visually impaired children also have gross motor delays, typically crawling at about 15 months and walking independently at 19.8 months. Age of walking is a better predictor of adaptive behavior than complexity or severity of medical problems in children with CHARGE (Salem-Hartshorne & Jacob, 2005). Delayed motor development and poor equilibrium are independent of whether there is a brain abnormality on MRI or CT (Abadie, et al., 2000; Salem-Hartshorne & Jacob, 2005).

Almost all children with CHARGE have atypical postural behavior. Most have abnormal or absent semicircular canals coexistent with hypotonia. Hypotonia adversely impacts the use of postural tone in controlling truncal movement. Activities requiring simultaneous balance and movement (such as walking) are particularly difficult. Moving from a "safe" position takes emotional and physical energy. Predictably, infants with CHARGE prefer a supine position for resting and often for activities such as looking at books (Figure 13-1). With age, children increasingly use compensatory mechanisms.

Visual stabilization by fixating on a distant point is impossible for an infant or child with significant visual acuity impairment. Specific orientation and mobility (O&M) training is helpful, as is vestibular rehabilitation in children who have poor balance, even in the absence of severe visual impairment or sensorineural hearing loss (Medeiros, et al., 2005; Rine, et al., 2004; see also Chapters 2, 4, 5, and 6).

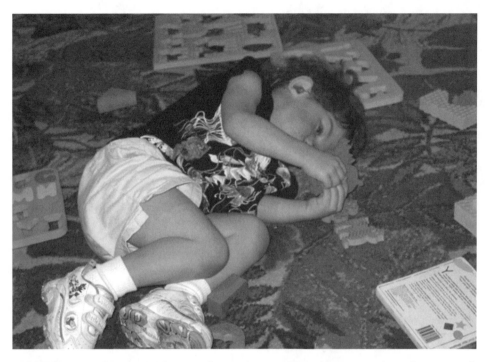

FIGURE 13–1. Many children prefer supine position when concentrating on work or objects.

Cranial Nerves: Manifestations

Some of the greatest disease burdens in CHARGE (beyond survival in infancy) come from the dysfunction of key cranial nerves (Table 13-1). Many articles report specific cranial nerve abnormalities based on symptoms alone without documentation of specific methodology. Certain parts of the neurologic examination, such as assessment of visual fields, smell, strength of muscles of mastication, and vestibular function, are particularly difficult to perform in infants and young children independent of the added difficulty of assessing the child with limited communication skills. Many cranial nerve deficits go unrecognized for months or even years.

Smell (CNI–olfactory) and Taste

See Chapter 7 on smell and Chapter 12 on feeding.

Vision (CNII–optic)

For more information on vision, see also Chapter 2.

Infants recognize bright spots and shadows at birth, bulls eyes and linear patterns in the first two months, and then add circular patterns sequentially, drawn faces and curved forms by four months. Color perception is present at

TABLE 13–1. Cranial Nerves

I	Olfactory	Smell
II	Optic	Vision
III	Oculomotor	Eyelid and eye movement inward, downward, and up
IV	Trochlear	Downward and lateral eye movement
V	Trigeminal	Chewing; head and face sensation and pain
VI	Abducens	Lateral eye movement
VII	Facial	Facial expression; taste
VIII	Vestibulocochlear	Balance and hearing
IX	Glossopharyngeal	Taste; swallowing
X	Vagus	Heart rate; swallowing; taste
XI	Spinal accessory	Lateral head movement and shoulder shrug
XII	Hypoglossal	Tongue movement

birth, but color discrimination develops around four months of age. It is not known whether children with CHARGE syndrome have abnormalities in color perception. Presumably, for those children with coloboma of the eye or optic nerve without central nervous system abnormalities, the remaining sensory retina and optic nerve still develop normally, but this has not been studied. Older children with associated cortical visual impairment typically prefer yellows and reds.

Trigeminal nerve (CNV)

Sensory function: The trigeminal nerve receives sensory information from the face, part of the scalp, membranes covering the brain (meninges), surface of the eyeball, sinuses, hard and soft palate, and inside the nose. The blink reflex (corneal reflex) is obtained by touching the cornea with a thin piece of cotton drawn from a cotton swab. This reflex involves the first branch of CNV (sensory) and CNVII (facial nerve) for the motor response.

Motor function: Children with oral motor apraxia, a disorder of incoordination of jaw, lips, and tongue, may or may not have weak muscles of mastication (see the section on dysphagia, later in this chapter).

No evidence indicates true CNV palsy or aberrant CNV brainstem nucleus development in CHARGE. Many individuals with CHARGE have dysfunction of oral motor coordination or weakness of chewing presenting as difficulty with sucking in infants and as oral motor dyspraxia in older children. Such incoordination is common in many infants and is seen in infants with numerous other syndromes.

Children fed by gastrostomy tube much of their young lives will have weak chewing muscles. This does not mean that they have trigeminal nerve palsy. Many children with CHARGE have oral sensitivity, indicating that sensory trigeminal function is present, although the quality of that experience is unknown (Dobbelsteyn, Marche, Blake, & Rashid, 2005). Aversion to oral stimulation also could be related to negative priming from previous aspiration, choking, regurgitating food into the oropharynx, or delayed introduction of oral feeds. Consistent with this is the observation that feeding improves with age (Harvey, Leaper, & Bankier, 1991).

Facial Nerve (CNVII)

The facial nerve has sensory and motor components. Sensory input to the central nervous system comes from the outer ear, hard and soft palates, and taste receptors from the anterior two thirds of the tongue. Motor output supplies muscles of facial expression, muscles involved in speech production, and muscles that stimulate tear and saliva production. The motor component is most commonly assessed.

Diagnosing facial weakness (paresis) involves more than just looking for facial asymmetry. One needs to look for the inability or compromised ability to initiate muscle contraction comparing one side of the face to the other. At rest, note whether there is any facial asymmetry such as drooping, sagging, or smoothing of normal facial creases (Figure 13–2). Initiation of facial movement should be symmetric. If the infant/child starts crying or closes their eyes, try to open the eyes and assess the relative strength of eye closure. Normally, the eyes cannot be opened against resistance.

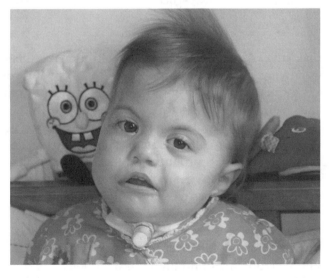

FIGURE 13–2. Unilateral facial palsy. Note smoothing of normal facial creases.

Children with CHARGE may have facial paresis or aplasia of the depressor angularis oris muscle (Lacombe, 1994). Unilateral or bilateral facial paresis or paralysis is quite common in CHARGE (32–54%) and results from aberrant CNVII nerve formation or migration (Strömland, et al., 2005). In infants with angularis oris aplasia (but without facial palsy), the lower lips are asymmetric with crying, but the nasolabial fold depth, forehead wrinkling, and eye closure are symmetric bilaterally

Hearing (CN VIII-auditory branch)

See Chapters 3 and 8.

Balance and Equilibrium (CN VIII-vestibular branch)

For more information on balance and equilibrium, see Chapters 4, 5, and 6.

It is especially difficult for children with both vestibular and visual impairment to estimate accurately their trajectory through space. Children with CHARGE often have difficulty walking on uneven surfaces (Souriau, et al., 2005). Frequent falls by infants and children may lead to significant reluctance to participate in gross motor activities. If a child has marginal vision, their visual field is moving, and their body sense in space is not stable, vision cannot be used to judge relative motion. Simply removing visual cues (e.g. moving from a hallway to a large open room) leads to errors in estimating trajectory (Fitzpatrick, Wardman, & Taylor, 1999). Individuals with CHARGE have described a feeling of "the world suddenly tipping at a 30-degree angle" (Meg Hefner, personal communication). Interestingly, parents report that many children with CHARGE like to move, especially as they age (Souriau, et al., 2005).

Feeding and Swallowing (CNIX–glossopharyngeal & CNX–vagus)

See Chapter 12.

Sialorrhea. Sialorrhea (drooling or excessive salivation) results from incoordination of swallowing, such that saliva pools in the front and spills from the mouth. Saliva is formed at a steady rate (up to a liter a day) from three pairs of salivary glands (submandibular, parotid, and lingual), with the great majority coming from the submandibular gland at rest and the parotid gland with ingestion of food. Drooling is really an abnormality of the oral phase of swallowing as opposed to an excess production of saliva.

In children with CHARGE syndrome, factors contributing to drooling may include poor oral-motor muscle control, mouth breathing or the inability to close the mouth, poor head control, body position, level of activity, and gastroesophageal reflux. Excessive drooling is stigmatizing socially in Western society and is distasteful for caregivers. Skin integrity also can be compromised with skin breakdown around the mouth and chin.

A wide spectrum exists, ranging from no drooling at all to severe sialorrhea in children with CHARGE (Blake, et al., 1998). A number of effective therapies exist that are certainly potentially useful in children with CHARGE. Behavioral therapies include prompting and cueing techniques, positive reinforcement, and biofeedback (Van der Burg, Didden, Jongerius & Rotteveel, 2007). Biofeedback, in particular, requires a level of cognitive development that precludes its use in many children with CHARGE and does not work well in very young children. Oral motor therapy is another useful intervention that employs techniques to increase sensory awareness of the gums and inner cheeks and to increase lip and cheek strength. Interestingly, increasingly lip and cheek strength may allow children with sialorrhea to better manage their saliva. Neither of these techniques has been studied in a systematic way in CHARGE.

Anticholinergics are medications that block a component of the autonomic nervous system (parasympathetic inhibitors). A side effect is to dry secretions. The most commonly used anticholinergics for sialorrhea are glycopyrrolate, scopolamine, and benztropine (Crysdale, et al., 2006; Meningaud, Pitak-Arnnop, Chikhani, & Bertrand, 2006). Glycopyrrolate most often is prescribed and appears to have fewer side effects (Tscheng, 2002).

Surgical management of drooling has evolved over time. Several approaches include submandibular duct relocation with excision of the sublingual glands, excision of the submandibular glands with parotid duct ligation, and ligation of the submandibular and parotid ducts (Stamataki, Behar, & Brodsky, 2008). Although this approach may sound drastic, sialorrhea has significant social consequences. We do not need all of the saliva we make. Because most children with CHARGE develop a fairly normal swallow over the first couple of years of life, these surgical techniques might best be reserved for those older children whose drooling has not stopped.

Literature is accumulating on the use of botulism toxin injected to the submandibular and parotid glands. Results are promising, but the effects rarely last more than a few months (Capaccio, et al., 2008). Most children require general anesthesia, and there are reports of adjacent muscle weakness after injection. This procedure is best done under ultrasound monitoring and by those physicians who have been specifically trained in this technique.

EMBRYOLOGY AND CLINICAL SIGNIFICANCE

It is now clear that CHARGE syndrome is the end result of anomalous neural crest formation, and for this reason, is considered to be a "neurocristopathy" (Aramaki, et al., 2007; Blake & Prasad, 2006). Neural crest cells are critical to the coordinated development of the forebrain and midbrain including the formation of craniofacial structures, with cranial ganglia developing from cranial neural crest cells (O'Rahilly, & Muller, 2007). Many of the neurologic abnormalities found in CHARGE, particularly the multiple cranial nerve dysfunctions, are best understood in the context of abnormalities of embryologic development (Adams, et al., 2007; Layman et al., 2009). It appears that the cranial nerves, sensory ganglia, and sensory end organs are most likely to be affected, with relative sparing of the brainstem cranial nerve nuclei (Adams, et al., 2007; Bosman, et al. 2005; Lalani et al., 2006).

NEUROIMAGING AND NEUROPATHOLOGY

A wide range of brain malformations can be found in individuals with CHARGE (Johansson, et al., 2006). The most commonly reported brain anomalies involve forebrain development with hindbrain abnormalities the next most frequent (Table 13-2) (Strömland, et al., 2005). With the exception of a single case report of facial nerve nucleus agenesis (Lin, Siebert, & Graham, 1990), there have been no reports (neuropathological or neuroimaging) that confirm abnormalities of cranial nerve nuclei within the brainstem in CHARGE syndrome. In fact, there have been no systematic neuropathologic or neuroradiologic

TABLE 13–2. Range of Central Nervous System Malformations

Forebrain defects
Arhinencephaly
Holoprosencephaly (lobar)
Encephalocele
Cerebral dysgenesis (migrational abnormalities)
Cerebral and cerebellar heterotopias
Lissencephaly
Other "gyral abnormalities" not specified
Cerebral asymmetry
Complete or partial agenesis or hypoplasia of the corpus callosum
Agenesis septum pellucidum
Hippocampal hypoplasia or under-rotation
Hindbrain defects
Cerebellar hypoplasia or asymmetry
Partial or complete agenesis of the vermis
Dandy-Walker malformation
Aqueductal stenosis
Small brainstem
Decreased white matter
Pituitary or hypothalamic hypoplasia

studies of brains of children or adults with CHARGE syndrome aside from those of the olfactory bulb and tract.

The forebrain is well-known for its role in learning and memory. The cerebellum is important in balance, equilibrium, and the coordination of voluntary motor movement as well as muscle tone. It is increasingly recognized as important in language and social development, especially learning, attention, visual-spatial regulation, language, and memory. Agenesis of the cerebellar vermis has been associated with decreased movement coordination, social adaptation, and verbal communication (Steinlin, 2008). Four studies to date have documented the almost universal olfactory abnormalities of bulbs and/ or sulci in CHARGE by MRI (Blustajn, Kirsch, Panigrahy,& Netchine, 2008; Chalouhi, et al., 2005).

When evaluating any infant or fetus with anomalies and normal chromosomes, noncontrast MRI of the brain is essential, preferably read by a pediatric neuroradiologist. Noncontrast MRI is the best way to evaluate for possible brain anomalies and to ascertain the presence or absence of olfactory bulbs and tracts. Hydrocephalus does occur occasionally, most commonly congential or after an intraventricular hemorrhage (in premature infants). When CHARGE is suspected, high-resolution CT scan also is strongly recommended. This study is preferred for evaluating inner ear anomalies, including the cochlea, vestibule, internal auditory canal, and vestibular vestibule (McClay, et al., 2002).

FUTURE DIRECTIONS

Much remains to be learned about the neurologic issues of children and adults with CHARGE syndrome. There is a need to develop and validate a standardized multidisciplinary assessment of infants and children with CHARGE that should be required for all prospective clinical studies of this complicated disorder. Defining a comprehensive neurologic evaluation protocol would be part of this multidisciplinary assessment. Further, a need exists for increased collaboration and communication between all specialties that have occasion to evaluate and treat these individuals. Standardization of the clinical and imaging assessment will facilitate interdisciplinary collaboration and optimize the care and treatment of individuals with this complicated condition. Ideally, a clinical registry would be established that would enable researchers to do prospective, hypothesis-driven studies that will optimize our ability to not only reach children with multisensory impairments but optimize their growth and development.

REFERENCES

Abadie, V., Wiener-Vacher, S., Morisseau-Durand, M. P., Poree, C., Amiel, J., Amanou, L., . . . Manac'h, Y. (2000). Vestibular anomalies in CHARGE syndrome: investigations on and consequences for postural development. *European Journal of Pediatrics*, *159*(8), 569–574.

Adams, M. E., Hurd, E. A., Beyer, L. A., Swiderski, D. L., Raphael, Y., & Martin, D. M. (2007). Defects in vestibular sensory epithelia and innervation in mice with loss of Chd7 function: implications for human CHARGE syndrome. *Journal of Comparative Neurology, 504*(5), 519-532.

Aramaki, M., Kimura, T., Udaka, T., Kosaki, R., Mitsuhashi, T., Okada, Y., . . . Kosaki, K. (2007). Embryonic expression profile of chicken CHD7, the ortholog of the causative gene for CHARGE syndrome. *Birth Defects Research Part A: Clinical and Molecular Teratology, 79*(1), 50-57.

Blake, K. D., Davenport, S. L., Hall, B. D., Hefner, M. A., Pagon, R. A., Williams, M. S., & Graham, J. M., Jr. (1998). CHARGE association: An update and review for the primary pediatrician. *Clinical Pediatrics, 37*, 159-174.

Blake, K. D., & Prasad, C. (2006). CHARGE syndrome. *Orphanet Journal of Rare Diseases, 1*, 34.

Blustajn, J., Kirsch, C. F., Panigrahy, A., & Netchine, I. (2008). Olfactory anomalies in CHARGE syndrome: imaging findings of a potential major diagnostic criterion. *AJNR. American Journal of Neuroradiology, 29*(7), 1266-1269.

Bosman, E. A., Penn, A. C., Ambrose, J. C., Kettleborough, R., Stemple, D. L., & Steel, K. P. (2005). Multiple mutations in mouse Chd7 provide models for CHARGE syndrome. *Human Molecular Genetics, 14*(22), 3463-3476.

Capaccio, P., Torretta, S., Osio, M., Minorati, D., Ottaviani, F., Sambataro, G., . . . Pignataro, L. (2008). Botulinum toxin therapy: a tempting tool in the management of salivary secretory disorders. *American Journal of Otolaryngology, 29*(5), 333-338.

Chalouhi, C., Faulcon, P., Le Bihan, C., Hertz-Pannier, L., Bonfils, P., & Abadie, V. (2005). Olfactory evaluation in children: application to the CHARGE syndrome. *Pediatrics, 116*(1), e81-e88.

Crysdale, W. S., McCann, C., Roske, L., Joseph, M., Semenuk, D., & Chait, P. (2006). Saliva control issues in the neurologically challenged. A 30 year experience in team management. *International Journal of Pediatric Otorhinolaryngology, 70*(3), 519-527.

Dobbelsteyn, C., Marche, D. M., Blake, K., & Rashid, M. (2005). Early oral sensory experiences and feeding development in children with CHARGE syndrome: A report of five cases. *Dysphagia, 20*(2), 89-100.

Fitzpatrick, R. C., Wardman, D. L., & Taylor, J. L. (1999). Effects of galvanic vestibular stimulation during human walking. *Journal of Physiology, 517*(Pt 3), 931-939.

Hartshorne, T. S., Nicholas, J., Grialou, T. L., & Russ, J. M. (2007). Executive function in CHARGE syndrome. *Child Neuropsychology, 13*(4), 333-344.

Harvey, A. S., Leaper, P. M., & Bankier, A. (1991). CHARGE association: clinical manifestations and developmental outcome. *American Journal of Medical Genetics, 39*(1), 48-55.

Johansson, M., Råstam, M., Billstedt, E., Danielsson, S., Strömland, K., Miller, M., et al. (2006). Autism spectrum disorders and underlying brain pathology in CHARGE association. *Developmental Medicine and Child Neurology, 48*(1), 40-50.

Lacombe, D. (1994). Facial palsy and cranial nerve abnormalities in CHARGE association. *American Journal of Medical Genetics, 49*(3), 351-353.

Lalani, S. R., Safiullah, A. M., Fernbach, S. D., Harutyunyan, K. G., Thaller, C., Peterson, L. E., et al., (2006). Spectrum of CHD7 mutations in 110 individuals with CHARGE syndrome and genotype-phenotype correlation. *American Journal of Human Genetics, 78*(2), 303-314.

Layman, W. S., McEwen, D. P., Beyer, L. A., Lalani, S. R., Fernbach, S. D., Oh, E., . . . Martin, D. M. 2009). Defects in neural stem cell proliferation and olfaction in Chd7 deficient mice indicate a mechanism for hyposmia in human CHARGE syndrome. *Human Molecular Genetics, 18*(11), 1909-1923.

Lin, A. E., Siebert, J. R., & Graham, J. M., Jr. (1990). Central nervous system malformations in the CHARGE association. *American Journal of Medical Genetics, 37*(3), 304-310.

McClay, J. E., Tandy, R., Grundfast, K., Choi, S., Vezina, G., Zalzal, G., . . . Wilner, A. (2002). Major and minor temporal bone abnormalities in children with and without congenital sensorineural hearing loss. *Archives of Otolaryngology-Head & Neck Surgery, 128*(6), 664-671.

Medeiros, I. R., Bittar, R. S., Pedalini, M. E., Lorenzi, M. C., Formigoni, L. G., & Bento, R. F. (2005). Vestibular rehabilitation therapy in children. *Otology and Neurotology, 26*(4), 699-703.

Meningaud, J. P., Pitak-Arnnop, P., Chikhani, L., & Bertrand, J. C. (2006). Drooling of saliva: a review of the etiology and management options. *Oral Surgery, Oral Medicine, Oral Pathology, Oral Radiology & Endodontics, 101*(1), 48-57.

O'Rahilly, R. & Muller, F. (2007). The development of the neural crest in the human. *Journal of Anatomy, 211*(3), 335-351.

Raqbi, F., Le Bihan, C., Morisseau-Durand, M. P., Dureau, P., Lyonnet, S., & Abadie, V. (2003). Early prognostic factors for intellectual outcome in CHARGE syndrome. *Developmental Medicine and Child Neurology, 45*(7), 483-488.

Rine, R. M., Braswell, J., Fisher, D., Joyce, K., Kalar, K., & Shaffer, M. (2004). Improvement of motor development and postural control following intervention in children with sensorineural hearing loss and vestibular impairment. *International Journal of Pediatric Otorhinolaryngology, 68*(9), 1141-1148.

Salem-Hartshorne, N., & Jacob, S. (2005). Adaptive behavior in children with CHARGE syndrome. *American Journal of Medical Genetics A, 133A*(3), 262-267.

Souriau, J., Gimenes, M., Blouin, C., Benbrik, I., Benbrik, E., Churakowskyi, A., Churakowskyi, B. (2005). CHARGE syndrome: developmental and behavioral data. *American Journal of Medical Genetics A, 133A*(3), 278-281.

Stamataki, S., Behar, P., & Brodsky, L. (2008). Surgical management of drooling: Clinical and caregiver satisfaction outcomes. *International Journal of Pediatric Otorhinolaryngology, 72*(12), 1801-1805.

Steinlin, M. (2008). Cerebellar disorders in childhood: Cognitive problems. *Cerebellum, 7*(4), 607-610.

Strömland, K., Sjogreen, L., Johansson, M., Ekman Joelsson, B. M., Miller, M., Danielsson, S., et al., (2005). CHARGE association in Sweden: malformations and functional deficits. *American Journal of Medical Genetics A, 133A*(3), 331-339.

Tscheng, D. Z. (2002). Sialorrhea—therapeutic drug options. *Annals of Pharmacotherapy, 36*(11), 1785-1790.

Van der Burg, J. J., Didden, R., Jongerius, P. H., & Rotteveel, J. J. (2007). Behavioral treatment of drooling: a methodological critique of the literature with clinical guidelines and suggestions for future research. *Behavior Modification, 31*(5), 573-594.

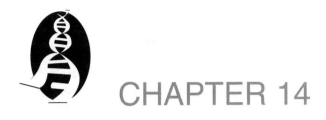

CHAPTER 14

The Heart of CHARGE or Congenital Heart Defects in CHARGE Syndrome

ANGELA E. LIN, M.D., AND
DANIELA BAUMGARTNER, M.D.

*C*ongenital heart defects are important features of CHARGE syndrome because of their frequent occurrence, implications for medical management, role in determining prognosis, and potential insight into developmental mechanisms. Their anatomic diversity ranges from the simplicity of a hole in the septum dividing the atria and/or ventricles to the complexity of a defect involving the outflow tract and aortic arch. As the criteria for diagnosing CHARGE evolved from the original mnemonic described by Pagon, Graham, Zonana, & Yong (1981) to that revised by Blake, et al., (1998), it was recognized that congenital heart defects (CHDs) were less specific and no longer considered a "major" diagnostic criterion. In the 2009 version of GeneReviews (Lalani, Hefner, Belmont, & Davenport, revised June, 2009), CHDs are considered a minor diagnostic criterion. Before reviewing the type and frequency of CHDs in CHARGE syndrome itself, it is worth reviewing a few aspects about the normal heart and the occurrence of CHDs in the general population.

DEFINITIONS

Although "heart disease" can encompass cardiomyopathy (heart muscle disease), arrhythmia, and coronary artery disease, a CHD refers more narrowly to a structural malformation. Readers are referred to a recent textbook of pediatric cardiology that provides comprehensive information about the structure, function, diagnostic methods, therapy, and genetic basis of CHDs from the fetus to the young adult (Allen, Driscoll, Shaddy, & Feltes, 2008). Included in this textbook is a chapter reviewing genetic aspects and featured among the syndromes with CHDs in CHARGE syndrome (Goldmuntz, & Lin, 2008). Also recommended is a text that provides a comprehensive clinical summary (Keane, Lock, & Fyler, 2006). Rather than provide a single illustrative diagram of heart anatomy, we encourage readers to visit several online educational resources sponsored by pediatric cardiology centers (Table 14–1). These excellent sites include the normal anatomy and a sample of CHDs.

Heart defects can be grouped according to severity (mild, severe, lethal). They also can be grouped by blood flow, too little (cyanotic, "blue"), or adequate (acyanotic, "pink"). Congenital heart defects also can be categorized broadly by the type of defect. Several CHDs are holes in the dividing walls: atrial septal defect (ASD) or a hole between the atria or upper chambers of the heart; ventricular septal defect (VSD) or a hole between the ventricles or lower chambers, and atrioventricular septal defect (AVSD), which is a large hole in the middle of the heart. Another common type of CHD concerns the adequacy of the blood flow in large blood vessels such as truncus arteriosus in which only one artery originates from the heart and tetralogy of Fallot (TOF), a complex but fairly common condition with four blood flow problems. All of these CHDs occur in CHARGE.

TABLE 14–1. Educational Websites Providing Information About Normal Heart Anatomy and Congenital Heart Defects

Children's Heart Institute Fairfax, VA	http://www.childrensheartinstitute.org/educate/heartwrk/hearthse.htm
Children's Hospital Boston, MA	http://www.childrenshospital.org/az/Site480/mainpageS480P0.html
Mayo Clinic Rochester, MN	http://www.mayoclinic.com/health/congenital-heart-defects/CC00026
Royal Children's Hospital Melbourne, Australia	http://www.rch.org.au/cardiology/defects.cfm?doc_id=3788

A classification based on postulated developmental mechanisms proposed 20 years ago has been useful for some clinical studies (Table 14–2) (Lin, Chin, Devine, Park, & Zackai, 1987). These categories are practical, although not completely verified.

TYPE AND FREQUENCY OF CONGENITAL HEART DEFECTS IN CHARGE

The reported frequency of CHDs in CHARGE syndrome varies from 65% to 85% of clinically diagnosed individuals among five case series and one population-based review (Table 14–3). All types of CHDs with the exception of heterotaxy have been reported in CHARGE, varying from mild to severe symptoms depending on the type and severity of the defect present. As a group, conotruncal and aortic arch CHDs have been reported more frequently when compared to a population-based study of newborns with CHD (Ferencz, Loffredo, Correa-Villaseñor, & Wilson, 1997).

The availability of molecular testing for *CHD7* has not altered these numbers significantly (Aramaki, et al., 2006; Jongmans, et al., 2006). In a comparative study, Lalani, et al., (2006) noted CHDs in 92% of those positive for the *CHD7* mutation but in only 71% of individuals clinically diagnosed, but without an identified mutation. Interestingly, no difference existed among the types of CHDs in those with and without identified mutations. Only patent ductus arteriosus was more common in mutation positive patients.

TABLE 14–2. Congenital Heart Defects and Their Approximate Timing in Gestation

A: CHDs, which occur only during early gestation (prior to 9 weeks)

    (1) Laterality and looping defects (situs inversus totalis, heterotaxy, l-transposition, complex single ventricle)

    (2) Conotruncal and/or aortic arch CHDs (truncus arteriosus, TOF, double outlet right ventricle, aberrant subclavian artery, right aortic arch, interrupted aortic arch, type B, conoventricular VSD)

    (3) Atrioventricular canal defect, complete; primum-type atrial septal defect, canal-type VSD

B: CHDs, which may occur early and later in gestation

    (4) Simple shunts (secundum-type ASD, VSD, patent ductus arteriosus)

    (5) Right and left heart obstruction (pulmonic stenosis, pulmonic atresia with intact ventricular septum, tricuspid atresia, aortic stenosis, mitral stenosis, coarctation, hypoplastic left heart syndrome)

    (6) Total anomalous pulmonary venous return

TABLE 14-3. Frequency of CHDs in CHARGE from the Literature

Study	Clinically Diagnosed (pre-CHD7)						CHD7 Testing			
	Cyran, et al., 1987	Lin, et al., 1987	Blake, et al., 1990	Wyse, et al., 1993	Tellier, et al., 1998	Issekutz, et al., 2005	Lalani, et al., 2006	Jongmans, et al., 2006	Aramaki, et al., 2006	Wincent, et al., 2008
Total Patients	55	53	50	59	47	77	101	107	17	30
Frequency of CHDs	36– 65%	34– 64%	42– 84%	47– 80%	40– 85%	65– 84%	+2% −71%	71 +66%	13 +76%	+15/21 −6/9 70%

Note. + = CHD7 mutation detected; − = CHD7 mutation not detected

Acknowledgements. Over many years, several authors of the preceding papers have helped me (A.E.L.) to monitor the type and frequency of CHDs in CHARGE syndrome. I extend my thanks to Drs. John Belmont, Kim Blake, Sandra Davenport, Kenjiro Kosaki, Seema Lalani, Stanislas Lyonnet, Alain Verloes, Josephine Wincent, Ms. Meg Hefner, and other colleagues.

CARDIOLOGY EVALUATION

At the time that CHARGE syndrome is first suspected, all patients should have a cardiology evaluation that, in children, should be done by a pediatric specialist. If a CHD was diagnosed or suspected by fetal echocardiography, it should have postnatal confirmation. In addition to a careful physical examination with auscultation and blood pressure measurement, chest radiography, and electrocardiography should be performed. Two-dimensional echocardiography with Doppler interrogation must be done, including evaluation of the aortic arch. As needed, MRI/MRA may be used to provide superior imaging of the distal pulmonary arteries and veins and descending aorta. Cardiac catheterization may provide additional information about pressures and anatomy. When appropriate, catheterization can be used for interventional procedures.

Occasionally, stress testing may be indicated to determine exercise capacity, especially as individuals with CHARGE syndrome with CHDs transition to adulthood. No late-onset heart problems are known to be unique to CHARGE syndrome and, thus, no recommendation for an additional cardiac evaluation in adult life for those who had a normal heart evaluation in childhood. There have been no reported concerns about degenerative valve disease, aortic dilation, valvular dysplasia or cardiomyopathy in CHARGE.

MANAGEMENT AND OUTCOME OF
CONGENITAL HEART DEFECTS

An individual with CHARGE syndrome with a CHD should be cared for by an experienced cardiology team, which may include a cardiac surgeon, nurse practitioner, and dietician. A genetics consult usually is obtained in all patients with suspected CHARGE syndrome at the time of diagnosis. Patients with interrupted aortic arch, type B, and truncus arteriosus, represent a subset who may have co-occurring DiGeorge sequence (without 22q deletion) as a developmental phenotype, and who should be evaluated by an endocrinologist and/or immunologist at the time of diagnosis (Shprintzen, 2005). Testing for B- and T-cell dysfunction and calcium likely would be advised in those cases.

A child with CHARGE syndrome who does not require cardiac surgery but needs pharmacologic support, might receive digoxin, diuretics, and/or vasodilators. When required, surgery will be timed based upon the anatomic defect, the child's overall health, and other surgical needs. In one study, 30/42 (71%) patients with CHARGE had a major CHD that required surgery (Blake, Russell-Eggitt, Morgan, Ratcliffe, & Wise, 1990). In general, CHDs with large shunts such as an AVSD are repaired before the second birthday to minimize pulmonary vascular disease. The outcome and risks associated with heart surgery in CHARGE syndrome depend on the type of CHD, the type of surgery, and on the presence of co-existing serious health problems, especially choanal atresia, tracheo-esophageal atresia, and/or cleft lip/palate.

Surgical Complications

Several observations about surgery and anesthesia in individuals with CHARGE syndrome should be kept in mind in the perioperative period. Children with CHARGE syndrome have had unusual reactions to anesthesia and should be monitored closely. Those with structurally abnormal airway (choanal atresia, stenosis, tracheo-esophageal fistula, malformed larynx) have an added risk for anesthesia, especially post operative complications (Blake, et al., 2008; Naito, et al., 2007). Cardiac procedures involving the aortic arch and mobilization of the recurrent laryngeal nerve (inferior branch of cranial nerve X) may pose a risk to swallowing dynamics. Swallowing problems, presumably due to involvement of cranial nerves IX and X, may lead to increased secretions and may present an additional risk of aspiration. These and other factors related to upper airway obstruction investigation and treatment were carefully studied by Naito, et al., (2007).

Some children have been reported to be resistant to chloral hydrate sedation which is sometimes used during echocardiography. Whether this is increased above the frequency of other children with dually diagnosed psychomotor and visual challenges is unknown. After CHD surgery, active coordination of diagnostic tests requiring general anesthetics (e.g., cardiac catheterization PE tube placement, and MRI of the temporal bone) can reduce the use of anaesthesia by at least 25% and may help to maintain feeding capabilities and reduce morbidity and mortality. Immunoprophylaxis against respiratory syncytial virus (RSV) is recommended in hemodynamically relevant shunts and in uncorrected cyanotic CHD (Cohen, et al., 2008).

POST-SURGICAL AND LONG-TERM MANAGEMENT

The child with CHARGE syndrome who is hospitalized for an extended period for cardiac surgery and the associated procedures generally experiences great stress (see Chapter 31). In particular, those children with significant visual impairments may have disturbances of their sleep cycle (see Chapter 23). Although most modern pediatric hospitals are progressive in their approach to the child with developmental and sensory challenges, there is always the possibility that milestones may be lost. Awareness by the family and caregivers of this situation, and recognition that setbacks may be temporary should be helpful in dealing with the developmental and psychological aspects of CHD surgery. Involvement of therapeutic services is integral to the postoperative process.

Individuals with CHARGE syndrome may experience slow growth especially when unrepaired CHDs are associated with congestive heart failure or chronic cyanosis. Even beyond the acute postoperative period failure to thrive may occur, but cardiac problems may not be the sole cause. Other causes may include feeding problems, frequent illnesses (especially chronic otitis media and respiratory infections), and possibly growth hormone deficiency.

Older individuals with CHARGE syndrome who have had surgical correction, or who are still being treated, must remain under the care of a cardiologist. Individuals diagnosed with a clinically mild CHD, such as a small ASD or VSD, should still have a cardiology evaluation even if they are apparently asymptomatic. Approaching adulthood, the pediatrician and parent or guardian should anticipate the transition from a pediatric to an adult cardiologist. The timing may vary based on institutions and regional health care delivery systems.

REFERENCES

Allen, H. D., Driscoll, D. J., Shaddy, R. E., & Feltes, T. F. (Eds.). (2008). *Moss and Adams' Heart Disease in Infants, Children, and Adolescents, including the Fetus and Young Adult* (7th ed.). Baltimore, MD: Williams and Wilkins.

Aramaki, M., Udaka, T., Kosaki, R., Makita, Y., Okamoto, N., Yoshihashi, H., . . . Kosaki, K. (2006). Phenotypic spectrum of CHARGE syndrome with *CHD7* mutations. *Journal of Pediatrics,148*, 410–414.

Blake, K., Maccuspie, J., Hartshorne, T. S., Roy, M., Davenport, S. L., & Corsten, G. (2008). Postoperative airway events of individuals with CHARGE syndrome. *International Journal of Pediatric Otorhinolaryngology*, *73*, 219–226.

Blake, K. D., Davenport, S. L. H., Hall, B., Hefner, M. A., Pagon, R., Williams, M. S., Lin, A. E., & Graham, J. M. (1998). CHARGE association. An update and review for the primary pediatrician. *Clinical Pediatrics*, *37*, 159–174.

Blake, K. D., Russell-Eggitt, I. M., Morgan, D. W., Ratcliffe, J. M., & Wyse, R. K. (1990). Who's in CHARGE? Multidisciplinary management of patients with CHARGE association. *Archives of Diseases of Childhood*, *65*, 217–223.

Cohen, S. A., Zanni, R., Cohen, A., Harrington, M., VanVeldhuisen, P., & Boron, M. L., (2008). Palivizumab use in subjects with congenital heart disease: Results from the 2000–2004 Palivizumab Outcomes Registry. *Pediatric Cardiology*, *29*, 382–387.

Cyran, S. E., Martinez, R., Daniels, S., Dignan, P. S., & Kaplan, S. (1987). Spectrum of congenital heart disease in CHARGE association. *Journal of Pediatrics*, *110*, 576–578.

Ferencz, C., Loffredo, C. A., Correa-Villaseñor, A., & Wilson, P. D. (1997). *Genetic and Environmental Risk Factors of Major Congenital heart defects: The Baltimore-Washington Infant Study: 1981-1989*. Armonk, NY: Futura.

Goldmuntz, E, & Lin, A. E. (2008). Genetics of congenital heart defects. In A. J. Moss, H. D. Allen, D. J. Driscoll, R. E. Shady, & T. F. Feltes (Eds.), *Moss and Adams' Heart Disease in Infants, Children, and Adolescents, including the Fetus and Young Adult* (7th ed., pp. 563–564). Baltimore, MD: Williams and Wilkins.

Issekutz, K. A., Graham, J. M. Jr, Prasad, C., Smith, I. M., & Blake, K. D. (2005). An epidemiological analysis of CHARGE syndrome: preliminary results from a Canadian study. *American Journal of Medical Genetics, 133A,* 309-317.

Jongmans, M. C., Admiraal, R. J., van der Donk, K. P., Vissers, L. E., Baas, A. F., Kapusta, L., . . . van Ravenswaaij, C. M. (2006). CHARGE syndrome: the phenotypic spectrum of mutations in the *CHD7* gene. *Journal of Medical Genetics, 43,* 306-314.

Keane, J. K., Lock, J. E., & Fyler, D. C. (Eds.). (2006). *Nadas' Pediatric Cardiology* (2nd ed.). Philadelphia, PA: Saunders Elsevier.

Lalani, S. R., Safiullah, A. M., Fernbach, S. D., Harutyunyan, K. G., Thaller, C., Peterson, L. E., . . . Belmont, J. W. (2006). Spectrum of *CHD7* mutations in 119 individuals with CHARGE syndrome and genotype-phenotype correlation. *American Journal of Human Genetics, 78,* 303-314.

Lalani, S. R., Hefner, M., Belmont, J. W., Davenport, S. L. H. (2009, June). CHARGE syndrome. *GeneReviews.* Retrieved June 21, 2009, from http://www.ncbi.nlm.nih.gov/bookshelf/br.fcgi?book=gene&part=charge.

Lin, A. E., Chin, A. J., Devine, W., Park, S. C., & Zackai, E. (1987). The pattern of cardiovascular malformations in the CHARGE association. *American Journal of Diseases in Childhood, 141,* 1010-1013.

Naito, Y., Higuchi, M., Koinuma, G., Aramaki, M., Takahashi, T., & Kosaki, K. (2007). Upper airway obstruction in neonates and infants with CHARGE syndrome. *American Journal of Medical Genetics, 143A,* 1815-1820.

Pagon, R. A., Graham, J. M. Jr, Zonana, J., & Yong, S. L. (1981). Coloboma, congenital heart disease and choanal atresia with multiple anomalies: CHARGE association. *Journal of Pediatrics, 99,* 223-227.

Shprintzen, R. J. (2005). Velo-cardio-facial syndrome. *Progress in Pediatric Cardiology, 20,* 187-193.

Tellier, A. L., Cormier-Daire, V., Abadie, V., Amiel, J., Sigaudy, S., Bonnet D., . . . Lyonnet, S. (1998). CHARGE Syndrome: report of 47 cases and review. *American Journal of Medical Genetics, 76,* 402-409.

Wincent, J., Holmberg, E., Strömland, K., Soller, M., Mirzaei, L., Djureinovic, T., . . . Schoumans, J. (2008). *CHD7* mutation spectrum in 28 Swedish patients diagnosed with CHARGE syndrome. *Clinical Genetics, 74,* 31-38.

Wyse, R., Al-Mahdawi, S., Burn, L., & Blake, K. D. (1993). Congenital heart disease in CHARGE association. *Pediatric Cardiology, 14,* 75-81.

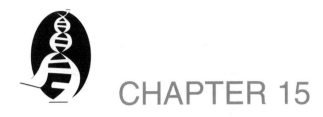

CHAPTER 15

Renal and Urinary Systems

MARC S. WILLIAMS, M.D.

THE NORMAL URINARY TRACT

The normal urinary tract consists of two kidneys. Urine is produced in the kidney and is drained by the renal pelvis. Urine then flows into the ureters. These tubes drain into the urinary bladder. When we urinate, the urine travels through another tube called the urethra. This tube is very short in females and longer in males (as it has to travel through the length of the penis). Normally, urine flows in only one direction.

Urinary Tract Abnormalities in CHARGE Syndrome

Abnormalities of the urinary tract are seen in 20% to 40% of children with CHARGE syndrome (Issekutz, Graham, Prasad, Smith, & Blake, 2005; Ragan, Casale, Rink, Cain, & Weaver, 1999; Tellier, et al., 1998;). They can be of two types, structural or functional. The structural anomalies are listed in Table 15–1. Facial palsy is significantly associated with structural renal anomalies, which are usually ipsilateral (on the same side) to the palsy (Blake, Russell-Eggitt, Morgan, Ratcliffe, & Wyse, 1990).

TABLE 15–1. Structural Anomalies of the Urinary Tract

Structural anomalies	Description
Absent or hypoplastic kidney	One kidney is not present or is small.
Ectopic, or pelvic kidney	Kidney is in an abnormal location.
Horseshoe kidney	Kidneys are fused together.
Duplications	Kidney, renal pelvis, and/or urethra are duplicated.
Hydronephrosis	Renal pelvis is enlarged.
Multicystic dysplastic kidney	Kidney is formed abnormally with many cysts.

Functional Abnormalities (Urine Doesn't Flow Properly)

Vesicoureteral reflux (hereafter referred to as reflux) is a very common problem. When the bladder contracts to assist urination, urine normally flows out the urethra. The bladder wall pinches off the ureters to prevent urine flowing backward toward the kidneys. If the ureters remain open during bladder contraction, urine can flow back toward the kidney. This is reflux. It can be mild to severe. Reflux can predispose to urinary tract infection (UTI). If severe, it can result in hydronephrosis and direct damage to the kidneys, which ultimately can lead to kidney failure. Somewhat less common is when the bladder does not empty completely. This is called *bladder residual* and can predispose to urinary tract infections.

IMPLICATIONS OF URINARY TRACT ABNORMALITIES ON PATIENTS

Although neither structural nor functional urologic abnormalities will have a direct impact on the development and therapy of individuals with CHARGE syndrome, it is important to recognize that the consequences of these abnormalities can have a dramatic impact.

Urinary Tract Infection

The most common consequence that a patient with urinary tract abnormalities is likely to experience is urinary tract infection (UTI). Signs and symptoms associated with UTI include fever, listlessness, irritability, increased frequency of urination, pain on urination, and blood in the urine. A patient with frequent UTIs could experience significant disruption of their health and well-being, which could interfere with education and therapy. Any child who has fever without an identifiable source on physical examination should have a clean urine specimen obtained looking for UTI. This may involve placing a catheter through the urethra to obtain a specimen or sticking a needle through the abdomen into the bladder (suprapubic or bladder tap). Bagged specimens are inadequate for this purpose. Older children may be able to provide a clean voided specimen. Urine culture must be done to confirm UTI. Standard medical therapy with antibiotics is acceptable for treatment of UTIs. Suppressive therapy (that is chronic use of low-dose antibiotics) may be necessary if infections are recurrent. Recurrent UTIs that are refractory to medical therapy may require surgical correction of the underlying structural or functional abnormality.

Voiding Abnormalities

The vast majority of alterations in voiding patterns will be secondary to UTIs. Ragan, et al., (1999) reported one patient in their series with a neurogenic bladder secondary to a spinal cord abnormality. No other reports of this problem exist in patients with CHARGE syndrome in the medical literature, so this is likely a very rare problem. A neurogenic bladder can result in build up and retention of urine in the bladder. This also can predispose to UTIs and may require medication or regular insertion of a catheter to assist the bladder to drain.

Renal Failure

No cases have been reported of kidney or renal failure in patients with CHARGE syndrome. However, it is well-known that chronic reflux, particularly if associated with chronic, recurrent UTIs, can cause progressive kidney damage that could ultimately lead to kidney failure (Blumenthal, 2006). Renal failure (uremia) can cause lethargy, poor appetite, and vomiting and negatively impact cognitive abilities. Treatment for renal failure involves medication and diet, dialysis, and in the final stages renal transplantation. These treatments are very disruptive for patients and families leading to a significant negative impact on the patient's health and well-being (Kutner, 1994). Therefore, it is important to aggressively ascertain and treat reflux and infection to avoid this outcome.

EVALUATION OF THE URINARY TRACT

A number of modalities can be used to assess the structural and functional abnormalities of the urinary tract. These include the following:

- Renal Ultrasound (US). Used to identify structural abnormalities.

■ Voiding Cystourethrogram (VCUG). This test is indicated if reflux is suspected. It involves placing a small tube (catheter) through the urethra into the bladder. The bladder is filled with a liquid (contrast) that can be seen on X-ray. X-rays are taken while the child urinates. This test is necessary to diagnose reflux or bladder residual.

■ Intravenous Pyelogram (IVP). This is another test primarily used to examine kidney structure. Because it involves the injection of contrast into a vein as well as X-ray exposure, this test has for the most part been replaced by the renal ultrasound. It does have the advantage of requiring intact blood supply to the kidneys and provides information regarding the kidney's ability to make urine (which renal US or VCUG do not). IVP can be used to determine whether duplicated kidneys are functioning.

■ Radionucleotide renal scan. This test involves the injection of a radioactive material into a vein that concentrates in the kidney. Indications for the test are similar to IVP, but this test gives more information about function and less information about structure than the IVP. The amount of radioactivity is small, and it is eliminated rapidly in the urine so the radioactive exposure is minimal.

■ Both Computerized Tomography (CT) and Magnetic Resonance Imaging (MRI) provide high-resolution images that allow much better definition of structure than the renal ultrasound. One of these would be indicated if the renal ultrasound was unable to resolve a complex structural abnormality of the urinary tract. The CT scan uses X-rays, but usually does not require sedation as it scans very rapidly. The MRI uses magnetic fields (which do not have harmful effects on body tissues) and has better resolution than CT scan. It also can be used to evaluate blood vessel anatomy (Magnetic Resonance Angiography or MRA). The scan time is longer, so young children frequently require sedation. This is an important issue in children with CHARGE due to the increased risk of airway compromise. We recommend full airway precautions if sedation is to be used. See sedation precautions; MRI precautions (e.g., cochlear implant, BAHA, metal rods).

SUMMARY

■ 20% to 40% of individuals with CHARGE have a urinary tract anomaly.

■ All types of structural problems (solitary kidney, hydronephrosis, renal hypoplasia, duplex kidney, posterior urethral valves, multicystic kidney, etc.) have been reported, as well as vesico-ureteral reflux.

■ Facial palsy is significantly associated with renal anomalies, which are usually on the same side as the palsy.

■ Children with CHARGE are at increased risk for urinary tract infection. Evaluation of a patient who has fever without an obvious source should include a urinalysis and urine culture.

■ Baseline renal and bladder ultrasounds to evaluate anatomy are warranted, as early identification and treatment may reduce long-term morbidity.

■ Functional studies (such as voiding cystourethrogram) may be indicated as follow-up to anatomic study, or if the patient develops urinary tract infection.

■ Standard medical therapy is acceptable for treatment of UTIs. Suppressive therapy may be necessary if infections are recurrent.

■ Surgical intervention is indicated for certain abnormalities. Indications for surgery are the same as for children who don't have CHARGE. Caveats for surgery include the following:

   ■ Anesthetic risk is increased in children with airway involvement such as choanal atresia or laryngotracheomalacia (both common in CHARGE). Children with choanal atresia and complex heart defects have the highest rate of serious complications and/or poor outcome.

   ■ Swallowing problems with increased secretions (presumably due to involvement of cranial nerves IX and X) may present an additional risk of aspiration.

REFERENCES

Blake, K. D., Russell-Eggitt, I. M., Morgan, D. W., Ratcliffe, J. M., & Wyse, R. K. (1990). Who's in CHARGE? Multidisciplinary management of patients with CHARGE association. *Archives of Disease in Childhood, 65,* 217–233.

Blumenthal, I. (2006). Vesicoureteric reflux and urinary tract infection in children. *Postgraduate Medical Journal, 82,* 31–35.

Issekutz, K. A., Graham, J. M., Prasad, C., Smith, I. M., & Blake K. D. (2005). An epidemiological analysis of CHARGE syndrome: Preliminary results from a Canadian study. *American Journal of Medical Genetics, 133A,* 309–317.

Kutner, N. G. (1994). Assessing end-stage renal disease patients' functioning and well-being: measurement approaches and implications for clinical practice. *American Journal of Kidney Diseases, 24,* 321–323.

Ragan, D. C., Casale, A. J., Rink, R. C., Cain, M. P., & Weaver, D. D. (1999). Genitourinary anomalies in the CHARGE association. *Journal of Urology, 161,* 622–625.

Tellier, A. L., Cormier-Daire, V., Abadie, V., Amiel, J., Sigaudy, S., Bonnet, D., . . . Lyonnet, S. (1998). CHARGE Syndrome: Report of 47 cases and review. *American Journal of Medical Genetics*, *76*, 402–409.

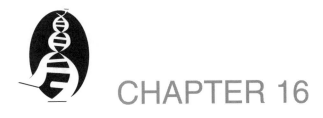

CHAPTER 16

Endocrinology

JEREMY KIRK, M.D.

*C*hildren with CHARGE syndrome often have problems with growth, puberty, or both. Careful evaluation, monitoring, and management is very important.

NORMAL GROWTH

Growth of a child occurs in three separate phases, which merge into each other, but which are under different controls, both hormonal and nutritional (Figure 16-1). All of these are affected in CHARGE syndrome.

Infantile phase: This occurs during the first two to three years of life and is a continuation of fetal growth (i.e., growth in the womb). This phase is almost completely nutritionally dependent.

Childhood phase: This occurs from about two years of age until puberty. This phase is dependent on both nutrition and also hormones such as growth hormone and thyroid hormone.

Pubertal phase: From puberty onward, which starts at an average of 10 years in girls and 10½ years in boys, this phase is under the control of growth hormone and sex hormones acting together. It also has different timing and strength in the two sexes and accounts for the sex differences in final height of around 5 inches (12.5 cm) between males and females.

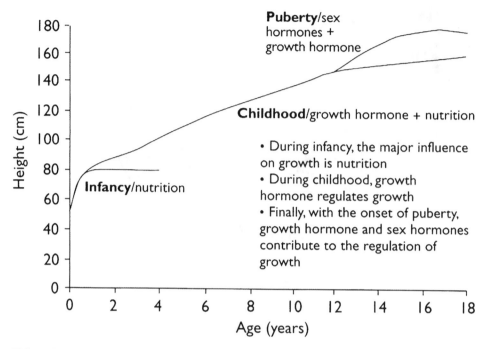

FIGURE 16–1. The Infancy–Childhood–Puberty (ICP) Model of Growth. Courtesy of Karlberg, J. (1987). On the modeling of human growth. *Statistics in Medicine*, *6*(2), 185–192. Use by permission of Wiley-Blackwell.

GROWTH PROBLEMS IN CHARGE SYNDROME

Failure of any of these three phases will lead to short stature, and all of these are seen in children with CHARGE, with about 75% having both height and weight at or below the lower end of the normal range. Although no disease-specific growth charts for CHARGE exist, we previously have described growth in a group of children with CHARGE syndrome (Blake, Kirk, & Ur, 1993) (Figures 16–2 and 16–3).

Infancy

Intra-uterine growth retardation (IUGR) may occur, as some children with CHARGE have a low birth weight, e.g., less than 6 lb 10 oz (3 kg) at term. Overall, however, average birth weight and birth length are on the 10th percentile in CHARGE syndrome.

More than 90 percent of children with CHARGE have difficulty swallowing foods of different textures. This can be due to both mechanical and neurological factors. Mechanical problems can include choanal atresia or stenosis (blockage or narrowing of posterior nasal passages), small or pos-

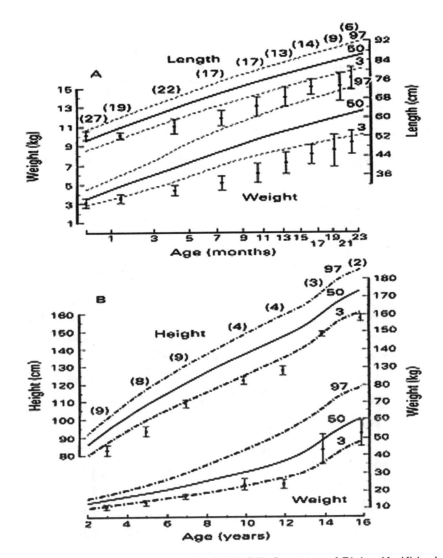

FIGURE 16–2. Growth in Boys with CHARGE. Courtesy of Blake, K., Kirk, J. M., & Ur, E. (1993). Growth in CHARGE association. *Archives of Disease in Childhood, 68*, 508–509. Used by permission of BMJ Publishing Group Ltd.

teriorly placed jaw, cleft lip and/or palate, tracheoesophageal fistula (either a join or block between the trachea [windpipe] and esophagus [gullet]), or gastroesophageal reflux. Neurological problems can include facial palsy and swallowing difficulties.

Growth in the first year of life (both height and weight) is characteristically poor in children with CHARGE (so called "failure to thrive" or "faltering growth"), and it has been shown that children are more likely to fail to thrive if they have feeding difficulties (including gastro-esophageal reflux and fundoplication), larynx/pharynx problems, facial palsy, and also have had major operations and prolonged hospitalization.

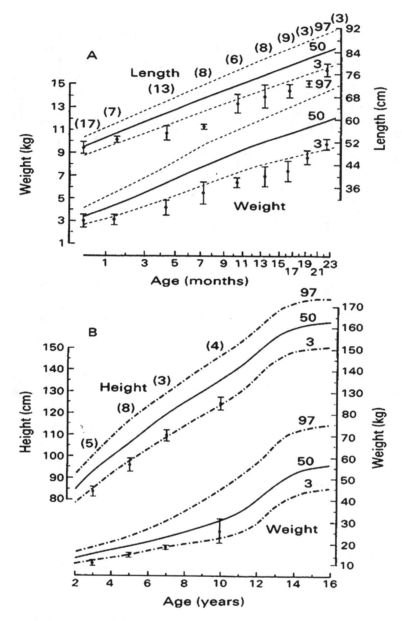

FIGURE 16–3. Growth in Girls with CHARGE. Courtesy of Blake, K., Kirk, J. M., & Ur, E. (1993). Growth in CHARGE association. *Archives of Disease in Childhood, 68,* 508–509. Used by permission of BMJ Publishing Group Ltd.

Childhood

Children with CHARGE often can grow normally during childhood and may even grow faster than usual during preschool years: so-called "catch-up" growth. Despite this, many children with CHARGE remain short.

Puberty

This pubertal phase is often delayed or absent in CHARGE. This is primarily due to problems with production of the sex hormones, both from the pituitary gland and in males from the testicles themselves. Data from a number of centers, including our own, indicate that very few males enter puberty spontaneously, whereas approximately 50% of girls will do so, including some who pass completely through puberty and menstruate spontaneously. Little data exists on fertility in either sex, although the authors know of both women and men with CHARGE who have had children.

Although short stature is well recognized in CHARGE, few data exists on final height. In one study (Blake, Salem-Hartshorne, Daoud, & Gradstein, 2005) of individuals 19 years or older, final height of five males averaged 5'6" (167.5 cm), with a range of 5'1"-6' (155-182 cm), and the average final height of six girls was 5'3" (161 cm), with a range of 4'11"-5'7" (150-170 cm). In my own clinic of 18 adolescents, half have heights above the 2nd centile (≥-2 SD), although four of those have received growth hormone therapy.

INVESTIGATION AND MANAGEMENT OF GROWTH PROBLEMS IN CHARGE

Children with CHARGE syndrome should be followed by a specialist in endocrine disorders: a pediatric endocrinologist. At each assessment the following measurements should be taken and plotted:

- Height

- Weight

- Weight for height (body mass index)

- Head circumference in younger children

- Pubertal assessment in older patients

Height should be measured lying down until 2 years of age, and then standing, when possible. The head needs to be positioned so that a line from lower edge of the eye to the ear canals is parallel to the surface: "the Frankfurt plane." Shoes should be removed, although thin socks can be worn. Weight should be measured ideally with electronic scales, with minimal clothing, and no diapers. Head circumference is measured with a nonstretcheable tape above the ears and eyes at the widest point on the head. Weight for height also should be calculated and can be useful to distinguish between nutritional problems, where weight is characteristically low for height, and hormonal problems, where weight tends to be greater than height. Body mass index is probably the most common way to assess weight for height. This is calculated as weight (in kilograms) divided by height (in meters) squared (wt/ht^2). Serial measures of height (ideally over at least 12 months) enables a height velocity to be calculated. Additional information on height potential also can be obtained by using the following methods:

- Midparental height, based on parental heights (ideally measured), can be used to calculate expected final height in their children. Children with CHARGE syndrome are often well outside their expected genetic target range.

- Biological age, rather than chronological age, is assessed using the "bone age," which is calculated by looking at the growing ends (epiphyses) of the bones. This is characteristically performed in a left wrist X-ray and assesses how much remaining time (and, therefore, remaining growth) there is before the bones fuse and no further growth will occur.

Puberty is assessed using a standardized staging system, looking at breast development in girls, genital development in boys, and pubic and axillary (armpit) hair in both sexes. Testicular volume in boys can be measured using special graduated beads (the orchidometer).

Hormones are chemicals secreted by specialized (endocrine) glands, which then pass round the body in the bloodstream to produce their actions (Figure 16-4). A number of different hormones are involved in growth, and several have been shown to be abnormal in children with CHARGE syndrome. It is worth remembering that some hormones, such as thyroid hormone or the insulin-like growth factor 1 (IGF1), are produced at a constant rate, while others are produced in a diurnal fashion, being highest at different times of the day (such as the stress hormone cortisol), or in a pulsatile fashion (such as growth hormone). As a result, patients require specialist advice for selection of tests, in performing the testing and also interpretation of tests, along with any decision regarding treatment.

MONITORING GROWTH

Many of the reasons for poor growth are clear, although, as with other syndromes, CHARGE itself also may be associated with reduction in height, as many children without feeding and hormonal problems are small in comparison with their siblings and parents. Investigation and management of growth problems in infancy often will require a multidisciplinary feeding team including a speech therapist, dietician, occupational therapist, physical thera-

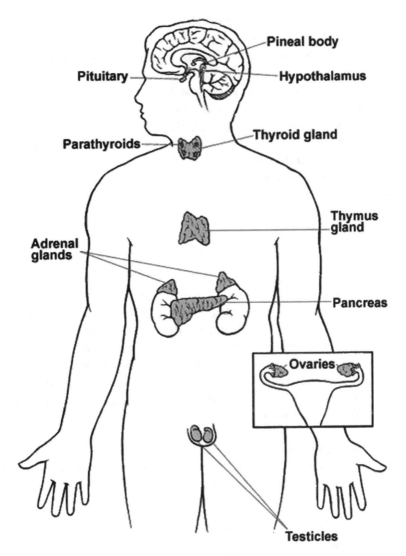

FIGURE 16–4. The Endocrine System. Courtesy of Current Procedural Terminology (CPT), used by permission of the American Medical Association.

pist, and behavioral psychologist (see Chapter 12). Medical input may be necessary from a general pediatrician, pediatric gastroenterologist, and pediatric surgeon. Optimizing nutritional input may also require medication to improve gastric emptying and reduce reflux, as well as tube feeding, naso-gastric feeding, or feeding directly via tube into the stomach (gastrostomy), or small bowel (jejunal).

There is currently little published evidence that children with CHARGE have increased problems with growth hormone secretion. If children are growing poorly, especially if nutritional problems have been resolved, then further specialist investigation of hormones is warranted.

A number of international databases include information on several dozen children with CHARGE who have been treated with growth hormone, including those who were growth hormone deficient and those who were not. Most patients have been treated for only short periods of time, and responses to treatment have been variable, which make it difficult to draw overall conclusions. This, along with the high cost of growth hormone (~$15,000/year), the lack of a product license in CHARGE syndrome, plus the fact that growth hormone needs to be given by daily injection undoubtedly limits its current use.

PUBERTY

Delayed puberty is taken as the absence of signs of puberty by 14 years in girls (initially breast development) and 14½ years in boys (initially testicular and scrotal enlargement). In addition, it is thought that some adolescents with CHARGE may have initial signs but not progress through puberty at an appropriate rate (arrested puberty). While other hormonal problems are relatively uncommon, individuals with CHARGE commonly have delayed or defective production of sex hormones from the gonads (testicles in boys and ovaries in girls). A number of reasons exist for this:

- Reduced central hormonal drive from the pituitary gland (hypogonadotrophic hypogonadism). These two pituitary hormones are called gonadotrophins: luteinizing hormone (LH) and follicle stimulating hormone (FSH).

- Reduced hormone production from gonads in boys arising from undescended testicles.

The nerve cells (neurons) involved in production of gonadotrophin hormones in the pituitary gland actually develop within the nose in early fetal life and migrate into the brain. Therefore, patients with CHARGE often also have absent or abnormal sense of smell (anosmia), and MRI scanning of the brain may show abnormally developed olfactory lobes. There is also cross-over with another condition that causes hypogonadotrophic hypogonadism, Kallmann syndrome, and some patients with the latter have now been shown to have mutations in the CHARGE gene (CHD7) (see Chapter 7).

In addition to baseline and stimulated hormone levels along with bone age estimation, in girls pelvic ultrasound can be used to assess the size of the ovaries and uterus (womb), and also, along with pubertal ratings, the response to sex hormone therapy.

Treatment of Delayed Puberty

In children with CHARGE, there are often potential concerns about administration of sex hormones, as they might produce worsening behavior, inappropriate sexual behavior, menstrual bleeding (in girls), or persistent erections (in boys). These concerns must be balanced against the long-term risk of osteoporosis (brittle bone disease), as much of the bone strength is laid down in late teens and early twenties under the influence of sex hormones. Increasing evidence exists of the latter in older patients with CHARGE, which will predispose to early fractures (Forward, Cummings, & Blake, 2007).

Unfortunately, there does not seem to be a dose of sex hormones that will protect against osteoporosis but not produce unacceptable behavior. In girls, a gradually increasing dose of the female hormone estrogen given by mouth is commonly used, and once full pubertal development has occurred, changing over to either hormone replacement therapy (HRT) or the low-dose oral contraceptive pill (OCP) is commonly used. To avoid frequent and distressing periods in the latter, the packs can be used without breaks between so that withdrawal bleeds occur only 2–3 times per year rather than monthly. In boys, gradually increasing doses of testosterone are given by monthly injection or daily capsule. The advantage of the latter is that if there are behavioral problems, then the dose can be cut back rapidly. When puberty is complete, testosterone also can be given as a gel, patch, or implant. It is likely that hormone replacement in both sexes will need to be given long-term.

GENITAL ABNORMALITIES SEEN IN CHARGE

Although genital abnormalities (a minor diagnostic criterion) are undoubtedly common in CHARGE, little information describes these problems or their treatment. More importantly, as children may have other potentially more serious problems (especially at birth), the genital abnormalities are often not noted or treated.

As with puberty, the genital abnormalities are due to abnormal production of hormones (chemical messengers) from the pituitary gland (a small pea-sized gland lying underneath the brain), which control the production of sex hormones from the testicles in boys and ovaries in girls.

In boys, undescended testicles (one or both) and small penis (micropenis; less than 1 inch [2.5 cm] stretched length) are present at birth. About three-quarters of boys with CHARGE will have micropenis, and approximately half will have undescended testes. Both problems are due to the fact that the descent of the testicles into the scrotum and growth of the penis in the last part of the pregnancy are dependent on the production of the sex hormone testosterone from the testicles (under the influence of pituitary hormones).

In girls, the clitoris and labia minora (inner vaginal lips) may be smaller than usual, but this will not be as obvious as micropenis is in boys. It is probably very common in girls with CHARGE.

It is likely, although not necessarily inevitable, that children with these genital abnormalities will also have pubertal problems, as the hormones involved from the pituitary are the same.

Investigation

The surge in sex hormones immediately after birth, which lasts for around six months, offers a "mini-puberty," a window of opportunity to investigate these hormones. As a result, baseline unstimulated hormones may be useful, although stimulation tests of the pituitary (LHRH or GnRH) and testicular axis (hCG stimulation) may be useful, and in the latter, may also have a therapeutic effect in producing testicular descent.

Undescended Testicles

As testes need to be situated at a lower temperature within the scrotum to function normally, if they are undescended, they need to be brought down. This can be done as follows:

■ Surgically, requiring one or more operations. Although ideally this should be done within the first months or years of life, other more pressing problems of CHARGE often mean that this surgery is performed when boys are older, often in conjunction with other procedures.

■ Medically, using a course of injections (usually twice weekly over 3–6 weeks), which mimics the hormone stimulus from the pituitary. These injections probably work best in testicles that are not completely undescended and in older patients.

Micropenis

A penis that at birth is less than 2.5 cm (1") (stretched) is defined as a micropenis. In addition, there are charts showing the normal range of stretched penile length during childhood.

Ideally, any treatment with male sex hormones (usually testosterone) should be given soon after birth to mimic the normal neonatal surge. Testosterone can be administered topically, as a gel or cream, usually applied twice daily for up to three months, or by injection, usually intramuscular for 3–4 months.

Although there have been theoretical worries that early treatment will affect the subsequent growth of the penis during puberty, this does not appear to happen. Testosterone can also cause fluid retention and should, therefore, be used with caution in children with heart failure.

CONCLUSIONS

Although growth problems are common in CHARGE syndrome, there is little evidence that in many patients this is due to primary hormone deficiencies. Genital abnormalities and delayed puberty, however, are commonly seen and are due to reduced hormonal drive from the pituitary gland.

REFERENCES

Blake, K., Kirk, J. M., & Ur, E. (1993). Growth in CHARGE association. *Archives of Disease in Childhood*, *68*, 508–509.

Blake, K. D., Salem-Hartshorne, N., Daoud, M. A., & Gradstein, J. (2005). Adolescent and adult issues in CHARGE syndrome. *Clinical Pediatrics*, *44*, 151–159.

Forward, K., Cummings, E. A., & Blake, K. D. (2007). Bone health in adolescents and adults with CHARGE syndrome. *American Journal of Medical Genetics*, *143A*, 839–845.

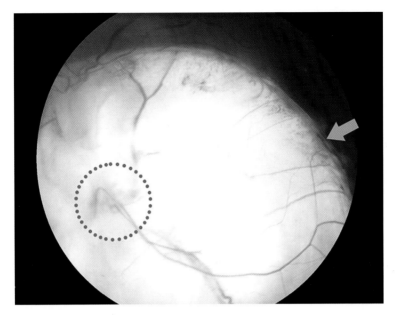

COLOR PLATE 1. The closure of the edges of the optic fissure has not happened and thus there is no retina and no choroid in the lower part of the inner eye. The area of the optic disc is marked with a dotted line and the location of the macula with an arrow.

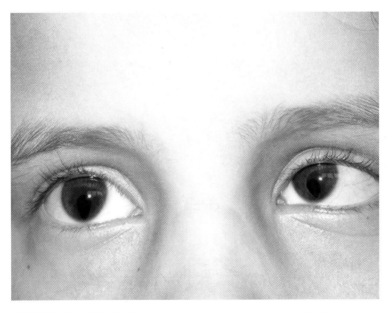

COLOR PLATE 2. Keyhole pupil in each eye. If the furrow remains open in the anterior, front part of the eye, there is a defect in the lower part of the iris, the key hole pupil.

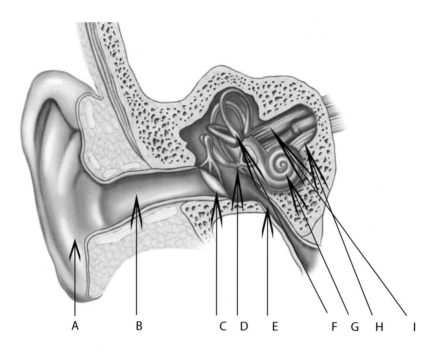

A external ear
B external auditory canal
C tympanic membrane
D ossicles of the middle ear
E eustachian tube

F semicircular canals (inner ear)
G cochlea
H auditory section of cranial nerve VIII
I vestibular section of cranial nerve VIII

COLOR PLATE 3. Structures of the auditory system. Adapted from Shutter-stock® image.

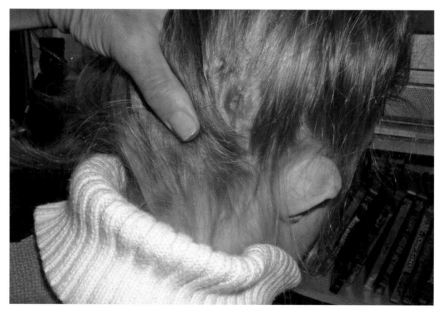

COLOR PLATE 4. The Baha is implanted surgically.

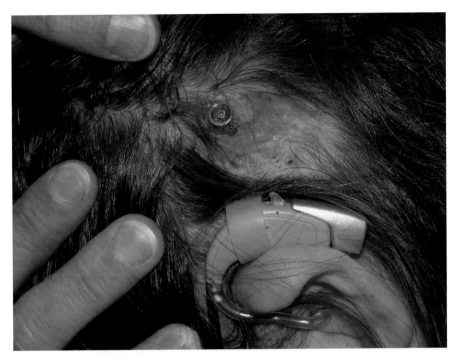

COLOR PLATE 5. Baha requires wound maintenance for life.

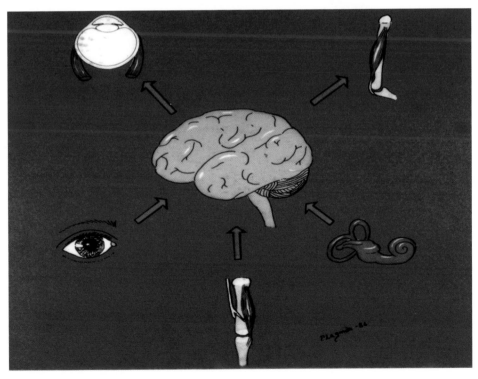

COLOR PLATE 6. Afferent and efferent systems of the eye, muscles, vestibular, and brain. Courtesy of Claes Möller.

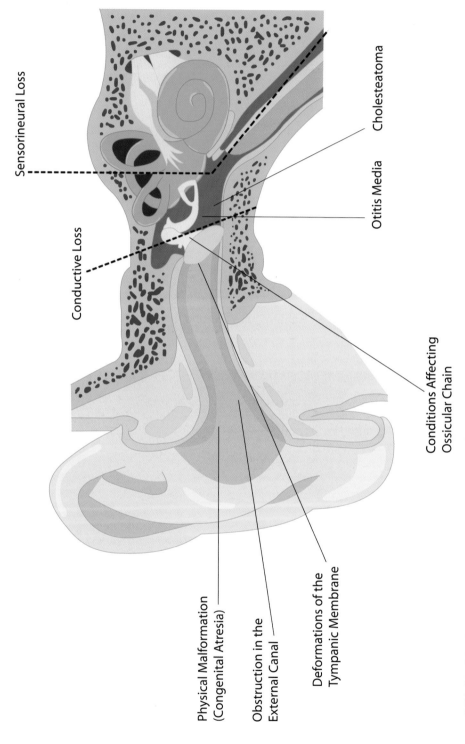

Sensorineural Loss

Conductive Loss

Cholesteatoma

Otitis Media

Conditions Affecting
Ossicular Chain

Physical Malformation
(Congenital Atresia)

Obstruction in the
External Canal

Deformations of the
Tympanic Membrane

COLOR PLATE 7. Conductive and sensorineural hearing loss. Photo adapted from Shutterstock®. All rights reserved.

CHARGE Outer Ears

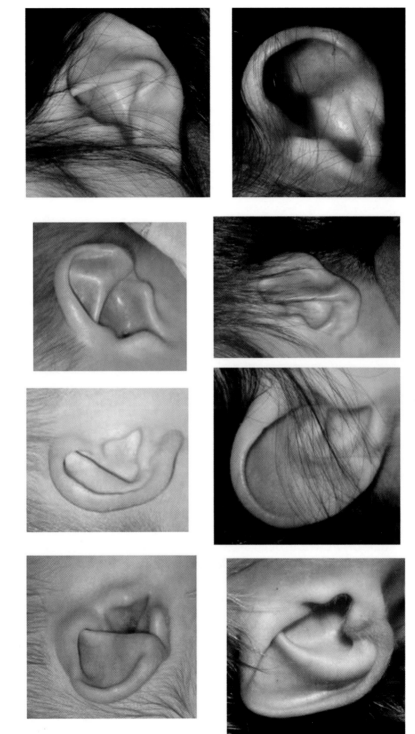

COLOR PLATE 8. Examples of CHARGE ears.

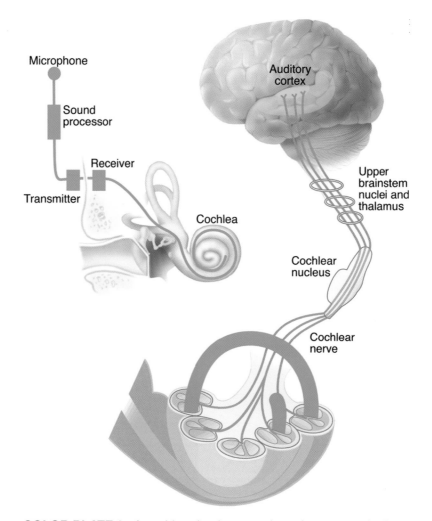

COLOR PLATE 9. A cochlear implant consists of an external microphone, which collects sound waves, and a speech processor, which converts the sound waves into electrical impulses that then are transmitted to a receiver implanted under the skin. The receiver sends the electrical impulses to a microelectrode array implanted within the cochlea. The electrodes directly stimulate the correct populations of auditory nerve fibers so that electrical signals are propagated to the appropriate (tonotopic) regions of the cochlear nucleus of the brainstem and then on to higher auditory processing centers. From Rauschecker, J. P., & Shannon, R. V. (2002). Sending sound to the brain. *Science, 295,* 1025–1029. Reprinted with permission from AAAS.

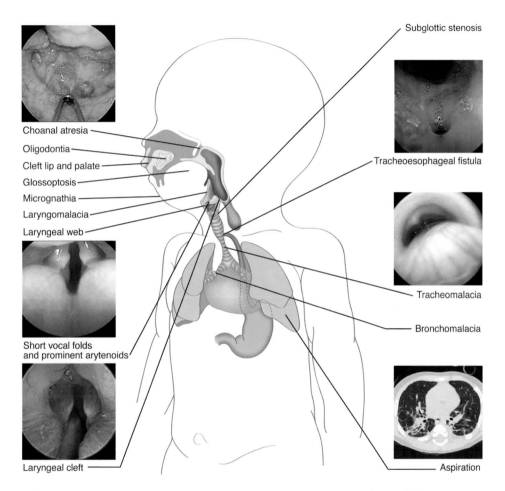

COLOR PLATE 10. Airway anomalies seen in children with CHARGE syndrome.

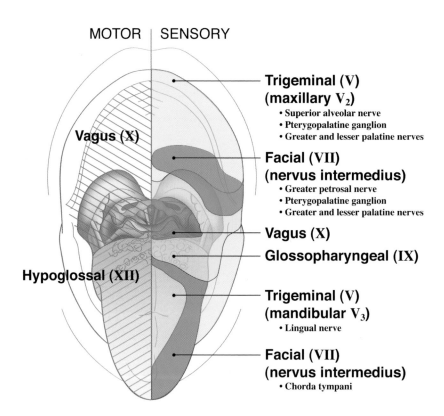

MOTOR | SENSORY

Trigeminal (V)
(maxillary V$_2$)
• Superior alveolar nerve
• Pterygopalatine ganglion
• Greater and lesser palatine nerves

Facial (VII)
(nervus intermedius)
• Greater petrosal nerve
• Pterygopalatine ganglion
• Greater and lesser palatine nerves

Vagus (X)

Glossopharyngeal (IX)

Trigeminal (V)
(mandibular V$_3$)
• Lingual nerve

Facial (VII)
(nervus intermedius)
• Chorda tympani

Vagus (X)

Hypoglossal (XII)

COLOR PLATE 11. Normal sensory and motor innervations of the oral cavity, pharynx, and larynx.

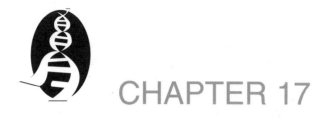

CHAPTER 17

Immune System

SANDRA L. H. DAVENPORT, M.D.

*I*n developing the outline for this book, we wanted to be certain that we addressed areas of emerging concern, even though our understanding of the problem in CHARGE is still developing. This is one such area.

The immune system is extremely complex and beyond the scope of this book to describe. The two major components, however, are cellular and humoral. The cellular system involves white blood cells that derive from the thymus (T cells) and the bone marrow (B cells) as well as others. The humoral system involves the so-called immunoglobulins and other factors that circulate in the blood.

Many individuals with CHARGE syndrome have multiple infections, and even the early literature documented cases that overlap with DiGeorge syndrome (hypocalcemia, heart disease, and immune deficiency). DiGeorge results from a deletion on chromosome 22, whereas we now know that a majority of those with CHARGE have a CHD7 mutation on chromosome 8. Since the CHD7 gene discovery in late 2004, several papers have been published that report significant problems with the immune system in 35 patients who had deletions in the CHD7 gene (Chopra, Baretto, Duddridge, & Browning, 2009; Gennery, et al., 2008; Hoover-Fong, et al., 2009; Jyonouchi, McDonald-McGinn, Bale, Zackai, & Sullivan, 2009; Theodoropoulos, D. S., & Theodoropoulos, G. A., 2003; Writzl, Cale, Pierce, Wilson, & Hennekam, 2007).

The largest study of 25 patients (Jyonouchi, et al., 2009) found that 18 had significantly low calcium, and of these, 14 had low lymphocyte counts, whereas only one of the seven with normal calcium levels had lymphopenia.

Eight died in infancy, three attributed to severe cardiovascular disease, two from infectious complications, and three from respiratory failure of whom two had severe combined immunodeficiency (SCID). Seven of the eight had severe lymphopenia. Nine patients had cell typing, including two of the deceased. Of these, five had normal T cells (derived from the thymus), whereas two had moderately low levels, and two had almost complete absence of T cells. Only one of nine had abnormally low levels of B cells (derived from the bone marrow stem cells). Eight patients had quantitative studies of immunoglobulins as well as specific antibody levels for vaccine antigens. One of those with complete absence of T cells also had severely low IgG levels and absent antibody response to vaccination. One with low IgG levels had had frequent pulmonary and sinus infections. Two had undetectable IgA levels at six and eight years of age. Two had low antibody titers to tetanus and one to diphteria. In summary, 72% had low calcium levels; 60% had cellular immunity problems; and half of the eight studied had documented defects in humoral immunity.

Ten other patients with CHD7 mutations have been reported. Gennery, et al., (2008) reported two with SCID and two with the Omenn syndrome (a SCID variant with eosinophia and elevated IgE). Writzl, et al., (2007) described two with significant T cell lymphopenia. Chopra, et al., (2009) reported an additional three with moderate to severe T-cell lymphopenia and one who had no thymus on X-ray. At three months he had a mononuclear cell transplant that seemed to improve function at first; however, ten months after transplant, he developed edema of the lungs and bowel with a viremia, which was successfully treated. At 14 months, he demonstrated no host thymic function and died suddenly of acute renal failure and untreatably high potassium for which no cause was found.

It should be kept in mind that initial reports of a syndrome or a major characteristic of a syndrome tend to emphasize the severe end of the spectrum since these cases tend to end up in academic centers where the medical staff are accustomed to writing up their findings. These cases demonstrate, however, that immune function can be mildly to severely impaired and that an immunological workup is warranted when the diagnosis of CHARGE is confirmed.

REFERENCES

Chopra, C., Baretto, R., Duddridge, M., & Browning, M. J. (2009). T-cell immunodeficiency in CHARGE syndrome. *Acta Paediatrica*, *98*(2), 408–410.

Gennery, A. R., Slatter, M. A., Rice, J., Hoefsloot, L. H., Barge, D., McLean-Tooke, A., . . . Johnson, D. (2008). Mutations in CHD7 in patients with CHARGE syndrome cause T − B + natural killer cell + severe combined immune deficiency and may cause Omenn-like syndrome. *Clinical and Experimental Immunology*, *153*(1), 75–80.

Hoover-Fong, J., Savage, W. J., Lisi, E., Winkelstein, J., Thomas, G. H., Hoefsloot, L. H., & Loeb, D. M. (2009). Congenital T cell deficiency in a patient with CHARGE syndrome. *The Journal of Pediatrics, 154*(1), 140–142.

Jyonouchi, S., McDonald-McGinn, D. M., Bale, S., Zackai, E. H., & Sullivan, K. E. (2009). CHARGE (coloboma, heart defect, atresia choanae, retarded growth and development, genital hypoplasia, ear anomalies/deafness) syndrome and chromosome 22q11.2 deletion syndrome: a comparison of immunologic and nonimmunologic phenotypic features. *Pediatrics, 123*(5), e871–877.

Theodoropoulos, D. S., & Theodoropoulos, G. A. (2003). Immune deficiency and hearing loss in CHARGE Association. *Pediatrics, 111*, 711–712.

Writzl, K., Cale, C. M., Pierce, C. M., Wilson, L. C., & Hennekam, R. C. (2007). Immunological abnormalities in CHARGE syndrome. *European Journal of Medical Genetics, 50*(5), 338–345.

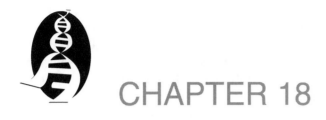

CHAPTER 18

Musculoskeletal System

MARC S. WILLIAMS, M.D.

*T*he musculoskeletal (MS) system consists of more than 200 bones and 500 muscles. Two aspects are critical: structure and function. Normal structure means that all of the components of the system (that is, the muscles and bones) are present and are in the proper relationships to one another. Normal function means that the bones are maintaining the normal structural integrity of the skeleton, and the muscles (through contraction) are able to move the portions of the skeleton that are supposed to move (the joints). All structural abnormalities lead to functional abnormalities (although the severity of the abnormality may not be clinically significant), but not all functional abnormalities lead to structural abnormalities. For example, a person who suffers a spinal cord injury has *structurally* normal muscles and bones, but the muscles are *functionally* abnormal because of the absence of nerve signals.

Two other important concepts are strength and tone. Strength is the ability of a muscle, or group of muscles, to work against a load. It can be measured objectively. Tone, however, is a subjective assessment of muscle function at rest and takes an experienced professional to assess. When we are resting, i.e., not moving a particular muscle or group of muscles, there is a baseline level of activity that can be detected, which we refer to as muscle tone. Muscle tone helps with posture and maintaining normal skeletal relationships. Low tone is also called hypotonia. Individuals with low muscle tone often are described as floppy and may have slumped posture, problems with head control, standing, etc. High tone is called hypertonia, or spasticity, and this can lead to abnormal joint positions and result in toe-walking, hip and knee flexion contractures, etc. Abnormalities in muscle tone can be due to abnormalities of the nervous system (brain, spinal cord, spinal nerves, peripheral nerves, or connections between the nerve and the muscle) or to abnormalities within the muscle itself (myopathy). It may be difficult to distinguish between these two causes on clinical examination.

TYPES OF MUSCULOSKELETAL ABNORMALITIES IN CHARGE SYNDROME

Between 30% and 50% of patients with CHARGE are born with some type of skeletal abnormality (Brock, Mathiason, Rooney, & Williams, 2003; Tellier, et al., 1998). Severity can range from clinically insignificant (minor changes of the creases of the palms due to short hand bones), to quite severe (missing fingers). Severe vertebral anomalies and rib fusions have been reported rarely in some patients categorized as atypical CHARGE. Strömland, et al., (2005) reported that 25% of patients in their series had "spine anomalies," but no structural or functional information was provided. An epidemiologic study from Canada (Issekutz, et al., 2005) noted that 35% of patients identified in their series have neck and shoulder anomalies, including short or webbed neck or sloping shoulders (Figure 18–1). No functional information was provided. In the best characterized series of patients that met diagnostic criteria and had a mutation in *CHD7*, the clinical description was limited to "hypoplastic vertebra" (Jongmans, et al., 2006).

Several patients have been reported to have fusion of fingers or toes (syndactyly) or clefting of the hand or foot. The underlying pathogenesis of the skeletal anomalies is not understood, although some authors have speculated on this (Van de Laar, et al., 2007; Williams, 2005).

Hypotonia

Low muscle tone (hypotonia) is very common in children with CHARGE syndrome, especially in the upper body (trunk). There have not been any patients with CHARGE syndrome known to have hypotonia due to a myopathy (abnormality of the muscles themselves). Unless new information becomes available, it is probably safe to assume that the hypotonia is due to a central nervous system abnormality (i.e., brain). Low muscle tone may have an effect on development: if the upper body is floppy, it will be more difficult to sit alone or stand. Combine weak tone with vision loss and balance problems, and you may have a child who does not walk until age 4 to 6 years. Presence of low muscle tone dramatically impacts the creation and implementation of plans for physical and occupational therapy. There is also some evidence from

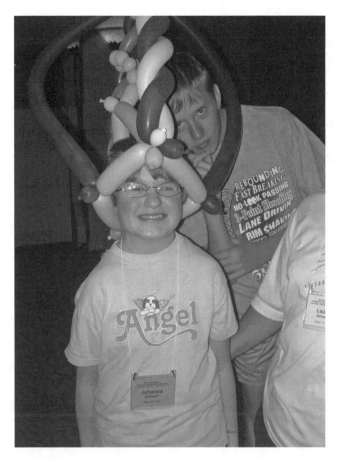

FIGURE 18–1. Short neck and sloping shoulders (also typical face).

work with children affected with cerebral palsy that recognition and adaptive treatment of abnormalities of tone can positively impact speech and feeding. Hulme, Bain, Hardin, McKinnon, and Waldron (1989) reported that adaptive seating for hypotonic children resulted in positive effects in language and feeding. A Cochrane Evidence Review that addressed the role of speech therapy in children with cerebral palsy (Pennington, Goldbart, & Marshall, 2003) while criticizing the lack of high-quality studies in this area did recognize that positive trends in communication change were shown. Therefore, they recommended continuation of current speech therapy practices in this population. Given that speech, occupational, and physical therapies are provided by different therapists and, at least for the first 3 years of life, are typically home-based rather than center-based, communication and coordination between therapists is critical to early recognition of problems and coordination of care plans to optimize developmental progress.

Scoliosis

Scoliosis (lateral curvature of the spine) and kyphosis (forward bending of the spine) are very common in children with CHARGE (Doyle and Blake, 2005). Although scoliosis (kyphosis and scoliosis will be referred to as scoliosis for the rest of the discussion) is generally thought of as a teenage problem, it has been seen in children as young as age three with CHARGE syndrome. By the teenage years, a majority of individuals with CHARGE syndrome (perhaps as high as 60% of patients) have scoliosis of some degree. This may be due, at least in part, to the low muscle tone in the upper body, although there is a single report that alterations in the *CHD7* gene are associated with idiopathic scoliosis (Gao et al., 2007). While preliminary, this suggests that *CHD7* may play a role in growth and orientation of the spine. Structural vertebral anomalies also could contribute, although this has not been well characterized in the literature.

The severity of the scoliosis can vary, but in some cases is severe enough to require therapy, bracing, or surgery. Early identification of the scoliosis is important as it may allow more effective treatment (Kotwicki & Jozwiak, 2008). Untreated, scoliosis can result in compromise of the lungs and heart that can result ultimately in cardio-respiratory failure and death. Progressive scoliosis can result in abnormal positioning that will compromise functional abilities (such as walking and the use of upper extremities) and rarely can result in progressive damage to the spinal cord leading to deterioration of muscular strength and tone as well as bowel and bladder control issues.

Osteoporosis

In a 2002 study, Brown and Josse identified risk factors for poor bone health and osteoporosis in the pediatric population. These included poor nutrition, inactivity, hypogonadism, and growth hormone deficiency—all of which are seen in CHARGE syndrome. The only study addressing this issue in individuals with CHARGE syndrome (Forward, Cummings, & Blake, 2007) confirmed the presence of these risk factors in a survey of 30 individuals. Bone density assessment (using a DEXA scan) had been done in 10 patients. All those tested had negative Z-scores (ranging from −0.9 to −4.7), suggesting low bone mineral density. To accurately interpret a DEXA scan, however, one must control for age, height, weight, gender, pubertal status, and race. Therefore, the authors caution about over-interpretation of these results given that the DEXA scans are difficult to interpret even in healthy adolescents, and these problems are magnified in individuals with CHARGE syndrome. The DEXA scan results in this paper were supplied by the individual or family so there was no opportunity to standardize the interpretations. It was interesting to note that in four individuals with low bone-mineral density that were treated with a variety of modalities including hormone replacement, calcium, Vitamin D, and bisphosphonates, there was at best modest improvement in bone density, a finding also noted in the patient reported by Searle, Graham, Prasad, and Blake (2005). There were no reports of pathologic fractures or chronic bone pain.

Osteoporosis surveillance for women (particularly postmenopausal women) is a well-established part of clinical care, but there are also concerns that males, particular those males at risk due to hormonal abnormalities, may not be detected in a timely fashion (Ebeling, 2004). Although no evidence exists for or against routine bone densitometry for patients with CHARGE syndrome (beyond those for routine preventive care in all patients), it seems reasonable to have an increased index of suspicion in individuals with CHARGE—particularly those with pituitary dysfunction. Densitometry can be considered based on clinical suspicion. Forward, Cummings, and Blake (2007) suggest that there may be a role for serial DEXA scans to document changes in bone density over time. The role of supplementation with calcium and Vitamin D is unknown, although in patients with documented inadequate intake, supplementation is indicated. Hormone replacement is indicated to correct deficiency and may have the added benefit of improving bone density. No studies address the use of bisphosphonates in individuals with CHARGE syndrome who have low bone mineral density. This is clearly an area that would benefit from prospective research.

EVALUATION FOR MUSCULOSKELETAL ABNORMALITIES

Table 18-1 lists diagnostic tests for the evaluation of the musculoskeletal system. The most important diagnostic test in very young children is a careful physical examination of the musculoskeletal system. Imaging studies (such as X-ray, ultrasound) are indicated if there is suspicion of an abnormality on

TABLE 18–1. Diagnostic Tests for Evaluation of Musculoskeletal Abnormalities

Test	Indication
Skeletal Survey	Never routinely indicated
Targeted X-ray, US, MRI	As indicated by specific finding on examination
Electromyography	Suspect primary muscle problem (rare in CHARGE)
Muscle Biopsy	Suspect primary muscle problem (rare in CHARGE)
MRI Spinal Cord	Suspect spinal cord injury or abnormality (changes in tone, reflexes, progressive weakness, changes in bowel/bladder function, asymmetry of neurologic examination

physical examination. A skeletal survey (to look at all the bones of the skeleton) is not indicated routinely nor are tests of muscle (muscle biopsy, electromyography [EMG]) generally indicated, unless a primary muscle problem is also suspected.

Regular physical exam for scoliosis is indicated. These examinations should begin as early as possible (no later than age 3 years) and should be repeated yearly—more frequently if the examination suggests scoliosis may be developing. If scoliosis is suspected, X-rays may be indicated to determine the extent of the scoliosis as well as to guide intervention. Routine bone densitometry is not indicated but could be considered in patients with hypogonadism particularly if there is a history of fractures.

Management of Musculoskeletal Abnormalities

Medical and/or surgical management is based on the type of anomaly. They are not managed differently whether or not the child has CHARGE syndrome. Outcome following intervention is generally good, but clearly depends on the severity of the problem and the treatment that is required. As noted previously, occupational and physical therapies are helpful in dealing with low muscle tone, although decreased stamina, which can be seen with hypotonia, may limit the individual's ability to tolerate the therapy. Communication and coordination between therapists, medical providers, and patients is essential.

SUMMARY

Prevalence of musculoskeletal anomalies is between 30% and 50%. This may increase as more cases of scoliosis are noted in older individuals.

Severity of anomalies has ranged from very minor (e.g., dermatoglyphic anomalies) to moderately severe (e.g., congenital hip dysplasia, syndactyly, polydactyly, club foot).

No consistent pattern of anomalies has been seen, although syndactyly of fingers or toes seems to be more frequent. Some of these patients have an atypical split-hand deformity. These hand anomalies could create challenges for fine motor activities that could benefit from adaptive devices and therapy. A specific palmar crease pattern often occurs with a so-called "hockey stick" distal palmar crease, which is considered by some a minor diagnostic criterion (Figure 18–2).

Hypotonia, particularly of the upper body, is frequent (Figure 18–3). This is likely to be a neurologically based problem. There have been no reported cases of a primary myopathy in individuals with CHARGE. Muscle biopsy would not be indicated, unless a second diagnosis is suspected.

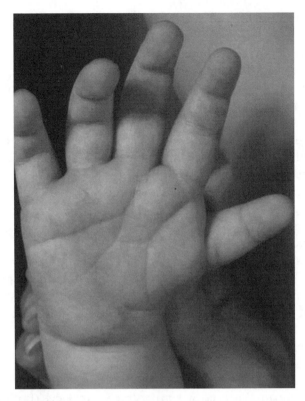

FIGURE 18–2. The "hockey stick" palmer crease.

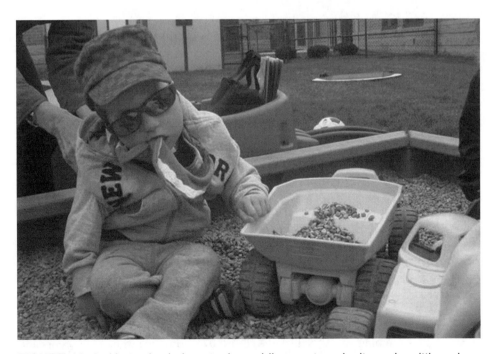

FIGURE 18–3. Upper body hypotonia and ligamentous laxity make sitting alone difficult.

Scoliosis is frequent (perhaps a high as 60% of patients), with a mean age of diagnosis between 8 and 9 years of age (range 3-19 years).

Osteoporosis may occur in adults with untreated hypogonadism and growth hormone deficiency. No data suggests patients with CHARGE syndrome are unusually susceptible to fractures.

Careful physical examination of the musculoskeletal system is the only "test" indicated in all patients. It is important to screen for scoliosis beginning as early as is feasible (no later than age 3).

Other diagnostic tests (X-ray, ultrasound, MRI) may be indicated based on physical findings.

X-rays obtained for other reasons (i.e., chest X-rays) should be examined carefully for skeletal abnormalities.

Routine assessment of bone mineral density is not recommended, however, it may be considered in individuals with documented hypogonadism or growth hormone deficiency, particularly if there is clinical suspicion.

Treatment is anomaly specific. No differences in therapy are necessary if the patient is diagnosed with CHARGE syndrome. If surgery or sedation is necessary, caveats include:

■ Anesthetic risk is increased in children with airway involvement such as choanal atresia or laryngotracheomalacia (both common in CHARGE). Children with choanal atresia and complex heart defects have the highest rate of serious complications and/or poor outcome.

■ Swallowing problems with increased secretions (presumably due to involvement of cranial nerves IX and X) may present an additional risk of aspiration.

REFERENCES

Brock, K. E., Mathiason, M. A., Rooney B. L., & Williams M. S. (2003). Quantitative analysis of limb anomalies in CHARGE syndrome: correlation with diagnosis and characteristic CHARGE anomalies. *American Journal of Medical Genetics, 123A*, 111-121.

Brown, J. P., & Josse, R. G. (2002) Clinical practice guidelines for the diagnosis and management of osteoporosis in Canada. *Canadian Medical Association Journal, 167*(10), S1-34.

Doyle, C., & Blake, K. D. (2005). Scoliosis in CHARGE: A prospective survey and two case reports. *American Journal of Medical Genetics, 133A*, 340-343.

Ebeling, P. R. (2004). Idiopathic or hypogonadal osteoporosis in men: Current and future treatment options. *Treatments in endocrinology, 3*, 381-391.

Forward, K., Cummings, E. A., & Blake, K. D. (2007). Bone health in adolescents and adults with CHARGE syndrome. *American Journal of Medical Genetics, 143A*, 839-845.

Gao, X., Gordon, D., Zhang, D., Browne, R., Helms, C., Gillum, J., . . . Wise, C. (2007). CHD7 gene polymorphisms are associated with susceptibility to idiopathic scoliosis. *American Journal of Human Genetics, 80*, 957–965.

Hulme, J. B., Bain, B., Hardin, M., McKinnon, A., & Waldron, D. (1989). The influence of adaptive seating devices on vocalization. *Journal of Communication Disorders, 22*, 137–145.

Issekutz, K. A., Graham, J. M., Prasad, C., Smith, I. M., & Blake, K. D. (2005). An epidemiological analysis of CHARGE syndrome: Preliminary results from a Canadian study. *American Journal of Medical Genetics, 133A*, 309–317.

Jongmans, M. C., Admiraal, R. J., van der Donk, K. P., Vissers, L. E., Baas, A. F., Kapusta, L., . . . van Ravenswaaij, C. M. (2006). CHARGE syndrome: the phenotypic spectrum of mutations in the CHD7 gene. *Journal of Medical Genetics, 43*, 306–314.

Kotwicki, T., & Jozwiak, M. (2008). Conservative management of neuromuscular scoliosis: Personal experience and review of the literature. *Disability and Rehabilitation, 30*, 792–798.

Pennington, L., Goldbart, J., & Marshall, J. (2003). Speech and language therapy to improve the communication skills of children with cerebral palsy. *Cochrane Database of Systematic Reviews*, Issue 3. Art. No.: CD003466.

Searle, L. C., Graham, J. M., Prasad, C., & Blake, K. D. (2005). CHARGE Syndrome from birth to adulthood: An individual reported on from 0 to 33 years. *American Journal of Medical Genetics, 133A*, 344–349.

Strömland, K., Sjögreen, L., Johansson, M., Joelsson, B. M. E., Miller, M., Danielsson, S., . . . Granström, G. (2005). CHARGE association in Sweden: Malformations and functional deficits. *American Journal of Medical Genetics, 133A*, 331–339.

Tellier, A. L., Cormier-Daire, V., Abadie, V., Amiel, J., Sigaudy, S., Bonnet, D., . . . Lyonnet, S. (1998). CHARGE Syndrome: Report of 47 cases and review. *American Journal of Medical Genetics, 76*, 402–409.

Van de Laar, I., Dooijes, D., Hoefsloot, L., Simon, M., Hoogeboom, J., & Devriendt, K. (2007). Limb anomalies in patients with CHARGE syndrome: An expansion of the phenotype. *American Journal of Medical Genetics, 143A*, 2712–2715.

Williams, M. S. (2005). Speculations on the pathogenesis of CHARGE syndrome. *American Journal of Medical Genetics, 133A*, 318–325.

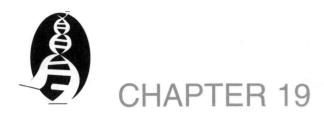

CHAPTER 19

Teenage and Adult Medical Issues

KIM D. BLAKE, M.D., AND NANCY SALEM-HARTSHORNE, PH.D.

*T*he adolescent or adult with CHARGE syndrome has to deal with many lingering medical problems (Blake & Prasad, 2006; Blake, Salem-Hartshorne, Daoud, & Gradstein, 2005). Table 19–1 gives an overview of some of these problems.

TABLE 19–1. Medical Problems To Be Considered in the Older Individual with CHARGE Syndrome

---

Gastroenterological reflux (gagging, coughing, hiccupping, refuses to eat)

Constipation (liquid stool may be overflow)

Celiac disease (Tissue Transglutaminase [tTG] screening is suggested)

Hypothyroidism (tiredness, lethargy, cold intolerance)

Heart disease (sweating, pallor, tiredness)

Deteriorating sensory issues (hearing and vision e.g., retinal detachment)

Delayed puberty and low bone mineral density

Antipsychotic medication (too high, wrong medication, too many medications)

The older individual with CHARGE syndrome may present with changes in behavior, a lag in school progress, or regression of skills that have been learned previously. It is important when there is any presenting complaint that the physician rule out a physical medical diagnosis. It is well known that the individual with CHARGE often has atypical reactions to pain and degrees of challenges in communication, which can add to the diagnostic dilemma. We suggest working through a head-to-toe approach both with a history and physical examination. We always find it helpful to revisit the past medical history. For example, Matthew is a 15-year-old who had been eating relatively normally to date but previously, as an infant and child, had been on tube feedings and regularly given large amounts of anti gastroesophageal reflux medication. Matthew is no longer on reflux medication, but two months ago he had a prolonged episode of gastroenteritis with vomiting. He presented with behavioral outbursts, coughing, hiccupping, and sleepless nights. Teachers were reporting significant poor behaviors at school and were asking whether he should be medicated with drugs to calm him down. After further investigation, it was found that Matthew was suffering from severe gastroesophageal reflux about which he was not able to communicate. He also had a breakdown of a previous fundoplication and a hiatus hernia. Matthew's situation of presenting with behavioral problems but having a physical diagnosis is not uncommon.

Individuals within the CHARGE population have vast past medical histories that need careful documentation. Tables 1 and 2 in the Introduction could be used as a template to check through common medical issues. Personal growing-up stories from older individuals explaining how medical concerns present are important, as they help the caregiver and youth with CHARGE traverse some of this uncharted territory. Searle, Graham, Prasad, and Blake (2005) give a comprehensive account of a young man and his medical issues up to 33 years of age.

Deterioration in vision and hearing need to be high on the list of concerns and probably will require specialist examination. However, a family doctor finding a foreign body lodged in the ear canal is not at all uncommon. Some cardiovascular concerns encountered in childhood can return as the adolescent or adult ages. Abnormalities in heart rhythm and structure should be ruled out in the individual who is having episodes of sweatiness, pallor, chest pain, or frequently, only fatigue.

Some conditions that originally were thought to be rare or occasional in CHARGE syndrome now have been found to be more prevalent. The adolescent or adult with CHARGE may not have been screened early on for certain conditions such as renal anomalies, problems with the immune system (Jyonouchi, McDonald-McGinn, Bale, Zackai & Sullivan, 2009), or spinal anomalies. Concerns about scoliosis may present as the older individual with CHARGE syndrome grows. Therefore, any obvious curvature of the back needs to be followed by an orthopedic surgeon (Doyle & Blake, 2005). Table 19–1 lists the more common medical problems that should be considered, along with those in Tables 1 and 2 of the Introduction, especially in the nonverbal child with a limited ability to express pain and discomfort.

Monitoring growth and wellness should start with prevention. Although a majority of doctors know little about CHARGE syndrome, they are still able to address areas of prevention, such as the following:

◾ Are all immunizations up to date? Have any been missed?

◾ Obesity is prominent in our society and this does not exclude the older CHARGE population (Figure 19–1). Recommendations include monitoring height, weight, and BMI and building a healthy lifestyle at school, during transition to adulthood, and in independent life as an adult.

◾ Finding physical activities in which the individual will be able to engage can prove challenging, given balance and sensory impairments (Figure 19–2). However, this is important not only for overall

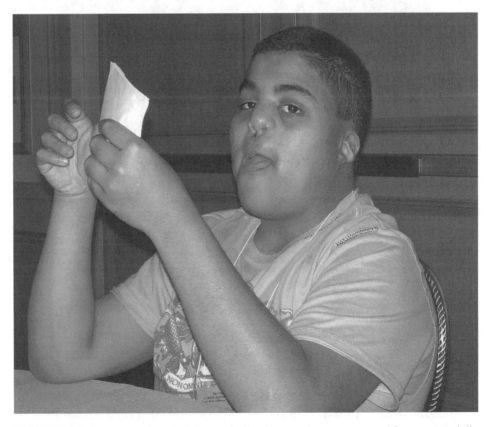

FIGURE 19–1. Increasing weight and obesity can become a problem, especially in the teen years and later.

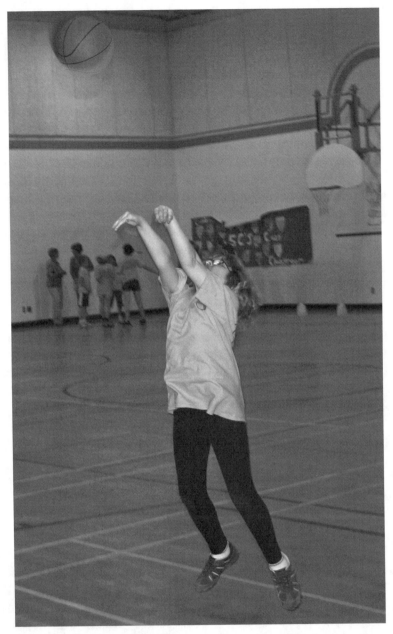

FIGURE 19–2. Regular organized physical activity is important.

health, but for bone mineral density, a frequent concern for individuals with CHARGE syndrome. Physical, occupational and recreational therapists can guide parents and educators in choosing the appropriate activities. (Forward, Cummings, & Blake, 2007).

■ Fatigue often can be due to simple non CHARGE conditions such as infectious mononucleosis or an underactive thyroid.

■ Lastly, do not forget depression and anxiety. All adolescents, with and without CHARGE, can be prone to depression and general melancholy.

REFERENCES

Blake, K. D., & Prasad, C. (2006). CHARGE syndrome. *Orphanet Journal of Rare Diseases, 1*, 34.

Blake, K. D., Salem-Hartshorne, N., Daoud, M. A., & Gradstein, J. (2005). Adolescent and adult issues in CHARGE syndrome. *Clinical Pediatrics, 44*, 151–159.

Doyle C., & Blake, K. D. (2005). Scoliosis in CHARGE: A prospective survey and two case reports. *American Journal of Medical Genetics, 133A*, 340–343.

Forward, K., Cummings, E. A., & Blake, K. D. (2007). Bone health in adolescents and adults with CHARGE syndrome. *American Journal of Medical Genetics, 143A*, 839–845.

Jyonouchi, S., McDonald-McGinn, D., Bale, S., Zackai, E. & Sullivan, K. (2009). CHARGE (Coloboma, Heart Defect, Atresia Choanae, Retarded Growth and Development, Genital Hypoplasia, Ear Anomalies/Deafness) Syndrome and Chromosome 22q11.2 Deletion Syndrome: A Comparison of Immunologic and Nonimmunologic Phenotypic Features. *Pediatrics, 123*, e871–e877.

Searle, L. C., Graham, J. M., Prasad, C., & Blake, K. D. (2005). CHARGE Syndrome from birth to adulthood: An individual reported on from 0 to 33 years. *American Journal of Medical Genetics, 133A*, 344–349.

PART III

Developmental Issues in CHARGE

*D*ue to the relatively recent identification of CHARGE syndrome, we often refer to "children with CHARGE." Of course, adolescents and adults also have CHARGE, but we simply do not know as much about them. Our knowledge is increasing rapidly as the cohort of young children we first began to follow in 1993 is entering adulthood. This section addresses several of the developmental challenges faced by individuals with CHARGE as they age. In particular, Chapter 24 (from the perspective of multiple authors as well as from stories directly from several young adults with CHARGE), reviews development from infancy through young adulthood.

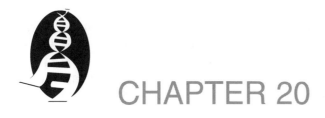

CHAPTER 20

Cognitive

NANCY SALEM-HARTSHORNE, PH.D.

*C*ognitive abilities, IQ, intelligence: these interchangeable terms, although relatively easy to assess in the general population, are particularly difficult to determine for the CHARGE syndrome population. Many factors contribute to this difficulty, especially the combination of sensory deficits and early severe medical complications.

RANGE OF COGNITIVE ABILITIES IN INDIVIDUALS WITH CHARGE

The population of individuals with CHARGE syndrome has been described in terms of intellectual outcome. About 50% of the population has been observed to have good intellectual outcomes, with 25% having expected moderate developmental outcomes and 25% having very poor outcomes (Blake, Russell-Eggitt, Morgan, Ratcliffe, & Wyse, 1990; Davenport, 1993). Formal measurement of intellectual outcomes has resulted in similar findings. Salem-Hartshorne and Jacob (2004, 2005) found that about half of a sample of 100 children with CHARGE had developmental abilities falling within the low average to average range, as assessed using an adaptive behavior scale administered to their parents. The other half of the sample had scores falling in the impaired range and spreading about equally across all possible scores. Longitudinally, these findings were found to be stable over time. Raqbi et al. (2003) found a similar ratio of 50% average, 25% low average, and 25% impaired in their assessments of 21 children with CHARGE syndrome.

Interestingly, although children with CHARGE syndrome most often are born with multiple complex medical conditions necessitating intense or long-term treatment, the severity of medical conditions does not seem to be a predictor of intellectual outcomes (Figure 20–1). However, vestibular difficulties *do* seem to be an important factor.

POSSIBLE PROGNOSTIC FACTORS

Salem-Hartshorne and Jacob (2005) found that children who walked earlier had better intellectual outcomes. In addition, early toilet training seemed to be correlated with better outcomes. Significant positive relationships also were found between the adaptive behavior measure (used in place of formal

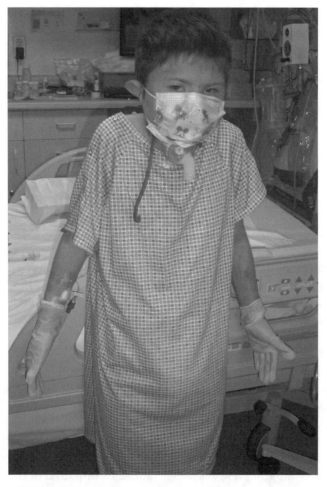

FIGURE 20–1. Children with CHARGE often have multiple illnesses and hospitalizations even beyond infancy.

intellectual assessment) and the following: (1) level of reading decoding and comprehension and (2) the number of friendships the individual enjoys.

Raqbi et al. (2003) lists three prognostic factors related to the intellectual outcomes. The first is extensive bilateral coloboma resulting in low vision. They explain that although vestibular difficulties can predict poorer intellectual outcome, having good vision can be a compensatory factor for vestibular impairment. Nearly all individuals with CHARGE have some (typically significant) impairment of the vestibular system, while the degree of vision loss is more variable. Raqbi, et al. (2003) purport that those individuals with CHARGE syndrome having both an impaired vestibular system and severe bilateral colobomas will have poorer intellectual outcomes than those with an impaired vestibular system and better vision.

The second and third prognostic factors suggested by Raqbi, et al. (2003) to predict poorer intellectual outcomes are microcephaly and brain malformations. They further suggest that although the half of their sample who seemed to do well intellectually still had motor delays, these could be attributed to sensory problems rather than central nervous system dysfunction. The one consensus among all of the researchers seems to be that intellectual ability in individuals with CHARGE syndrome is underestimated.

CHALLENGES IN ASSESSMENT

Several factors may account for the difficulty in accurately determining the abilities of these individuals. First, individuals with CHARGE have sensory impairments, either visual or auditory, and most of the time, both. Although accurate cognitive assessment of children with hearing impairment or visual impairments has been standardized, cognitive assessment of individuals with dual sensory impairment is more elusive. Some assessment instruments can be useful, but they must be used cautiously, especially when attempting to report an actual score. The validity of these methods with this population has not been well established, and therefore, scores from these instruments should not be used for decision-making purposes (i.e., eligibility for programs) unless the examiner has confidence that the individual understood the process of assessment, and the examiner understood the individual's responses to an adequate degree.

Second, the overwhelming majority of individuals with CHARGE syndrome have some sort of difficulty with their vestibular sense (see Chapters 4, 5, and 6). Therefore, it is imperative that an individual's vestibular functioning be taken into account when administering any kind of assessment. For example, some individuals with CHARGE feel the need to rock or move when asked to stand in one place. This movement may be giving input into their joints, telling their brain where they are in space, and allowing them to remain stable. Some individuals with CHARGE have difficulty with stability of their heads, and thus, their usable vision. These individuals may prefer to lie on their sides or lay their heads down in order to read, write, or examine and manipulate objects adequately. Because of these stability issues, formal assessment of intellectual ability must be conducted taking these factors into account.

Third, individuals with CHARGE syndrome often have strong sensory integration needs. Many have low muscle tone and/or spinal anomalies, both of which can cause fatigue. During assessment sessions, preferred sensory items should be made available with frequent breaks. If these needs are not recognized, a score from a formalized assessment is likely to underestimate the individual's intellectual abilities.

Fourth, children with CHARGE syndrome frequently are born with multiple physical and medical needs that are quite intense, most often including heart defects, breathing, and eating difficulties. The first months, and even years, of life often are spent merely trying to survive. Until homeostasis is achieved in the infant/toddler, learning about the outside world is unlikely to take place. For others, the amount of time spent in hospitals and recovering from major surgeries can make them unavailable for learning. In the same sense that examiners and early interventionists frequently correct for prematurity when scoring assessments, the fact that a child with CHARGE was not *available* for learning for some months or years should be taken into account when evaluating a child's overall intellectual development.

Fifth, individuals with CHARGE syndrome are unique in their instructional needs. Most early intervention and school programs are not prepared to meet the needs adequately without support and consultation. The fact that consultation is available (in the United States) through state DeafBlind projects often is not widely recognized (see Sidebar 24–2 in Chapter 24). Because of this, some individuals with CHARGE merely may have lost out on appropriate learning opportunities, resulting in a lag in their achievement and perceived intellectual abilities.

Finally, family and caregiver input is an essential ingredient in assessment. Often, children with CHARGE will display ability in one setting that they do not in another. Therefore, it is imperative that family members and caregivers be an integral part of conducting an assessment on a child with CHARGE syndrome in order to ensure that valuable and useful information is not missed.

CONCLUSIONS

No *typical* individual with CHARGE syndrome exists. The range of abilities found in this population is large and varied. For example, the author has met individuals with CHARGE who need 24-hour care and supervision and others who are working on graduate degrees. The range of abilities also is changing. The studies done by Salem-Hartshorne and Jacob followed a sample of children who were born in the 1980s and early 1990s. Because medical care for these individuals, as well as general knowledge about both their medical and educational needs, has improved and increased significantly over the past 20 years, it is likely that those born after the early 1990s will enjoy better outcomes.

It is increasingly clear that the complexity of these individuals makes individualized, standardized assessment of intellectual ability a challenging endeavor. Therefore, the author suggests that formal intellectual assessment is not the assessment of choice for individuals with CHARGE syndrome. In essence, it becomes merely a score—a score that follows the individual, accurate or not, throughout his or her lifetime. It is absolutely more important to determine each individual's strengths and needs, through both formal and informal assessment, consultation, interview, and observation. In doing this, practitioners will be able to create a school, work, and/or home environment that not only builds on the unique needs and strengths of the person, but also responds specifically to the individual's preferences, sensory needs, and communication gaps, thus promoting social integration into the natural community.

RECOMMENDATIONS

An IQ score simply cannot provide sufficient information to create a supportive learning environment. Several assessment techniques *can* provide such useful information. Choosing Options and Accommodations for Children (COACH) (Giangreco, Cloniger, & Iverson, 1998) is a tool used by assessment teams to assist families in choosing priorities for learning for their child, leading to meaningful goals and objectives in the Individualized Education Plan (IEP). Hometalk (Harris, et al., no date) provides families with the means to present the school with a comprehensive report about their child from the family perspective. The Supports Intensity Scale (Thompson, et al., 2004) assesses the intensity and frequency of support needs of the individual in various domains. Adaptive behavior scales can assist with planning for real-life learning needs that, when met, will lead to more independence. Person-Centered Planning techniques (MAPS, Personal Futures Planning) use a holistic, person-and family-centered approach to brainstorming, which results in a more complete picture of the individual's characteristics, relationships, dreams, needs, and desired outcomes. These instruments used individually or in combination will provide a much richer representation of the individual with CHARGE syndrome

REFERENCES

Blake, K. D., Russell-Eggitt, J. M., Morgan, D. W., Ratcliffe, J. M., & Wyse, R. K. H. (1990). Who's in CHARGE? Multidisciplinary management of patients with CHARGE Association. *Archives of Disorders in Childhood, 65,* 217–223.

Davenport, S. L. H. (1993, July). *R = Retardation of growth and/or development.* Paper presented at the First International CHARGE Syndrome Conference for Families, St. Louis, MO.

Giangreco, M. F., Cloniger, C. J., & Iverson, V. S. (1998). *Choosing Outcomes and Accommodations for Children: A guide to Educational Planning for Students with Disabilities* (2nd ed.). Baltimore, MD: Paul H. Brookes.

Harris, J., Hartshorne, N., Jess, T., Mar, H., Rowland, C., Sall, N., . . . Wolf, T. (No Date). *HomeTalk: A family assessment of children who are deafblind.* Portland: Oregon Institute on Disability and Development.

Raqbi, F., Le Bihan, C. L., Morisseau-Durand, M. P., Dureau, P., Lyonnet, S., & Abadie, V. (2003). Early prognostic factors for early intellectual outcome in CHARGE syndrome. *Developmental Medicine and Child Neurology, 45*, 483–488.

Salem-Hartshorne, N., & Jacob, S. (2004). Characteristics and development of children with CHARGE association/syndrome. *Journal of Early Intervention, 26*, 292–301.

Salem-Hartshorne, N., & Jacob, S. (2005). Adaptive behavior in children with CHARGE syndrome. *American Journal of Medical Genetics, 133A*, 262–267.

Thompson, J. R., Bryant, B. R., Campbell, E. M., Craig, E. M., Hughes, C. M., Rotholz, D. A., . . . Wehmeyer, M. L. (2004). *Supports Intensity Scale.* Washington, DC: American Association on Mental Retardation.

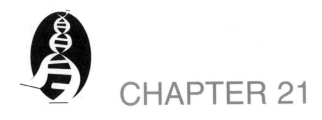

CHAPTER 21

Social/Emotional

TIMOTHY S. HARTSHORNE, PH.D. AND NANCY SALEM-HARTSHORNE, PH.D.

*S*ocial-emotional development is a term used to describe growing children's ability to form close, secure relationships and to use their emotions productively in interactions with others. This requires the development of social skills such as initiating, sharing, responding, supporting, and engaging. It further requires the ability to regulate one's emotions so that they do not overwhelm interactions with others in ways that can hurt or destroy relationships. Social-emotional development begins in infancy with attachment to the parent or primary caregiver and then extends to the development of social skills as the child's world moves out to social groups. Emotion regulation is learned through the reactions of others, modeling, and parental discipline. In this section, we review attachment, social skills, and emotion regulation in CHARGE.

ATTACHMENT

Shortly after birth, or sometimes even before, parents develop a sense of being bonded with their child. This initial bonding is followed somewhat later by signs that the child feels attached to the parents. Attachment is a relational construct, meaning it involves a reciprocal interaction between parent and child. This suggests that anything interfering with the interaction has the potential to create difficulties. Some literature suggests that caregiver sensitivity, responsiveness, emotional availability, acceptance toward child, and predictability are all associated with the quality of the attachment relationship (Mullen, 1998). Establishing these conditions can be problematic with a child who does not have disabilities; CHARGE complicates matters exponentially (Figure 21-1).

Reda and Hartshorne (2008) obtained information from the parents of 25 children between the ages of 12 and 54 months with CHARGE regarding attachment and bonding. About half of the children, based on parent report, experienced some problems with normal attachment. The longer it took for the child to give evidence of attachment was related to how long it took the parent to feel bonded. The experience of having your child smile at you can influence how bonded you feel with your child. Due to multiple surgeries, frequent hospitalizations, facial palsy, coloboma, and deafness, it may take a child with CHARGE longer to smile at a parent or for the parent to detect the smile in the child. Simple experiences such as being able to hold the baby and bringing the baby home relatively soon after birth were related to more

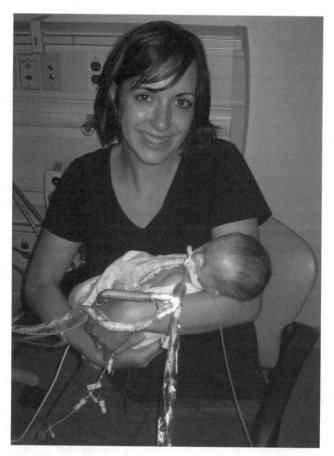

FIGURE 21–1. Even being able to hold your child after birth may be difficult for some infants with CHARGE.

secure attachment. About half the parents showed significant stress on the *Parenting Stress Index Short Form* (Abidin, 1995). The degree of stress was related to problems with bonding. Again, attachment is a reciprocal, relational construct. It is important for infant mental health workers and other professionals to be sensitive to the attachment problems inherent in raising a child with CHARGE, and that all professionals working with families encourage the development of that attachment (Figure 21–2).

SOCIAL SKILLS

Social relationships seem to be difficult for many children with CHARGE syndrome. Their odd looks due to facial palsy, floppy ears, mismatched eyes, etc., may be off-putting for some peers. Some children with CHARGE utter strange sounds and engage in odd movements that may be tics or self-stimulation.

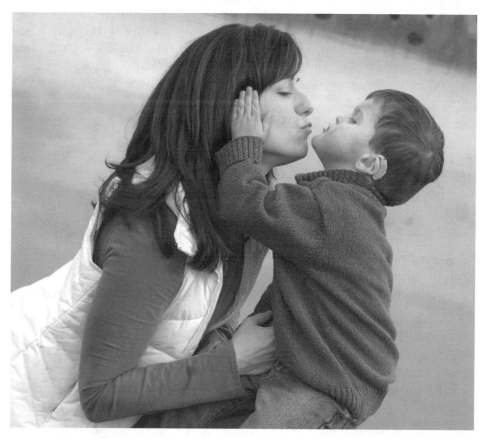

FIGURE 21–2. Professionals working with the family should do what they can to facilitate bonding and attachment.

The unusual behaviors or appearance can hinder other's ability to interact in typical ways with individuals with CHARGE. Individuals with CHARGE may have sensory impairments, and in some cases, intellectual disability that impede their ability to understand the social situations in which they interact. Within the small "communication bubble" (see Chapter 1), the individual with CHARGE is missing visual and auditory clues that typical children have for learning appropriate social interaction. Misunderstanding, or not recognizing, social cues may cause these children to appear self-absorbed and disinterested in their peers.

Hartshorne, Grialou, and Parker (2005) used the *Autism Behavior Checklist* (Krug, Arick, & Almond, 1993) to compare children with CHARGE to the instrument's norms for children with autism and deafblindness. On four of the five subtests, CHARGE scores fell between those for deafblindness and autism, meaning that they showed more indicators of autism than those who were deafblind, but fewer than those with autism. However, on the "relating" subtest, average scores for those with CHARGE were considerably different from the other two groups. The children with CHARGE were much less likely to avoid eye contact, avoid touch, or look through someone, than either the autism or deafblind groups. In fact, in our experience, children with CHARGE are very often socially interested, but not always socially appropriate. They are quite likely to walk up to you and grab at you. They may ask you the same question over and over. They may have difficulty modulating the volume of their voice. And most troubling, they suddenly may become aggressive and hit, scratch, or pull hair.

It is apparent that many children with CHARGE struggle to behave in a manner that promotes social relationships; however, we know of many situations in which they have been accepted by some peer groups. One high school girl, for example, very enthusiastically participated in cheerleading with the support of some of her cheerleading friends. Peer acceptance of a child with CHARGE is not guaranteed, and in most cases, must be fostered by school and family (Figure 21–3). One method of creating peer acceptance among peers is to establish a Circle of Friends (Forest, Pearpoint, & O'Brien (1996). A Circle of Friends is an inclusion tool to help build support for the child in the school, community, and workplace (Hartshorne, 2003) and has been found to positively impact the child's social acceptance (Frederickson & Turner, 2003).

EMOTION REGULATION

Emotion regulation can be defined as what a person does to manage his or her emotional states. One can do some things prior to experiencing intense emotions, such as avoiding certain situations or changing the internal cognitive messages they are giving themselves. One also can do some things dur-

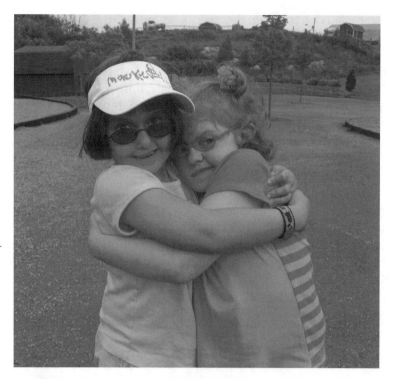

FIGURE 21–3. Friends often are easier to make in elementary school than later.

ing an intense emotional state to try to remain calm or to keep from losing control, such as trying to change the environment, modifying social interactions, engaging in various distractions, or by changing thinking (Endrerud & Vikan, 2007). Campos, Frankel, and Camras (2004) note that emotions and their regulation "reflect the attempt by the person to adapt to the problems he or she encounters in the world" (p. 379). We have observed that many children with CHARGE syndrome have difficulty controlling their emotions. Some of the most challenging behavior happens when they lose control and experience "melt downs," often harming themselves or others in the process. What is confusing to parents and teachers is that they cannot always understand what perceived problem led to the behavior. It can appear to come out of the blue.

Emotional control is thought to involve executive functions (Spinrad, Eisenberg, & Gaertner, 2007). Executive functions are the abilities needed to monitor, control, and regulate thought and action. This includes processes that serve to coordinate the execution of cognitive abilities such as attention and memory, planning, and decision-making (Hartshorne, Nicholas, Grialou, & Russ, 2007). Thus far, no studies of emotion regulation in CHARGE exist; however, Hartshorne, et al. (2007) looked at the presence of executive dysfunction in 98 children with CHARGE syndrome. Using the *Behavior Rating*

Inventory of Executive Function (Gioia, Isquith, Guy, & Kenworthy, 2000) about half had difficulty with tasks such as making transitions and flexible problem solving, monitoring their behavior and its effect on others, and refraining from acting on impulse. Only about a third, however, had significant difficulty on the subtest of "emotional control," which was the most direct measure of emotion regulation. However, half had clinically significant scores on the Behavioral Regulation Index, a composite score measuring the ability to inhibit behaviors, shift cognitive set, and emotional control.

Research on emotion regulation in CHARGE is needed. However, we can draw some inferences and recommendations from the preceding research findings. Because it is apparent that individuals with CHARGE are not always able to make the necessary adaptations themselves, it is up to professionals and family members to assist them with these tasks. People working with these individuals should watch for signs of impending emotional dysregulation, and take action before it occurs by changing the environment, modifying social interactions, engaging in various distractions, helping the individuals to change the way they are thinking, and making transitions smooth and predictable.

REFERENCES

Abidin, R. R. (1995). *Parenting stress index* (3rd ed.). Lutz, FL: PAR.

Campos, J. J., Frankel, C. B., & Camras, L. (2004). On the nature of emotion regulation. *Child Development*, 75, 377–394.

Endrerud, M. S., & Vikan, A. (2007). Five to seven year old children's strategies for regulating anger, sadness, and fear. *Nordic Psychology*, 59, 127–134.

Forest, M., Pearpoint, J., & O'Brien, J. (1996). MAPs, Circles of Friends, and PATH: Powerful tools to help build caring communities. In S. Stainback and W. Stainback (Eds.), *Inclusion: A guide for educators* (pp 67–86). Baltimore, MD: Paul H. Brookes.

Frederickson, N., & Turner, J. (2003). Utilizing the classroom peer group to address children's social needs: An evaluation of the Circle of Friends intervention approach. *Journal of Special Education*, 36, 234–245.

Gioia, G. A., Isquith P. K., Guy, S. C., & Kenworthy, L. (2000). *Behavior Rating of Executive Function*. Lutz, FL: Psychological Assessment Resources.

Hartshorne, T. S. (2003). Positive behavioral supports and social relationships. *Deafblind International Review*. July–December, Number 32, 4–6.

Hartshorne, T. S., Grialou, T. L., & Parker, K. R. (2005). Autistic-Like Behavior in CHARGE Syndrome. *American Journal of Medical Genetics*, 133A, 257–261.

Hartshorne, T. S., Nicholas, J., Grialou, T. L., & Russ, J. M. (2007). Executive function in CHARGE syndrome. *Child Neuropsychology*, 13, 333–344.

Krug, D. A., Arick, J. R., & Almond, P. J. (1993). *Autism Screening Instrument for Educational Planning* (2nd ed.). Austin, TX: Pro-Ed.

Mullen, S. W. (1998). The impact of child disability on marriage, parenting, and attachment: Relationships in families with a child with cerebral palsy. (Doctoral dissertation, University of Virginia, 1998). *Dissertation Abstracts International Section B*, 58, 3969.

Reda, N. M., & Hartshorne, T. S. (2008). Attachment, bonding, and parental stress in CHARGE syndrome. *Mental Health Aspects of Developmental Disabilities, 11,* 10-21.

Spinrad, T. L., Eisenberg, N., & Gaertner, B. M. (2007). Measures of effortful regulation for young children. *Infant Mental Health Journal, 28,* 606-626.

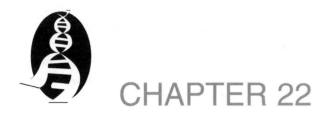

CHAPTER 22

Toileting

LAURIE DENNO, M.A.

*T*oilet training is a rite of passage for many children, families, and educational staff. It is a milestone in development and independence. Although toilet training may be somewhat delayed in children with CHARGE syndrome due to physical, sensory, and communication issues, it remains an important step for all youngsters.

BACKGROUND

Bowel and bladder control is influenced by physiological factors that include a complex set of muscles that must be developed sufficiently to ensure holding and releasing urine and stool. In addition, toilet training is influenced by culture and social customs. Toilet training in the United States usually is initiated at 24–30 months. The two main approaches to toilet training are the "wait until the child is ready" approach advocated by Brazelton (1962) and the "rapid training" approach advocated by Azrin and Foxx (1974).

Both approaches work with typically developing children. The Azrin and Foxx approach may result in faster training with fewer accidents. Although it has not been studied in children with CHARGE, this approach has been used extensively with developmentally delayed individuals. However, the Azrin and Foxx approach may be more successful for children with CHARGE syndrome because it is more structured. A multidisciplinary team approach to toilet training also is advised. To learn more about research in toilet training, read Berk and Friman (1990) or Klassen, et al. (2006).

Toilet training should be about success, learning, and increasing independence. It never should be forced or coercive, involve threats, punishment, or reprimands. These things lead to resistance, crying, tantrums, and other problem behaviors that are best avoided.

Although toileting is a central concern for many parents of children with CHARGE, little research exists on this. Blake, Salem-Hartshorne, Daoud, and Gradstein (2005) reported on 30 individuals with CHARGE ages 13 to 30 years of age. Based on interview questions, 10 of these individuals had no independent toileting skills, 4 had some, 2 were mostly independent, and 14 were completely independent.

Salem-Hartshorne, Blake, and Hartshorne (see Chapter 24), included questions on toileting in their study of 44 children with CHARGE, ages 9–21. For urine, 73% were independent, but 5% did not use the toilet; 10% needed reminders and assistance; 2% required physical help only; and 10% needed only reminders. For bowels, 65% were independent, and 5% did not use the toilet; 15% needed reminders and help; 10% required physical help only; and 5% reminders only. Overnight, 54% were independent, while 39% required protective undergarments, 1% reminders and help, 1% physical help only, and 3% reminders only.

Toileting is clearly a problem not only for the children, but also for parents and caregivers (Figure 22–1). Because toilet training often is delayed in children with CHARGE syndrome, it is important for everyone working with the child to be aware of the status of toilet training and be certain that the classroom setting, other therapies, and interventions all take this into account.

PREREQUISITES FOR TOILET TRAINING

For toilet training to be complete, the child must be able to recognize physical sensations that indicate the need to eliminate, walk to the bathroom, pull down pants and underpants, sit on toilet, eliminate in toilet, use toilet paper, put toilet paper in toilet, stand up, pull up underpants and pants, flush toilet, wash hands, dry hands, and exit bathroom. Some of the physical limitations of children with CHARGE can make completion of these tasks difficult. Also, toilet training is a highly social activity. Children who have limited social skills due to sensory impairments, communication issues, or health concerns (lengthy hospitalizations), as is the case with many children with CHARGE syndrome, may be less motivated by the usual social aspects of toilet training. There is additionally a question as to whether some children with CHARGE may have limited sensation and/or control due to structural or functional abnormalities that impair function of the nerves and muscles that allow release of urine and feces. Hearing loss (inability to hear urine stream) and

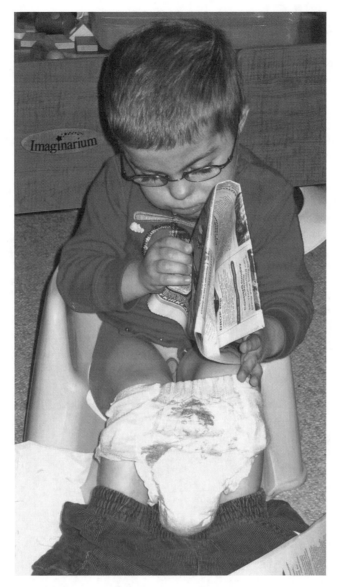

FIGURE 22–1. Potty training and exploring the news-
paper.

lack of sense of smell (soiled pants may not be particularly unpleasant) further complicate the picture.

Toilet training is a complex and time-intensive enterprise. When toilet
training children with CHARGE syndrome, one must consider hearing, vision,
balance, physical development, and physiological anomalies. Children with
CHARGE syndrome are individually unique. Toilet training is likely to happen
at an older age and take longer to complete than with typical children. However, first and foremost, toilet training is a *teaching* opportunity.

REFERENCES

Azrin, N. H., & Foxx, R. M. (1974). *Toilet Training in Less Than A Day*. New York, NY: Simon & Schuster.

Berk, L. B., & Friman, P. C. (1990). Epidemiologic aspects of toilet training. *Clinical Pediatrics, 29*, 278–282.

Blake, K. D., Salem-Hartshorne, N., Daoud. M. A., & Gradstein, J. (2005). Adolescent and adult issues in CHARGE syndrome. *Clinical Pediatrics, 44*, 151–159.

Brazelton, T. B. (1962). A child-oriented approach to toilet training. *Pediatrics, 29*, 121–129.

Klassen, T. P., Kiddoo, D., Lang, M. E., Friesen, C., Russell, K., Spooner, C., & Vandermeer, B. (2006). The effectiveness of different methods of toilet training for bowel and bladder control. *Evidence Report/Technology Assessment No. 147*. (Prepared by the University of Alberta Evidence-based Practice Center.) AHRQ Publication No. 07-E003. Rockville, MD. Agency for Health Care Research and Quality.

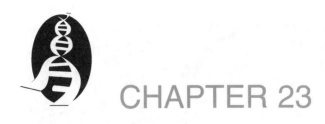

CHAPTER 23

Sleep

HELEN S. HEUSSLER, M.B., B.S., FRACP, MRCPCH, D.M.

*S*leep problems in children have strong relationships to behavior and function. In the general population approximately 20% to 25% of children will have a sleeping problem. The proportion can be much higher in a population of children with disabilities (Quine, 2000; Wiggs & Stores, 1996).

SLEEP PROBLEMS IN CHARGE

Parent reports indicate more than 50% of children with CHARGE syndrome as having a sleep problem, but importantly, nearly half do not (Hartshorne, et al., 2009) (Figure 23-1). That many children with CHARGE have sleep problems is not particularly surprising given the difficulties these children face. In a study of 87 children with CHARGE syndrome older than 6 years (Hartshorne, et al., 2009), being deafblind was associated with higher scores (more problems) on a sleep questionnaire. No correlation exists between sleep problems and choanal atresia or cleft palate (which can both cause breathing changes). A relationship *was* found with middle ear infections, which are very common in CHARGE (see Chapter 8), and those children with repaired clefts and choanal atresia may be subject to more middle ear pathology leading to ear infections (Samadi, Shah, & Handler, 2003). It is not known whether this relationship between ear infections and sleep is related to pain or to a long-standing problem with the upper airway. A relationship also existed with

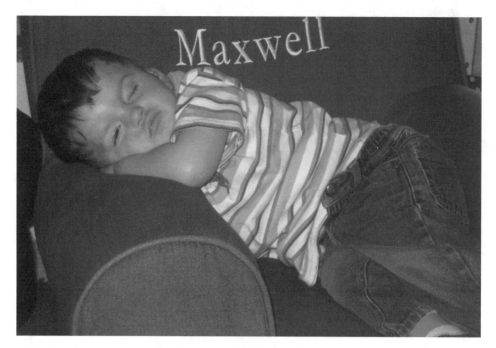

FIGURE 23–1. Some children with CHARGE sleep with one eye somewhat open.

delay in walking; however, this may be related to general brain development. It is well known that children's sleep patterns reflect their general developmental maturity. There was no relationship to age. Behavioral and sleep difficulties were correlated, and given the research in the general population, it is hard to know how much the sleep difficulties contribute to behavior or the behavioral difficulties contribute to sleep difficulties, particularly those of settling at night. On the Developmental Behavior Checklist (Einfeld & Tonge, 2002), sleep difficulties were most strongly associated with total behavioral scores, self-absorbed behavior, anxiety, and social relating behaviors. In the general pediatric population, sleep problems are more strongly related to hyperactivity, concentration, and memory.

POSSIBLE EXPLANATIONS

Many possible explanations can be given for sleep problems in children with CHARGE. These include abnormal upper airways predisposing to obstructive sleep apnea, poor vision predisposing to circadian or sleep rhythm abnormalities, and behavioral traits associated with sleep initiation and maintenance disorders. Early hospital experiences also might help set the stage for sleep difficulties.

Obstructive Sleep Apnea

All children with craniofacial abnormalities are at risk of sleep disruption from obstructive sleep apnea. Children with large tonsils and adenoids, clefts, choanal atresia, and the other craniofacial aspects of CHARGE are no different. Any obstruction should be managed as early as possible to avoid the compounding effects of obstructive sleep apnea. Known effects of obstructive sleep apnea include poor concentration, hyperactivity, alterations in mood, impulsivity, and other problems that have an impact on learning and cognition. Many of these effects can be ameliorated by treatment of the obstruction (Friedman, et al., 2003). Obstructive sleep apnea also can fragment sleep, making it difficult to maintain sleep. Relieving an obstruction on its own may affect daytime function.

Visual Impairment

It is also common for children with significant visual impairment to have difficulty with sleep rhythm (Stores & Ramchandani, 1999). Melatonin is produced by the pineal gland in the brain in response to low light, and production is stopped by bright light exposure. When children are not exposed to these visual cues, melatonin secretion cycles tend to be disrupted. It is, therefore, not surprising that children with CHARGE often have abnormal, free-running, or irregular sleep cycles. In these circumstances using extraneous methods such as strict adherence to routine, food, etc., is important to help entrain the sleep cycle. If consistent routine does not allow for a regular sleep cycle, the use of melatonin has been advocated in children with visual impairment with anecdotal success (Brennan, Jan, & Lyons, 2007).

Initiation and Maintenance

The study by Hartshorne et al., (2009) demonstrated that many of the problems were with sleep initiation and maintenance. These are difficulties that also have been commonly identified in other children with developmental disabilities due to genetic syndromes (Didden & Sigafoos, 2001). Many theories abound as to why children with disabilities may have problems with sleep initiation and maintenance. Some of these relate to various clock genes that drive our rhythm while others invoke purely behavioral traits causing children to have difficulty settling. High levels of anxiety or sensory processing difficulties may compound the underlying cause, as they certainly have been implicated in more general sleep problems in children (Shochat, Tzischinsky, & Engel-Yeger, 2009). These facets of settling issues often need to be explored in depth, particularly where the child has difficulty communicating.

DIAGNOSIS AND MANAGEMENT

The first step in management of sleep issues involves diagnosis and treatment of any physical obstruction such as choanal stenosis or adenotonsillar hypertrophy. Secondly, children should be encouraged into good sleep hygiene practices. These principles involve regular routine and settling practices with day/night contrast (activity/quiet and light/dark). Good sleep hygiene includes regular bed and wake times with appropriate sleep associations such as routines (e.g., bath) and security objects (e.g., blanket). Exploration of what allows a particular child to settle and relax is important and may vary in children with CHARGE who may have different sensory experiences and preferences. This may involve heavy covers, temperature management, vibratory toys, etc. It is important to try to avoid light at night and to try to maximize night-day (dark-light) contrast as much as possible. Those children who develop significant circadian scheduling problems relating to visual impairment or poor routines may benefit from a trial of melatonin (Jan & Freeman, 2004).

REFERENCES

Brennan, R., Jan, J. E., & Lyons, C. J. (2007). Light, dark, and melatonin: emerging evidence for the importance of melatonin in ocular physiology. *Eye (London, England)*, *21*, 901-908.

Didden, R., & Sigafoos, J. (2001). A review of the nature and treatment of sleep disorders in individuals with developmental disabilities. *Research in Developmental Disabilities*, *22*, 255-72.

Einfeld, S. L., & Tonge, B. J. (2002). *Manual for the Developmental Behaviour Checklist* (2nd ed.). University of New South Wales and Monash University.

Friedman, B. C., Hendeles-Amitai, A., Kozminsky, E., Leiberman, A., Friger, M., Tarasiuk, A., & Tal, A. (2003). Adenotonsillectomy improves neurocognitive function in children with obstructive sleep apnea syndrome. *Sleep*, *26*, 999-1005.

Hartshorne, T. S., Heussler, H. S., Dailor, A. N., Williams, G. L., Papadopoulos, D., & Brandt, K. K. (2009) Sleep Disturbances in CHARGE Syndrome. (2009) *Developmental Medicine and Child Neurology*, *51*, 143-150.

Jan, J. E., & Freeman, R. D. (2004). Melatonin therapy for circadian rhythm sleep disorders in children with multiple disabilities: What have we learned in the last decade? *Developmental Medicine and Child Neurology*, *46*, 776-782.

Quine, S. (2000) Sleep problems in primary school children: Comparison between mainstream and special school children. *Child: Care, Health, and Development*, *27*, 201-211.

Samadi, D. S., Shah, U. K., & Handler, S. D. (2003). Choanal atresia: A twenty-year review of medical comorbidities and surgical outcomes. *The Laryngoscope*, *113*, 254-258.

Shochat, T., Tzischinsky, O., & Engel-Yeger, B. (2009). Sensory hypersensitivity as a contributing factor in the relationship between sleep and behavioral disorders in normal schoolchildren. *Behavioral Sleep Medicine*, *7*, 53-62.

Stores. G., & Ramchandani, B. M. (1999). Sleep disorders in visually impaired children. *Developmental Medicine and Child Neurology, 41,* 348–352.

Wiggs, L., & Stores, G. (1996). Severe sleep disturbance and daytime challenging behaviour in children with severe learning disabilities. *Journal of Intellectual Disability Research, 40,* 518–528.

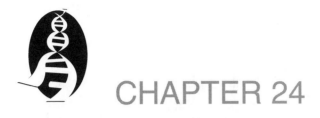

CHAPTER 24

Changes over the Life Cycle

*T*his chapter addresses the primary life cycle tasks faced by individuals with CHARGE from infancy to adulthood (Figure 24-1). Our knowledge of these changes has developed along with the children we have known for many years. At the first International CHARGE Syndrome Conference for Families and Professionals in 1993, most of the children in attendance were under six years of age. Today, this group is entering adulthood. In the final section of this chapter, some of these young adults speak for themselves.

INFANCY

SANDRA L. H. DAVENPORT, M.D.

Infants born with CHARGE syndrome can have a large number of problems, not all of which are evident at birth (see Tables 1 and 2 in the Introduction). Because the expression of each symptom can be mild to severe, each child has a unique set of circumstances that needs to be addressed (Figure 24-2). Many infants with CHARGE are extremely ill and, in fact, about 20% do not make it to their second birthday. Many remain medically fragile throughout their lives.

The physical influences on development are many. Figure 24-3 is a schematic diagram of some of these influences. When multiple body functions do not work properly, a great many factors impinge on development.

CHARGE: 7 to 19 years

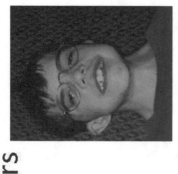

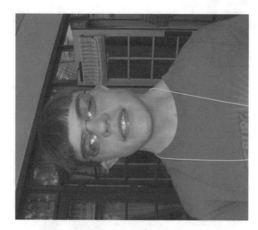

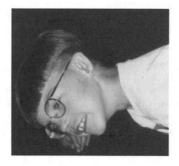

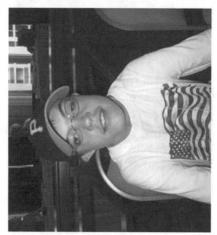

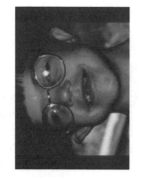

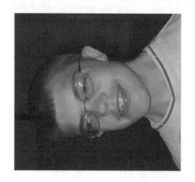

FIGURE 24–1. CHARGE 7 to 19 years.

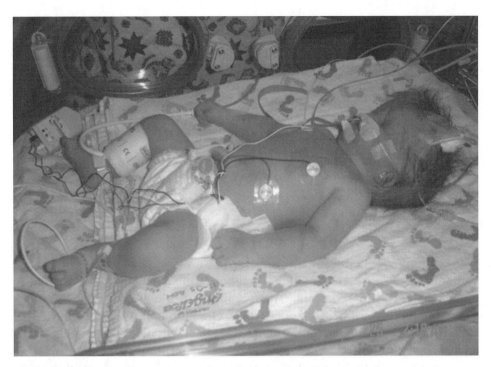

FIGURE 24–2. Many medical issues must be addressed at birth and for the next several years.

Physical Influences on Development in CHARGE

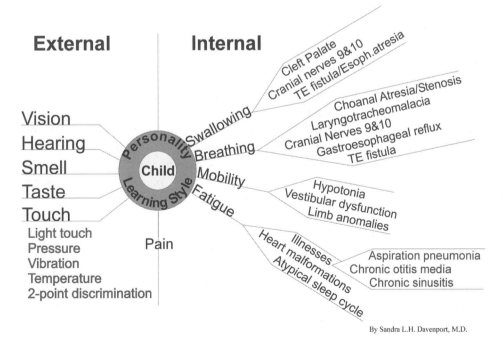

By Sandra L.H. Davenport, M.D.

FIGURE 24–3. Physical influences on development in CHARGE.

Figure 24–3 breaks these influences down into those that are *external* (vision, hearing, touch, etc.) and those that are *internal* (swallowing, breathing, mobility, etc.). In one way all are internal since the five input senses are all part of the body; however, these senses require outside stimuli. Pain is placed between the two because it can occur as a result of external or internal events (see Chapter 30). Every child also has, of course, his or her own personality and learning style. With so many physical and sensory challenges, it may be difficult to figure out just what the underlying personality and learning style may be.

Physical Issues

The many physical abnormalities result in swallowing problems, breathing difficulties, mobility constraints, and fatigue, all of which are addressed in other chapters. This constant fatigue can cause a child to not have much energy to put towards learning new skills. The problems listed on Figure 24–3 do not even constitute a comprehensive list. Just when one issue seems to be under control, another one arises. The first one to three years of life are often devoted to dealing with medical concerns. Not much time is left in the days of some families to devote to developmental stimulation, yet this is the very thing that will produce the most functional adult. If possible, members of the medical team, particularly the therapists, should communicate with their counterparts on the educational team so that a consistent and integrated program can be developed.

Sensory Issues

The sensory issues in CHARGE were addressed in Part I. Quite a bit is known about vision and hearing, which are the primary senses for learning about the environment and for language development. The sense of smell is probably more important than previously appreciated and needs further study, especially when its absence is combined with deafblindness. Individuals who are lacking most or part of those three primary senses are left with taste, touch, and the internal senses which help control balance, namely vestibular sense and proprioception. Taste requires something being put in the mouth and many young children with CHARGE seem to mouth objects for longer periods than other children (anecdotal observations). Touch is far more complex than it appears, since different neurological pathways serve different aspects of touch. More research needs to be done on touch, as it is a very important avenue for learning. Some individuals with CHARGE report that light touch can be very annoying and they prefer a firmer approach. Sensory integration techniques such as using weighted vests are often found to be a calming influence for many of these children. These considerations should be explored starting in infancy.

One of the most important developmental considerations is for the infant or child to anticipate what will come next. The usual approaches in a medical setting are to talk soothingly or to show the child something to interest and distract them and then proceed with the examination. These approaches do not work well when the child can neither see nor hear well. Therefore, approaching the child in a consistent way using touch is important (see Project Salute, http://www.projectsalute.net/). For instance, placing a hand on the leg or arm and leaving it there, encouraging the child to lay his/her hand on top of the examiner's hand and moving it to the place of interest (e.g., otoscope or other instrument) and then allowing some exploration, can be useful strategies. Waiting is not something busy medical professions usually have time for, but children and even infants who are deafblind need to be allowed more time to understand what is going on and to develop a response.

Developmental Milestones

The first few years in the life of a child with CHARGE are filled with hospitalizations and medical appointments. Children at the very least do not develop and in fact probably regress when in hospital for prolonged stays. Developmental delay is almost always an issue and can be misinterpreted as representing mental retardation if the extent of the medical involvement and sensory losses are not appreciated. Gross motor milestones are delayed due to vestibular dysfunction, the often-present truncal hypotonia, chronic fatigue due to heart disease and/or intermittent illnesses, and unusual sleeping patterns. If large retinal colobomas are present, large portions of the upper visual field are absent. This, too, has an effect on gross motor development, since infants in a prone position will not have any incentive to lift their heads. They only see what is, literally, in front of their noses. If central vision is also affected, fine motor performance will also be delayed since manipulation of objects will be dependent on the tactile experience. Hearing loss will cause delay in establishing a formal communication system unless nonauditory approaches are integrated into the learning process. Personal-social skills will also be affected if parents and other care givers are not aware of the profound effect of multiple sensory losses on accessing information from people and the setting the infant is in.

Involvement of Multiple Specialists

CHARGE syndrome is a condition which requires the involvement of many specialists both in the immediate newborn period and periodically throughout life. Families are often overwhelmed with the enormity of the task ahead and a frequent question is, "Who's in charge? Who can coordinate these appointments for us?" While in the newborn nursery, the neonatologist is in charge of making sure that all organ systems are properly assessed and that the infant becomes medically stable enough to be discharged home. After discharge, the primary care pediatrician and nurse are frequently hard-pressed to spend adequate time to serve as care coordinators. Occasionally this role is taken on by geneticists, though they are more often consultants. Developmental pediatricians in chronic care clinics may be available (usually within a university setting) to fill this need. But most often the parents end up as the coordinators, a difficult task for the most experienced of parents and often complicated by new problems periodically being added to the list of issues. Keeping track of the number of specialists and procedures can be challenging (see Sidebar 24–1). Parents may find they are spending a great deal of their time at medical visits, consuming much of what was once family or even work time (Davenport, Kloos, Prouty, 2003). From the beginning, a seemingly endless stream of physicians, nurses, therapists and counselors interact with the child with CHARGE and the family (Table 24–1). The sheer number of people involved can have a profound impact on the family and child and there is often a high degree of turnover of the particular specialists interacting with any one child. Most of these professionals look only at the organ systems within their specialty and have little understanding of the profound problems presented by having multiple sensory losses. Communication is done through the parents, as is appropriate for young children, but the effect on examiners' interaction with a child who has limited distance senses of sight and hearing is rarely understood. As a consequence, children are examined, poked, and prodded without understanding what is happening or will happen to them. This can lead to more than the usual aversion to white coats, hospitals, and procedures and can result in significant tactile and oral defensiveness. This, too, needs rigorous study and development of model programs for educating medical professionals on how to approach children with significant sensory losses.

Sidebar 24–1

To help keep track of the many appointments with a range of specialists, families should keep a notebook with sections divided by specialty and a listing at the front of the notebook with the date and specialist visited, noting any procedures such as surgery. This appointments listing can be shown to each specialist who wants more of the child and family's time so that appointments can be coordinated or even minimized. When possible, team meetings involving the various specialists (or at least consultations among the specialists) can be very helpful.

TABLE 24–1. Possible Members of a Medical Team

Specialties Involved Initially	
Neonatology	Audiology
Primary Care	Ophthalmology
ENT	Radiology
Genetics	Medical social worker
Cardiology	Developmental Pediatrician
Neurology	

Other Consultants	
Urology	Psychology
Endocrinology	Feeding team
Gastroenterology	Physical therapy
Plastic surgery (cleft palate team)	Occupational therapy
	Cardiothoracic surgery
Immunology	Pediatric surgery
Infectious disease	Speech therapy
Psychiatry	Respiratory therapy

Management

Referral to the early childhood educational team occurs when developmental delay is obvious or, sometimes, as soon as the diagnosis of CHARGE syndrome is made. The Early Childhood team is usually limited to three or four people who provide services in the home. Once again, however, many specialists may become involved with a child with CHARGE (Table 24-2). Like medical consultants, most education consultants (educators, therapists, psychologists, and others) have had little exposure to the issues involved in combined sensory losses. This can result in misleading assessments and program development. Referral to a Deafblind Project consultant can be helpful (see Sidebar 24-2). Unless in a specialized classroom setting, the teachers for the deaf/hard of hearing and the blind/visually impaired do not do hands-on teaching but, rather, provide indirect service (technical assistance) through information for and training of the early childhood or classroom teacher. One study (Petroff, 1999) showed that students who are deafblind had an average of 13 people on their education team and that half of the team rotated out each year. At this rate, there is a whole new team every third year.

TABLE 24–2. Possible Members of an Education Team

Early childhood teacher	Physical education/recreation teacher
Physical therapist	Art teacher
Occupational therapist	Music teacher
Speech and language therapist	Counselor
Deaf/hard of hearing teacher	Psychologist
Blind/visually impaired teacher	Social worker
Orientation and mobility specialist	Behavior specialist
Deafblind project consultant	School nurse/health services
Classroom teacher	Special education director
Special education teacher	Principal
Classroom aide	Assistive technology specialist
Sign language interpreter	Parent training
Intervener	Transportation

Sidebar 24–2

Deafblind projects are available in every state and territory funded by the U.S. Department of Education, Office of Special Education Programs. A list of projects is available at http://nationaldb.org/pp StateDBProjects.php. These projects provide consultation to schools, trainings on deafblindness, and support to families, for children who are deafblind, from birth through age 21. Most projects will work to support children with CHARGE even without the formal deafblind diagnosis. Parents should contact their state project as early as possible.

Finally, parents need time to simply be parents and to bond with their child as well as some time to themselves (see Chapter 32). This is hard to do when so many people are requesting time and making suggestions for their child, who has so many different needs. Someone needs to help the parents prioritize the many issues. Helping the parents identify respite services which are prepared to deal with a child with complex medical issues can help provide parents a break from the nonstop, stressful routine. Anyone who works with a child who has CHARGE needs to be aware of the multiple confusing bits of advice and instruction given to the child and family. Trying to keep instructions and other communications clear, simple, and in writing will help.

CHILDHOOD

NANCY SALEM-HARTSHORNE, Ph.D., AND
TIMOTHY S. HARTSHORNE, Ph.D.

Longitudinal and cross sectional studies of the development of children with CHARGE syndrome are scarce. Salem-Hartshorne and Jacob (2005) provided some longitudinal data on characteristics, abilities, and adaptive behavior in individuals with CHARGE over time. Adaptive behavior scores were found to remain relatively stable over the developmental years, with age at walking being the strongest predictor of later ability levels. Those children who walked earlier tended to have higher scores. Hartshorne, Grialou, and Parker (2005) provided some data regarding autistic-like behaviors in different age groups. The group with the highest scores was the three- to four-year-olds, and their scores were moderately correlated with the number of surgeries they experienced. From these and other studies, and from our experiences working with children with CHARGE and their families, some common themes in development can be generated. Table 24-3 summarizes some of these major issues of childhood for children with CHARGE (Figure 24-4).

Physiological Instability

Infants and young children with CHARGE syndrome are typically faced with multiple physical difficulties. Swallowing incoordination, ear infections, breathing difficulties, excess secretions, heart irregularities, multiple surgical interventions, and difficulties with achieving homeostasis in sleeping, breathing, and eating patterns are among this myriad of problems. Because of this, these children spend a majority of their waking hours attempting to regulate their internal systems and health. This is a major task in infancy and early childhood, and the child's struggles will inevitably take most of their energy, thus not allowing the child to be as available for typical physical and cognitive developmental milestones early on. It is important to respect this inner struggle when attempting physical or educational interventions that require dedicated concentration and attention.

TABLE 24–3. Major Childhood Issues

Early Childhood: 2–6 yrs	Middle Childhood: 7–12 yrs
Achieving physiological stability Learning to walk	Keeping up
Where and when to start school	Finding the right program
They like me; they really like me.	Where do I fit?

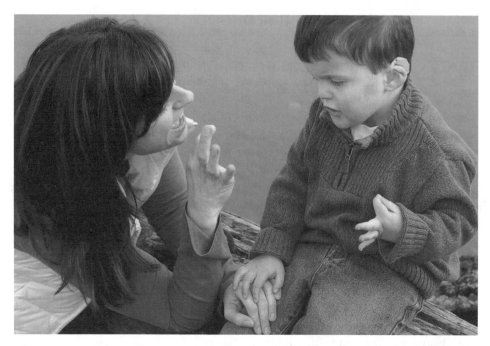

FIGURE 24–4. With major medical issues behind them, children with CHARGE must now learn to interact with their world.

The vestibular problems that delay walking are addressed in Chapter 4. But walking is a function also of some of the other senses, such as vision and proprioceptive feedback, as well as low muscle tone. Given these problems, it is surprising the children with CHARGE learn to walk at all (Brown, 2007). But they do. While some children learn to walk under 18 months, some are older than seven. Hartshorne, Grialou, and Parker (2005) report that of 117 participants, the average age of walking was 3 years, 1 month, and half walked between the ages of two and three.

What is the significance of learning to walk? A later age of walking is correlated with more challenging behavior (Hartshorne & Cypher, 2004), more autistic-like behavior (Hartshorne, Grialou, & Parker, 2005), poor adaptive behavior skills (Salem-Hartshorne & Jacob, 2005), more executive dysfunction (Hartshorne, Nicholas, Grialou, & Russ, 2007), number of psychotropic medications taken (Wachtel, Hartshorne, & Dailor, 2007), communication difficulties (Thelin & Fussner, 2005), and sleep problems (Hartshorne, et al., 2009). In other words, age of walking is a marker for more serious developmental complications of CHARGE syndrome.

It is not clear what it is about walking that makes it such an important marker. It may because being able to walk is related to so many other functions and early walking implies the other abilities are not as impaired. It may be that being upright facilitates more accurate perceptions of the world, improved breathing, and an opportunity for more social interaction. It is likely that the vestibular challenges associated with late walking also affect other important systems for learning.

Mastering walking is a huge achievement, but many children with CHARGE progress beyond that to pursue other motor activities, such as running, jumping, skipping, swimming, and even bike riding and rock climbing. Not all are successful, but some are. Finding ways to keep up with siblings and peers seems to be a huge motivator for children as they move through school.

School

The transition from home-based services to school-based services can be a difficult one for parents and children with CHARGE syndrome. The intensity of interventions typically provided by the parents during the first years of life creates clear ownership of child health and educational outcomes for the family. To relinquish this into the hands of educators who seemingly know little about the child or the syndrome is a difficult process of letting go (Figure 24–5).

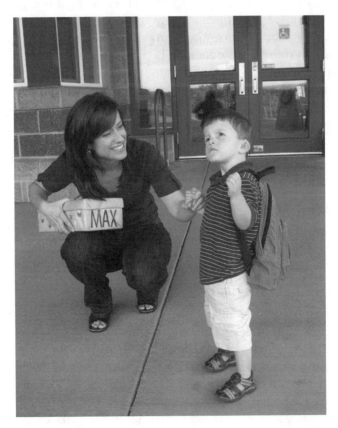

FIGURE 24–5. Families are faced with relinquishing some of their care to the schools.

Additionally, related services that the child may have been receiving in the home are likely to become school-based as well, with less allowance for parent observation and consultation during the service. Therefore, it is important for educators to allow for a gradual and smooth transition from home-based to school-based services, in order to provide comfort for the parents and child. In addition, regular contact between therapists and parents should take place after this transition, to maintain consistency between home and school. The wide variety of specialists involved in infancy and school are listed in Tables 24–1 and 24–2. Any or all of these should be considered for a child with CHARGE.

It is imperative that a student's program plan be written *before* a placement decision is made. It is somewhat typical of school districts to automatically group students into classrooms that match the students' labels. For example, a child labeled as having autism could be placed in a classroom for children with autism, based upon the label, instead of the child's specific needs. Children with CHARGE often have multiple "labels" and multiple needs. Prioritizing these complex educational needs may be helpful in identifying the most appropriate setting. Children with CHARGE have been successful in a wide variety of educational setting types. In the earlier years, it is especially important to consider inclusive education for the child to facilitate connections with nondisabled peers that can last throughout the school career. Research has indicated that individuals educated in more inclusive educational settings meet a greater number of their IEP goals, are more motivated, have natural models for appropriate behavior, and have sustained interactions with peers without disabilities (Stengle, 1996). These factors alone should make educators stop and think before eliminating this possibility.

Many children with CHARGE syndrome are accompanied throughout school by one-on-one personnel. Interpreters, intervenors, and health-care aides can seem attached like glue to the student. This can have a backfiring effect socially on the child's ability to connect on a personal level with other students. Other students may tend to ignore the child because the child is always with an adult. One-on-one adult aides need to be aware of this effect, and find ways to include peers with what the child is doing. For example, peers can be encouraged to eat with the child, to push the child's wheel chair or help to guide the child down hallways, to play during recess, and to sit with the child during class activities.

We have spoken with many parents of children with CHARGE who report that their child managed to stay on grade level at school until about third grade. This is when academics transition from being largely based on rote learning and memory to more abstract concepts, children are expected to spend more time in seat work and are given more homework. Given their sensory issues, extended seat work time is very difficult for children with CHARGE. It takes enormous powers of concentration to keep their hearing and vision focused on academic tasks while managing their vestibular and proprioceptive issues. The resulting exhaustion and frustration, along with the more challenging academic work, create considerable stress that can develop into more challenging behavior along with academic stagnation (see Chapter 31).

Children with CHARGE have been found to have more difficulty with reading comprehension than with decoding. In a recent study of 44 individuals with CHARGE (age 9 to 21 years), (Salem-Hartshorne, Blake, & J. Hartshorne, next section) reading existed in a range from no reading ability to college reading ability. Sixty percent of parents reported that their children understood what they read most or all of the time. The other 40% reported that their students understood "a little" to "half" of what they read. The complexity and diversity of children with CHARGE syndrome is such that many factors should be taken into account when providing them with reading and other instruction. Educators should become familiar with each child's needs (medical, cognitive, and sensory), and pay close attention to learning style, when providing instruction.

Utilizing a team approach to educating children with CHARGE is extremely helpful. The team gathers to collaboratively design and carry out plans for the student. Each team member has a different perspective and specific knowledge about certain areas of a child's education (for example, a physical therapist has knowledge of a child's gross motor abilities). When all members come together and share knowledge, everyone's expertise on the child is enhanced.

Social Issues, Friendships

Making and keeping friends in school is challenging for children with CHARGE syndrome. When first entering school, if in an inclusive setting, they may find friends and even be invited to birthday parties. As they move to middle childhood, this happens less often. In the same study of 44 individuals with CHARGE syndrome (see next section), 44% had no friends to report, 23% had only friends with disabilities, and 8% had friends without disabilities. Part of the difficulty seems to be problems with keeping up in terms of their peers' physical, cognitive, and social-emotional development. Because of the combination of varying developmental ability levels, personality and psychological quirks, asymmetrical facial features, appearance, walking gait, incontinence issues, educational placements, and lack of free time, children with CHARGE are less likely to be successful in making friends with students without disabilities.

Service providers can make a difference in the lives of these children. The keys to building friendships are proximity and shared experiences. Getting children with CHARGE involved in groups which include children without disabilities on a regular basis helps them to connect with same-age peers. Even if a child is educated in a segregated setting, he or she can participate in recreational sports, scouts, religious education, and neighborhood play dates.

These attempts at connection will help the child practice social skills, assist them in forming meaningful bonds, and help them to fit in. In addition, nondisabled peers often become strong advocates for their friends with CHARGE, assisting them to continue to fit in as they enter adolescence, and learn themselves about respecting and caring about others in a way they otherwise may not have.

TEENAGE YEARS

NANCY SALEM-HARTSHORNE, Ph.D., KIM D. BLAKE, M.D. and JOSHUA K. HARTSHORNE, Ph.D. CANDIDATE

The teenage years are a time of physical and psychological change for all adolescents, which parents approach with apprehension! A simplified timeline (Table 24-4) can help navigate these issues. Although the teenager with CHARGE syndrome may show physical and developmental delays, they will still travel through these psychological developmental stages. The time line may be shifted to the right; i.e. an adolescent who is 15 with CHARGE may be in early puberty and in the early developmental adolescent stage.

Little has been written about the teenage years for children with CHARGE. Surveys were sent to parents of 80 children with CHARGE who were also surveyed in two previous studies (Salem-Hartshorne & Jacob, 2004, 2005). The parents were asked for updates to the health history, and asked to complete the Adaptive Behavior Evaluation Scale (McCarney, 1983) and the Supports Intensity Scale (Thompson, et al., 2004). Data was returned regarding 51 individuals with CHARGE, ages 9 to 21, 24 male, 27 female. The results of this longitudinal study reveal that adaptive behavior scores for this sample appear to split equally between (1) moderate to severe impairment and (2) low

TABLE 24–4. A Timeline for Typical Adolescent Development

Early Adolescent 10–13 yrs	Middle Adolescent 14–16 yrs	Late Adolescent 17+ yrs
Appearance "How do I look"	Friends "Who are my friends"	Separation from Parents "I want my independence"
Conforming "I want to wear similar clothes"	Peer Approval "Do I fit in with the group"	Closer Relationships "I would like to hook up"
	Wanting to be Accepted	The Future and Transition "What is my future—I'm worried"
Anxiety "I'm afraid I don't fit in"		

average to average developmental abilities. Scores on the Adaptive Behavior Evaluation Scale over time show good test-retest reliability ($r = .68, .74, .84$, $p < .01$), and good stability, which increases as participants get nearer to adult age. Correlations between the ABES and other survey items reveal that those who walked and were toilet trained at an earlier age tend to score higher on the ABES. Significant relationships were also found with the ABES for number of friendships and degree of reading ability, including reading comprehension. The Supports Intensity Scale (SIS) was administered to those 18 and older (N = 15). The SIS is designed to measure the amount of support an individual with developmental disabilities needs. Mean scores for these participants for total and individual subscale scores clustered around "intermittent" and "limited" needs for supports (vs. "extensive" or "pervasive" needs). Adaptive behavior scores at Time 1 for these 15 participants were found to predict SIS scores in adulthood.

Early Adolescent (10–13 yrs)

The younger teenager with CHARGE syndrome will be concerned about their appearance. This concern can involve the clothes they wear, the changes in their body when puberty starts (or does not start!) and their distinct CHARGE features, which can significantly set them apart and engender peer assumptions about their abilities. Following trends and conforming to the "teenage look of the time" will be important.

Another challenge may arise when a teenager with CHARGE requires significant one-on-one attention. Interpreters and intervenors in close proximity to students all of the time are likely to have a stifling effect, socially, on the adolescent's ability to connect on a personal and more intimate level with other teenagers. Other students may see the student with CHARGE syndrome as unapproachable or even undesirable because an adult is always around. Educators and one-on-one providers should take steps to allow the student to be able to conform, to be as independent as possible, and to have some natural support from peers.

Anxiety and depression are common in teenagers with chronic illnesses going through the transitions of puberty, but even more so for teens with CHARGE syndrome. There is a paucity of literature in this area. Cognitive behavioral therapy and drug treatment may be necessary.

Middle Adolescent (14–16 yrs)

In the middle of the adolescent spectrum it is still very important for teenagers with CHARGE syndrome to fit in with their peers.

Social issues and friendships are among the most important developmental tasks of adolescence. However, for several reasons, these are more challenging for individuals with CHARGE syndrome, with many having few if any friends. As stated above, half of the children in our study were friendless, and one-fourth only had friends who had disabilities themselves.

Why are friendships so difficult? There may be multiple reasons, including the teens' developmental level, associated conditions such as ADHD, obsessive compulsive behavior, autistic-like behavior, delayed puberty, and appearance. Additionally, the necessity for assistance in getting around, and a more segregated educational placement add to the challenges of making friends without disabilities for these individuals.

It is important to attempt to consciously provide opportunities for friendships to emerge. The keys to building connections and friendships are proximity and opportunity. In order to form bonds, people must have frequent access to one another. Ways to enhance these opportunities include attendance at school with nondisabled peers and gaining memberships in extracurricular groups with others of their age. If a teenager becomes involved in extracurricular activities with peers, they are likely to make connections with others and develop closer friendships. If these attempts are less than successful, a formal Circle of Friends (Pearpoint, Forest, & O'Brien, 1996) may be necessary to assist the individual (see Sidebar 24–3).

Segregated classrooms may also be a culprit in the difficulty of adolescents with CHARGE to form friendships with nondisabled peers. In our study we found that only half of our sample spent any time in a general education classroom where they had access to nondisabled peers. Forty percent attended a segregated setting full-time, and 10% did not attend an educational setting at all. Again, in inclusive educational settings, there are more natural models for appropriate behavior, and more sustained interactions with peers without disabilities (Stengle, 1996).

Late Adolescent (17+ yrs)

For individuals with multi-sensory impairments, learning to be independent can be a challenge. Repetition and routine are essential in order for adoles-

---

Sidebar 24–3

A Circle of Friends is a group of people that forms around a person with a disability. Its purpose is to support the individual's inclusion into the school, community, and workplaces, always taking into account the individual's personal dreams, wishes, and needs. The individual invites those whom they feel support them in their lives to be involved in the circle. Circles may be formed around adults and also in schools, where they are made up primarily of the individual's nondisabled peers.

cents with CHARGE syndrome to learn how to take care of themselves. The constant presence of parents, interpreters, interveners and others can result in learned helplessness or at least passivity in everyday life. Promoting independence can be a difficult task for both educators and parents. Blake, Salem-Hartshorne, Daoud, and Gradstein (2005) found that about one-third of their adolescent and adult CHARGE sample exhibited no independence in personal care, in the community, or in taking care of their homes and finances. However, independence was achieved in other areas. See Table 24-5.

Although many individuals with CHARGE syndrome have some independence in self-care, higher order skills of independence are lacking for most of these individuals. This is an important finding, as it likely reveals at least in part a lack of instruction in these areas for adolescents and adults still attending school or in transitional programs. This may help explain why so few of these individuals move out of their family homes. Because so much of the instruction for home care, finances, and shopping takes place *in* the home for typical adolescents, it is expected that individuals with CHARGE will receive that instruction at home as well. However, families with teens with CHARGE are often ill-equipped, both instructionally and time-wise, to provide the intensity of instruction needed at home to foster independence in their children. Schools and transition programs should step forward to meet this important need for these individuals and their families.

Transition

Transition from school to work and from home to a living situation outside of the home is a natural step for older adolescents and young adults. For individuals with CHARGE syndrome, there seem to be fewer opportunities to find their paths through that transition. All but one of adults in our sample (12/13) were still living at home, with one living in a supported living arrangement.

When parents of younger adolescents were asked about the living arrangements they had envisioned for their children, one quarter of the parents envisioned their child living independently. The disconnection between parents'

TABLE 24–5. Independence in a CHARGE Syndrome Adolescent and Adult Population (*n* = 30)

Dressing and toileting independently	66%
Washing themselves independently	43%
Independent mobility in the community	30%
Independence in cleaning the house	20%
Independence in shopping	13%

visions for their child's future and what is actually happening at transition age is something that needs to be addressed.

Finding work in an appropriate setting as an adult can be challenging for individuals with CHARGE. Our current, though limited, data (N = 9) reveal that three individuals work in the community with some support, two split their time between school and a sheltered workshop, two split their time between a sheltered workshop and community work with support, and two had no school or work placement. This is not an atypical situation for individuals with more severe disabilities. Waiting lists and limited funding for vocational placements are significant barriers.

It is important for those working with individuals with CHARGE syndrome to assist them in their transition planning. This is most easily and effectively accomplished through the use of person-centered-planning techniques (Pearpoint, Forest, & O'Brien, 1996). These are a set of activities centered around the individual that take into account their needs, preferences, and interests when planning for the future. Outcomes of a good person-centered plan can include finding ways for individuals to have access to post-secondary education, vocational training, integrated employment (including supported employment), continuing and adult education, adult services, independent living (including supported living), and equally important, social connection and community participation. A person centered-plan can also include finding ways for older individuals with CHARGE syndrome to have access to various opportunities. Figure 24–6 illustrates the issues confronting the adolescent with CHARGE.

Summary

Plan early for the adolescent and adult stages of life. Start working with young teenagers on appearance. Help children and adolescents work on forming friendships and fostering peer approval. Plan for the independence that they seek but may not communicate. These growing up steps may not come naturally for individuals with CHARGE syndrome, but they are important steps, nonetheless, on the path to successful adulthood.

YOUNG ADULTHOOD

KASEE K. STRATTON, Ph.D. CANDIDATE

What is it like to be a young adult with CHARGE syndrome dealing with issues of independence, family and friend relationships, school and work experiences, challenges, and successes (Figure 24–7)? And what would young adults want others to know? Interviews were conducted with four young adults to

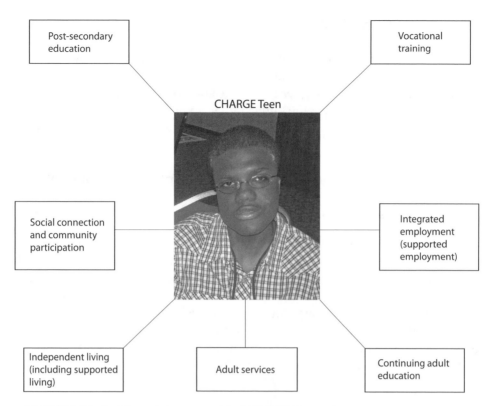

FIGURE 24–6. The adolescent with CHARGE is confronted by many issues.

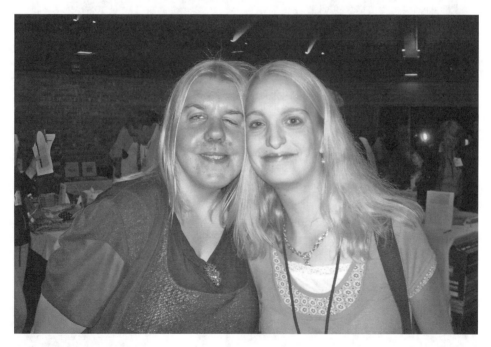

FIGURE 24–7. Some young adults with CHARGE get to know each other through conferences and Facebook.

describe their experiences. All responses are presented in their own words. There is a wide range of ability among individuals with CHARGE, and these young adults represent the higher end of the spectrum. Not all individuals with CHARGE syndrome will have the same kinds of experiences. Nevertheless, their insights are useful when considering the future for all persons with CHARGE.

Keith—19 years old—California, USA (College sophomore)

What I Want People To Know:

I find being a young adult with CHARGE relatively easy compared to my younger years (Figure 24–8). Relationships, however, have remained a challenge for me. In grade school, I faced many challenges from peers. I had a few great friends in high school; however, I found several of my really good friends in the CHARGE group. Although I have had a personal relationship that has failed, I have also found a very happy relationship with lovely girl with CHARGE syndrome. Social relationships and long-lasting friendships continue to remain a challenge for me into adulthood.

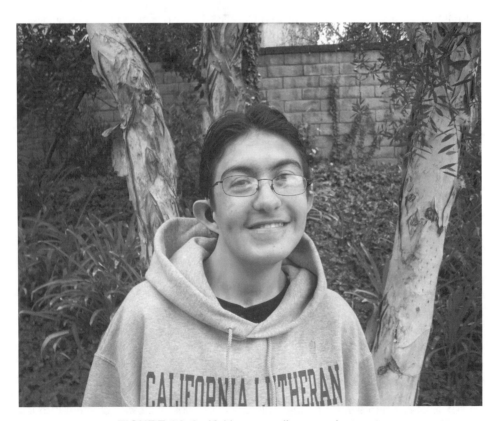

FIGURE 24–8. Keith as a college sophomore.

My emotional state is quite different from when I was a teenager. When I was a teenager, I was in emotional turmoil. I was carrying a lot of pain from having a stressful situation from 4th through 6th grade. I had a teacher and health aid that were very controlling and strict and quick to yell. I also got picked on in junior high. In my high school years, I slowly recovered and now I am much happier than I used to be. In high school, I wouldn't be able to make myself laugh, but now I am completely able to do that on my own.

Independence

I experienced a wave of independence upon my entrance into college. I have lived on the college campus for the past two years in a dorm. I plan to live in the dorms for the four years I have left. I live ten minutes from my home, so my parents can get to me if they need to and they can easily get me to doctor appointments, etc. I am currently a psychology major and I plan to become a family counselor to help families that need help.

Challenges

Some of the major issues I face as a young adult vary from social relationships to maintaining my health. I am nostalgic for high school; I miss two of my great best friends. I had another friend who pushed me away. The other major issue is my back brace. I had one for three years. In high school, I needed a brace that went from my hip to my neck, making moving very hard. When I entered college, I only needed a brace that covered my abdomen. Now, I only have to wear it at night. I also have Prilosec pills and a blended diet. My parents bring in more food every week, since I don't have the facilities to make more food. I am slowing moving from a g-tube to an oral diet during my breaks from school.

Successes

I have found many successes as I enter adulthood. I was Homecoming Prince last year as a freshman in college, and I finally figured out what I wanted to do in life. In high school I was also vice president of student council and received several scholarships in my senior year to use for college.

Ellen—24 years old—Sydney, Australia

What I Want People To Know

I'd like people to know that just because we (individuals with CHARGE syndrome) are grown up and have become adults, it doesn't mean we might not need the help and supports that we received as kids. It can be challenging when those supports are taken away and we have to find them on our own.

In school I had several supports and it was okay for me. I was mainstreamed for some of the classes, as a fairly high functioning person I was able to cope with most of what I was given. I was in a support unit with other kids my own age and often received hearing and vision assistance during the week. I needed a scribe in class at the main school. If a scribe was not provided for one lesson, I would be very behind in that day's work. My teachers were understanding and did their best to do everything they could for me.

Independence

While school was generally positive, finding work was very hard. People see someone who is deafblind and in a wheelchair as someone who can't function—which isn't always the case! I was doing a course in floristry once and I had trouble focusing. They said I was disruptive because I'd ask too many questions or not do the work properly but the way they talked to me I just lost faith in doing it properly. I didn't see any point. When I tried to take another course the next year, they wouldn't accept me because of how I was the previous year—they wouldn't even give me a fresh start.

Currently, I attend a program for people like me, which has goals set for individual needs. I'm working on improving social skills and other skills. I'm finding some volunteer work. At this program, I get one day a week at the Sheltered Workshop. This is a place for people like me who can't really go into the normal work because of their disabilities. They have supports and stuff. I do packaging of all different kinds. For example, today I packaged those bathroom detergents into little boxes. I also do labeling sometimes.

Currently, I live with my mum and dad. One day, I'd like a house with my friends (Figure 24-9).

Challenges

One of the major issues I have as a young Charger is lack of services for people like me. The closest one is based an hour away. I'm lucky my program is half an hour away and is part of the larger service housed farther away. Compared to being a teenager some challenges as a young adult are different. I have medical issues like hormonal problems and worrying whether I'm doing the right stuff with it all. I also have reflux. Socially, I still have challenges that I'm trying to overcome slowly. I am still very touchy feely. I have trouble controlling what I eat which is difficult with the reflux. Heat is also a challenge but I am doing good overall.

Successes

As a young adult, one of my successes was getting my HAC, High School Certificate. I am also getting healthier.

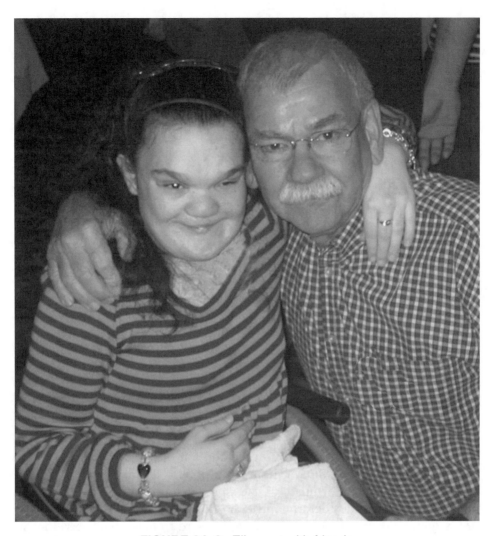

FIGURE 24–9. Ellen out with friends.

Anonymous, age 25

What I Would Like People To Know:

I would like people to know that I am not my disability. It is only a part of what makes me who I am. Just because I have a disability does not mean I cannot achieve a lot. People assume so many things about me are due to my disability. They assume if something "bad" happens to me it's because my disability makes me vulnerable when it is not the case. On the other hand, if something "good" happens, they assume I used my disability to get it. Remember, I'm not my disability.

People with CHARGE are as smart as anyone. Physical and sensory problems may limit us somewhat, but in the end we all seem to have determination which makes us strive for our best. CHARGE has so many different "defects" attached to it that scare people. People shouldn't expect us to be different when we are not. Some people with CHARGE have mental impairment and some do not. Even those who do seem to always have lots of determination and are just as bright as any other person, "D" should be added to the end of acronym for "determination" I think!

Independence

Within the last year, I have been able to get a full-time job but it was after a long time and lots of hard work. I have found, though, even within my job it took time to get them to trust me to do some things. I had to take my own initiative to just start taking phone enquires the other week when the boss was away. Once my boss saw that I could do it he was fine with it. People think because I have a vision impairment and CHARGE that it affects my abilities to do things such as communicate. I suppose to some extent it does, but I can be just as assertive, stand up for myself, and be as good as anyone else.

Currently, I live in a suburb with my parents. I know I am capable of living independently someday if I wanted to.

Challenges

Vision has been my main problem in life and a hearing impairment has also hindered me somewhat. One of the main problems during school was reading the blackboard, but fortunately I had an integration aide to assist me. I also have trouble sometimes determining who people are. My hearing has been pretty good; however I have always found it hard to follow conversations in loud places where lots of people are around. Additionally, I have to rely on public transportation as I cannot drive.

Successes

I have been able to overcome many of the obstacles that my disability has brought up. I have been able to learn to travel independently. I've even been overseas a few times by myself and also on an organized tour to visit relatives and friends.

I have been able to successfully finish high school and continue to study at a university. I have been studying a degree for longer then most people but I am determined to keep going until I get it.

As previously mentioned, I have been able to get a full time job in the past year. I have been able to adapt to the workplace just as anyone else can.

Paul—28 years old—Washington D.C., USA

What I Want People To Know

Many people who first read about CHARGE syndrome often have this picture of a person that is severely disabled and cannot function properly in society. Having CHARGE syndrome does not mean having a limited life. In addition, people who have CHARGE are not all the same.

Independence

Some aspects of independence have been challenging. An example of this is when I applied as a volunteer for an international program. There were two stages, an interview and a health evaluation. I passed the interview with flying colors. The health evaluator later called me and asked me what CHARGE syndrome was. I basically explained what each letter meant, thinking nothing of it. The evaluator decided to do her own research on the Internet. From this point on, her perspective of me changed and I was denied. In response to this, I made an appeal and had all my doctors send letters and I myself wrote a letter explaining how I have lived in places where there was no running water or electricity for weeks and was able to survive. In addition, I added how I've become an avid kayaker and rock climber and have traveled to thirteen countries (Figure 24–10). Again I was denied. Was I upset? Of course! The important point is I have not let this deter me from finding other places to volunteer.

I currently live on my own in one my of parents' homes. Living on my own has its positives and negatives. One of the positive aspects of living alone is that I have to keep track of bills and maintain the house, e.g., yard work and keeping the house clean. I feel doing this will prepare me for the future when I have my own apartment or house. In moving from one of the positives to one of the negatives is groceries! I am lucky that I live in Washington D.C., where everything is close by and there is major transportation, such as the Metro and buses. I am not able to drive, however, so I have to depend on neighbors or friends when I need to buy a lot of groceries which cannot be easily transported on the Metro. Although I live on my own, my family does contact me often through emails and phone calls. I do the same as well.

Challenges

One of the major issues I have as a young adult is making friends. In the Deaf world, this is simple; however, in the hearing world it is extremely difficult. I have a hard time trying to get people to understand that I don't hear as well as they do. On the other hand, I do have close friends from college that I keep in contact with. As for my family relationships, my family consists of five sisters

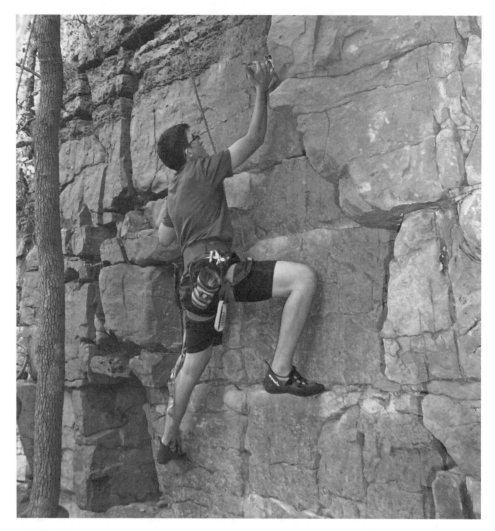

FIGURE 24–10. Paul rock climbing, one of his many outdoor adventure activities.

and me. I would consider my family close-knit. When problems arise, I always consult them for advice.

Throughout elementary and middle school I attended a mainstream private school. A major challenge I had there was trying to get teachers to understand that I was hard of hearing. A lot of my teachers would brush it off as if I were trying to gain attention. I could list countless examples of this but one stands out in my mind. As a hard of hearing person, I have to watch what people are saying to fully understand what is going on. As a child, I did not realize that I was actually reading people's lips. During class, I was watching my teacher speak and all of a sudden she walked up to me and asked me why I was staring at her. I don't blame the teacher for not understanding, but it does upset me that they would allow individuals to become teachers without learning how to deal with people that have disabilities.

Successes

During my time as an undergraduate student at Gallaudet University, I started the first chapter for Best Buddies International. The purpose of this chapter was to create friendships between people with Down syndrome and college students. As the director of the organization, I felt that I had made a step that had not been made before by matching deaf college students with people who had Down syndrome and were deaf as well.

REFERENCES

Blake, K. D., Salem-Hartshorne, N., Daoud. M. A., & Gradstein, J. (2005). Adolescent and adult issues in CHARGE syndrome. *Clinical Pediatrics 44*, 151–159.

Davenport S. L. H., Kloos, E., & Prouty, S. (2003). *Minnesota Developmental Timeline.* Retrieved December 28, 2009, from http://www.dbproject.mn.org/mntime line.html

Hartshorne, T. S., & Cypher, A. D. (2004). Challenging behavior in CHARGE syndrome. *Mental Health Aspects of Developmental Disabilities*, 7(2), 41–52.

Hartshorne, T. S., Grialou, T. L., & Parker, K. R. (2005). Autistic-Like Behavior in CHARGE Syndrome. *American Journal of Medical Genetics, 133A*, 257-261.

Hartshorne, T. S., Heussler, H. S., Dailor, A. N., Williams, G. L., Papadopopoulos, D., & Brandt, K. K. (2009). Sleep disturbances in CHARGE syndrome. *Developmental Medicine and Child Neurology, 51*(2), 143–150.

Hartshorne, T. S., Nicholas, J., Grialou, T. L., & Russ, J. M. (2007). Executive function in CHARGE syndrome. *Child Neuropsychology, 13*, 333–344.

McCarney, S. B. (1995). *The Adaptive Behavior Evaluation Scale Home Version-Revised.* Columbia, MO: Hawthorne Educational Services.

Pearpoint, J., Forest, M., & O'Brien, J. (1996). MAPs, Circles of Friends, and PATH: Powerful tools to help build caring communities. In S. Stainback & W. Stainback (Eds.), *Inclusion: A guide for educators.* Baltimore, MD: Paul Brookes.

Petroff, J. G. (1999). *A national transition follow-up study of youth identified as deaf-blind: Parent perspectives.* Doctoral Dissertation, Temple University, Philadelphia.

Salem-Hartshorne, N., & Jacob, S. (2005). Adaptive behavior in children with CHARGE syndrome. *American Journal of Medical Genetics, 133A*, 262–267.

Stengle, L. J. (1996). *Laying Community Foundations: For your Child with a Disability: How to Establish Relationships That Will Support Your Child After You're Gone.* Bethesda, MD: Woodbine House.

Thelin, J. W., & Fussner, J. C. (2005) Factors related to the development of communication in CHARGE syndrome. *American Journal of Medical Genetics, 133A*, 282–290.

Thompson, J. R., Bryant, B. R., Campbell, E. M., Craig, E. M., Huges, C. M., Rotholz, D. A., . . . Wehmeyer, M. L. (2004). *Supports Intensity Scale.* Washington, DC: American Association on Mental Retardation.

Wachtel, L. E., Hartshorne, T. S., & Dailor, A. N. (2007). Psychiatric diagnoses and psychotropic medications in CHARGE syndrome: A pediatric survey. *Journal of Developmental and Physical Disabilities, 19*, 471–483.

PART IV

Communication Systems and Language Development in CHARGE

*I*n the introduction, we used the phrase "Communication, communication, communication." Individuals with CHARGE syndrome have multisensory impairment. The loss experienced within each sensory system reduces input from the environment, impairing the ability of the child to explore and comprehend the world. The inability to smell may seem somewhat trivial until one considers that this is a major way to learn about the environment. Couple this with visual and auditory impairments and an unstable world due to vestibular and proprioceptive impairments, and the result can be significant isolation. Understanding the fundamentals of developing communication in this situation is challenging and imperative. Lack of communication skills can not only lead to mental health and behavioral complications but also can make it challenging to know when the person is in pain, stressed, or ill. This section provides the foundation for understanding the communication challenges in CHARGE and how to address them.

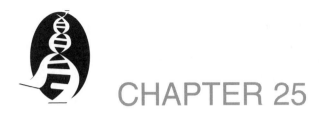

CHAPTER 25

Communication Skills

LORI A. SWANSON, PH.D.

*P*ublished and/or formal research on communication skills in individuals with CHARGE syndrome is limited (Peltokorpi & Huttunen, 2008). Thus, the bulk of the information presented here is based on personal observations or anecdotal reports from other professionals and parents. At this stage in the development of the understanding of communication in CHARGE, the anecdotal information and parental reports constitute some of the best information available. This chapter focuses on modes of communication, factors affecting communication development, and finally communication skills of individuals with CHARGE.

MODES OF COMMUNICATION

1. Manual Signs

Manual signs often are used with children with CHARGE. Because of their visual impairments, these children often require manual signs to be perceived tactually as well as visually. Although there is controversy, some believe signs should be delivered to the child in a "coactive" or "hand–under-hand" manner, in which the child's hands rest on top of the caregiver's hands, which are forming the signs. Proponents of "coactive" signing believe the caregiver should sit behind the child so the child feels the signs in the same manner in which they will be formed. Another form of tactual signing is "interactive" signing in which those interacting sit face-to-face and sign hand-under-hand. Some tactile component in learning manual signs is critical for children with limited visual skills. It is also imperative that the signs be produced within the child's limited visual field (see Chapter 2). One mother consistently signed approximately 6 inches in front of her son's face. Although this child had very limited vision, he did imitate the manual signs modeled for him. His mother signed to him consistently during daily routines (e.g., changing diaper, meal times) in the sign equivalent of "mom chatter" done instinctually with an infant or toddler. This repetitive modeling of signs during daily routines is what this child needed to eventually acquire spontaneous use of signs. The mother's input also allowed this child to interpret his environment, in that she provided signs for people, objects, and actions that he could not see or hear.

Children with CHARGE sometimes produce manual signs in a simplified or idiosyncratic manner. Caregivers need to recognize, respond to, and reinforce these communication attempts (Figure 25–1). If these communication

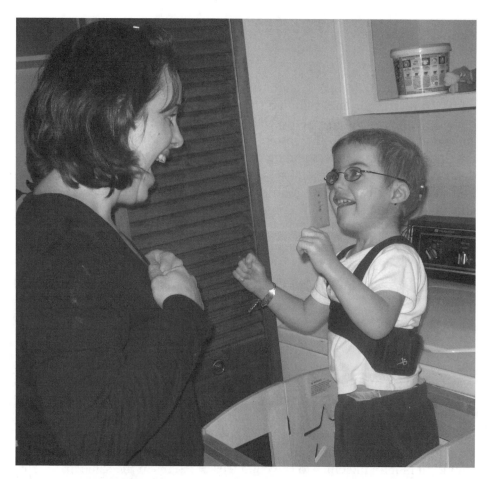

FIGURE 25–1. This mother is trying to shape the sign for "bath."

attempts go unnoticed, the child likely will go on to develop maladaptive behaviors to be noticed or to get their needs met. Making a video of the child's particular expression of signs can assist caregivers in understanding the child.

2. Visual Symbols and Voice Output Communication Aids (VOCAs)

Two-dimensional visual symbols such as photographs, Picture Communication Symbols (PCS, Johnson, 2001) and object symbols are used with some children with CHARGE. In one case report, a boy with CHARGE successfully used object symbols to express his wants (Lauger, Cornelius, & Keedy, 2005). Object symbols are a more direct avenue to symbolism than line drawings or manual signs because they are more concrete. In another study, 10 of 21 participants' parents reported using visual symbols with their child (one used a VOCA) to facilitate symbolic communication, but none of them reported using a visual system as the primary mode of communication (King, 2009; see also Chapter 27). This was an unexpected finding given the large number of participants who were presymbolic (8/21) or at the transitional level (7/21). Teachers and speech-language pathologists may be hesitant to recommend the use of visual symbols because of the visual impairments. However, most children with CHARGE are capable of recognizing and using visual symbols, especially when presented at close range, within their usable visual field. The advantage of visual symbols over signs is that the child only needs to recognize and "point to" or "exchange" (as in picture exchange communication system, PECS, Bondy & Frost, 2002) the symbol. In PECS, the child exchanges a graphic symbol for an object. The use of manual signs is more complex, because the sign must be first retrieved from memory and then produced.

VOCAs rarely are used with children with CHARGE because of the nearly ubiquitous hearing impairments (Figure 25–2). In King's investigation (2009), only 1 of 21 participants used a VOCA. It is possible that parents, teachers, and speech-language pathologists underestimate these children's ability to use VOCAs. In addition, children with CHARGE are categorized as deafblind for educational purposes, and classrooms for deafblind children are likely to favor the use of signs as opposed to visual symbols and VOCAs. Our observation is that many parents of (and even many educators working with) children with CHARGE have marginal signing skills, which also has been found to be the case with parents of other children who are deaf (e.g., Strong & Prinz, 1997). One advantage of VOCAs is that they can be understood by the child's parents as well as other interactants. A second advantage of VOCAs is that the child is using English for language production and is, therefore, more ready to become literate. Children who use American Sign Language (or some other sign language system) must learn English as a second language to acquire literacy skills. Some children with CHARGE use ASL, while others use Signing Exact English (SEE), which is a manual form of English.

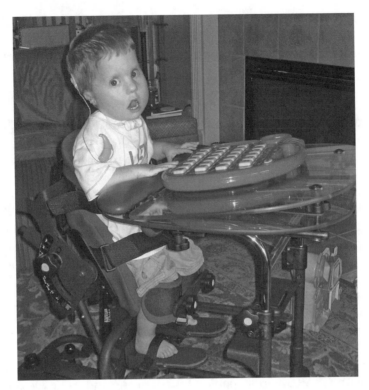

FIGURE 25–2. The use of VOCAs has several advantages.

One child with CHARGE in the Deafblind Program at *Perkins School for the Blind* started with an alphabet board and then was equipped with a voice output via Intellitools, which she learned with ease. She currently is being upgraded to a more powerful VOCA and uses a computer with enlargements for reading and formulating simple sentences. Children with CHARGE who have adequate hearing should be considered for VOCAs in order to fully participate in classroom activities, to be understood by unfamiliar listeners, and to be given the opportunity to more fully participate in literacy activities.

3. Speech

Approximately 40% of individuals with CHARGE use speech as their primary mode of communication (Thelin & Fussner, 2005). Significant hearing impairments are the primary barrier to speech. The frequent use of tracheostomies (approximately 30% of children with CHARGE have tracheostomies) also prevents this population from using speech, at least while the trach is in place. When a child has a tracheostomy stoma, that child is able to make only faint vocalizations. After the tracheostomy stoma is removed, or a Passy-Muir valve is in place, oral communication becomes an option. When children with CHARGE use speech to communicate, it is typically intelligible to both familiar and unfamiliar listeners. Their speech, however, is often loud and overanimated due to their hearing loss, poor pragmatic skills, and limited attention span. They are excited easily and often blurt out comments without restraint. In a survey study of 71 individuals with CHARGE, "only 3 children (4%) were capable of waiting for their turn to speak." (Souriau, et al., 2005, p. 279).

To our knowledge, the Tadoma method has not been employed with children who have CHARGE but could be used to allow them to perceive speech tactually. In the Tadoma method, the child is allowed to touch the speaker's lips using the thumb and to rest fingers on the speaker's face and laryngeal area. This method is important for children with low vision and limited residual hearing. It is questionable how many children with CHARGE would tolerate this method due to hypersensitivity to touch. Furthermore, only individuals familiar with the deafblind population are likely to feel comfortable with the Tadoma method and appreciate its value.

4. Gestures and Vocalizations

Assessment of prelinguistic communication is described by Bashinski in Chapter 26, including valuable information on the development of gestures in children with CHARGE. In addition, a procedure for evaluating form (e.g., gestures) and function use is given in Chapter 27. In general, contact gestures that involve touching an object are developed prior to distal gestures. Analysis of gestures is useful in evaluating the child's developmental level (Bruce, Mann, Jones, & Gavin, 2007; Crais, Watson, & Baranek, 2009). King (2009) examined the gestures and vocalizations used by 21 individuals with CHARGE. Findings indicated that gestures (e.g., give, show, reaching, contact pointing, distal pointing) and vocalizations (i.e., vocal productions of vowels and/or consonants) were used primarily by participants in the presymbolic stage of development, but participants in the transitional and symbolic stages also used them to express some intentional acts.

Facial gestures often are compromised due to facial paralysis, which occurs in approximately half of all individuals with CHARGE (Blake, Hartshorne, Lawand, Dailor, & Thelin, 2008). The complete lack of facial expression in children with bilateral facial palsy makes it difficult for the child to convey emotion. Thelin and Swanson (2006) observed one child to push the corners of her mouth upward to form a smile. She was observed to do this when a photograph was being taken.

5. Idiosyncratic Behaviors

Idiosyncratic behaviors most frequently are used by children with CHARGE who communicate at a presymbolic level. These children use unconventional behaviors rather than "symbols" to convey their needs. Some idiosyncratic behaviors may be considered challenging (kicking, head banging), and some subtle behaviors (slight movement of arm) may be difficult for others to recognize as communicative. *Communication dictionaries* created by family members and professionals working with a child can be extremely useful. The adults identify and describe the communication function for each of the child's idiosyncratic behaviors. They decide which behaviors will be retained and which will be replaced with more conventional behaviors (e.g., kicking replaced with sign for "more").

6. Total Communication

Total Communication (TC) involves the use of more than one mode of communication, often including voice, sign, gestures, pictures, etc. TC is the most common form of communication among children with CHARGE (Thelin & Fussner, 2005), and many parents choose it as a way to communicate with their children, even though the child may not yet use TC expressively. As children become more sophisticated in their use of language, the use of symbolic modes of communication increases (King, 2009). Children in the presymbolic stage of communication use idiosyncratic behaviors, gestures, and vocalizations. Children in the transitional stage of communication also use idiosyncratic behaviors, vocalizations, and gestures, but add manual signs and a limited number of spoken words to their repertoire. Those in the symbolic stage of communication continue to use the earlier developing forms but have functional use of signs and oral communication. Depending on the individual child, either manual signs or spoken words will become the primary mode of communication with the other serving as the secondary mode. Despite their apparent usefulness, visual symbols and VOCAs are not often used with this population in the public schools. They tend to be used only in settings in which professionals are familiar with CHARGE.

In summary, children with CHARGE use many different modes of communication. The speech-language pathologist carefully should select the modes in the child's total (TC) system. The ultimate goal is for children to communicate with all persons in their environment with minimal effort.

FACTORS AFFECTING LANGUAGE DEVELOPMENT

1. Vision and Mobility

Children with CHARGE typically are able to compensate for much of their visual impairments, resulting in visual functioning at higher than predicted levels (see Chapter 2). Nevertheless, the "communication bubble" for children experiencing CHARGE nearly always is restricted. The child's "communication bubble" is the area in which the child's vision and hearing are optimal for communicating. When signs are presented within the child's "communication bubble" (Davenport, 2002), they are able to interpret and imitate them. For children with limited mobility, caregivers need to be consistently mindful of the child's restricted visual field. Caregivers must be in close proximity to the child as well as positioned at the best angle. For example, a child with a retinal coloboma will have no upper visual field (see Chapter 2) and may have poor visual acuity. Signs need to be presented to such a child down low (in the lap) and up close (Figure 25–3). If central vision loss exists, children use their peripheral vision and prefer the listener to be positioned at their right or left side. When being guided, they may prefer to have the guide on the side with the best peripheral vision.

Thelin and Fussner (2005) used a parent questionnaire to determine factors correlated with symbolic language development. They found that the ability to walk independently was directly correlated with symbolic language development. Children who can position themselves and use their best visual field may be at an advantage. They are able to focus on the speaker's face,

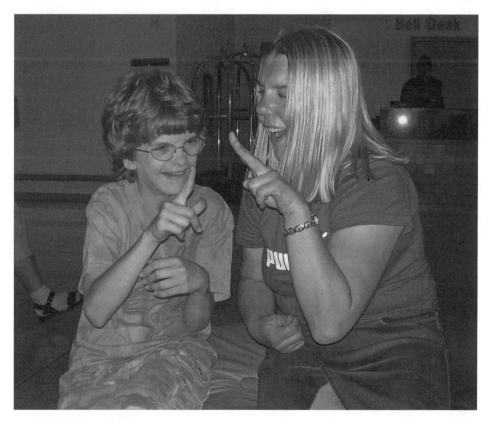

FIGURE 25–3. Signing must occur in the visual bubble, close to the face.

manual signs, and/or object of attention, which are crucial to joint referencing. The ability to pair a word with its referent is important for developing symbolic language skills. Unfortunately, children with CHARGE often have underdeveloped or absent semicircular canals, which can make mobility difficult due to balance problems (see Chapters 4, 5, & 6). However, the potential of these children to develop motor skills is underestimated. Most of these children with absent semicircular canals learn to walk, and many even ride a bicycle. Mobility, therefore, should be an important consideration and priority for facilitating communication development.

2. Hearing Loss

Some type of bilateral hearing loss (sensorineural, conductive, mixed) is present in most, but not all, children with CHARGE (e.g., Edwards, Kileny, & Van Riper, 2002). Thelin and Fussner (2005) found that children with CHARGE who have early successful amplification paired with good cognitive abilities have better language outcomes. The ability to make the best use of residual hearing is critical to later language development. Parents who find an audiologist familiar with children with CHARGE syndrome are more likely to obtain satisfactory results. Audiological assessments, amplification, and follow up are challenging with this population of children (see Chapter 3).

Cochlear implants recently have become an option for children with CHARGE (see Chapter 9). The early results of implants with deafblind children, including some with CHARGE, have been mixed (Soper, 2006; three small studies cited by Stremel & Malloy, 2006, p. 3; Taylor, Stremel, & Bashinski, 2005). Children with CHARGE *typically* continue to rely on manual signs after they have been implanted. Implants appear to allow children to have more perception of environmental sounds and speech, but, in many cases, not enough input to allow speech to develop. In contrast, Last (2007) reported that "Brent has a cochlear implant and has acquired speech but also relies on sign language to assist in his understanding when the listening environment is poor or when he is tired and needs a rest from listening." The percentage of children with CHARGE who develop speech after implantation(s) will need further study.

In a few cases, children with CHARGE did not appear to benefit from the cochlear implant until years after the surgery. Their neurological systems took an extended period of time to adjust to the implant. This anecdotal data should be verified with systematic research.

Bone anchored hearing aids (Baha) have been used to treat the conductive hearing loss in children with CHARGE (see Figures 3-2 and 3-3). Bahas are surgically implanted hearing aids that utilize bone conduction to carry sound to the cochlea. They typically are introduced at 9 to 10 years of age. Some children with CHARGE have benefitted from the improved hearing thresholds provided by Bahas.

3. Tracheostomy

Early communication development often is affected by prolonged use of a tracheostomy (Abraham, 2003). Children with CHARGE have been known to have had a tracheostomy with the stoma left in place for 15+ years. When the child first receives a tracheostomy, parents and professionals do not know the length of time the stoma will be in place. Unfortunately, the child is capable of producing only a "whispered" voice when the tracheotomy is in place and needs to rely on an augmentative form of communication even if there is relatively little hearing loss. If the child is to use signs, the parents and educators must become fluent signers to allow their child's language production skills to progress. In one case, a child with a tracheostomy stoma had fluent sign input because his mother used manual signs at her work. This rich input apparently allowed him to produce signs fluently as well. When his tracheostomy was removed, his transition from sign to oral communication was accomplished with ease. Use of manual signs allowed him to continue to develop expressive language skills while his tracheostomy tube was in place.

4. Early Language Stimulation

The key to the development of symbolic language in this population is early language stimulation. The frequent surgical procedures required by these children (typically 10 surgeries prior to age 3), however, often preclude early language intervention (Thelin & Swanson, 2006). Parents and professionals are so focused on the child's fragile medical state that communication needs often go unnoticed. Although this is understandable, speech-language pathologists must find means to intervene during the child's first three years of life. In two cases, children with CHARGE were born into ideal language environments. One girl had an aunt, who was a teacher of the hearing impaired, as her full-time caregiver, and one boy had a mother who worked in special education. These children had fluent manual sign and speech input from birth. Although these children had numerous medical issues during the early years, their language development was addressed as well. A deafblind specialist in Minnesota who has a son with CHARGE encourages parents to develop communication systems with their children as soon as possible (Prouty, 2001, Section I-D, p. 26). She states that her son's "communication" was first addressed when he was two months of age. He is currently fluent in American Sign Language and literate in English. All three of these children developed symbolic language early in part because of the increased input of multiple modes of communication early in their development (Figure 25–4).

One mother was observed reading storybooks with her toddler during one of his tube feedings. The child used manual signs to spontaneously label items in the storybook. He also responded to his mother's questions. Vocalizations were minimal due to a tracheostomy. The child's rate of productions was

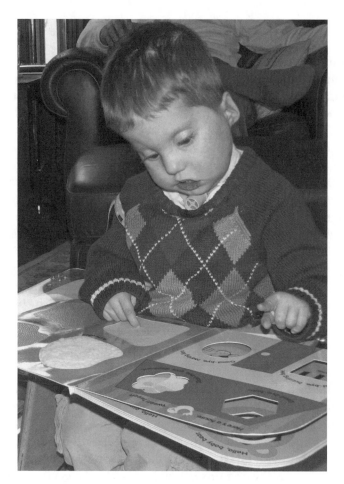

FIGURE 25–4. Child exploring a book.

4.4 acts per minute throughout this interaction, which is almost equivalent to the rate of typically developing toddlers (5 acts per minute, Paul, 2007). He produced a wide variety of signs and used language for many different purposes. When the first book was completed, the child signed "more book!" It is important to use books and other literacy-related items to facilitate language development, even if a child's vision and hearing levels are unknown or low. Fifty-seven of 71 (80%) individuals with CHARGE were reported to "like books" (Souriau, et al., 2005).

5. Cognitive Skills

Children with CHARGE display a range of cognitive skills (see Chapter 20), from above normal to cognitively impaired. Given the multiple sensory impairments, it is impossible to assess the cognitive skills of children with CHARGE using standardized measures (Hartshorne, N., 2002). It must be assumed from birth that cognitive skills are normal. These children are at risk for additional developmental delays, if appropriate input is not provided. Children need rich sensory input to develop their cognitive skills. Early language stimulation in children with CHARGE is as essential to preventing cognitive delays (Davenport, 1999; Gregory, 2001), as it is in children living in poverty (Roseberry-McKibbin, 2001).

6. Parent-Child Interactions

Reda and Hartshorne (2008) found that 7 of 14 parents indicated that bonding with their child with CHARGE was different than with their other children (see Chapter 21). These parents stated that bonding was different due to emotions associated with the diagnosis of CHARGE, lack of physical contact, and other related issues. Compromised parent-child interactions are likely to negatively affect early communication development due to the lack of synchrony in the parent-child interaction, the lack of mutual enjoyment, and the decreased amount of parental-child input. The ability of medical intervention to limit the debilitating effects of sensory impairments and life-threatening illnesses is crucial. Less time spent on medical issues translates to more time available to focus on early language development. Parents and professionals must strive to provide as many typical language models and normal interactions starting from birth (or as early as possible) to promote typical language development.

In conclusion, multiple factors appear to affect the communication skills of children with CHARGE, including sensory impairments (vision, hearing, smell, balance), lack of mobility, presence of a tracheostomy, limited early language stimulation, atypical parent-child bonding, and compromised cognitive skills. Future research is needed to document the relative impact of each of these factors. To date, there is only one study (Thelin & Fussner, 2005), which examined factors related to development of symbolic language in individuals with CHARGE. These researchers employed a parent questionnaire and identified only three factors that were correlated with symbolic language development: adequate audiologic management, ability to walk, and language intervention prior to age three. King (2009) also found that ability to walk and the presence of language intervention correlated with her participants' language skills. Audiologic management prior to age three was not examined.

COMMUNICATION SKILLS

1. Prelinguistic Skills

During the birth- to three-year-old period, most children with CHARGE do not proceed through the normal stages of prelinguistic development. Prelinguistic vocalizations and primitive gestures are delayed due to multiple factors, especially the numerous hospitalizations and medical procedures these children require. As previously stated, the typical baby with CHARGE has undergone 10 surgical procedures prior to age three. Early vocalizations are often made difficult by tracheostomies. Furthermore, the presence and severity of audiological and visual impairments are often unknown in these early stages. Certainly, some prelinguistic skills and primitive gestures will be produced, but the child will lag behind typically developing infants and toddlers (Brady & Bashinski, 2009).

2. Language Skills

Language Comprehension

The language comprehension skills of children with CHARGE typically exceed their language production skills. When given appropriate input, many are able to comprehend language at age-appropriate levels. Experience with one's environment is a vital part of receptive language development, and children with CHARGE often lack that environmental input due to their visual, hearing, and other sensory impairments. Unfortunately, these children often have very limited access to language and the world around them due to health or safety concerns. Starting very early, these children must be provided with opportunities to explore objects and their environment tactually. Then, special accommodations must be made for students to gain world knowledge. In summary, these children's language comprehension skills range from severely delayed to age appropriate depending on their ability, input, and experiences. Children who receive rich input (i.e., real life experiences, multisensory input, language presented in a variety of modes) from early on tend to have higher language comprehension skills (Figure 25–5).

A unique behavioral phenotype is believed to be part of CHARGE syndrome (see Chapter 28). As with the other features of CHARGE, the behavioral phenotype is more striking in some individuals than in others. They may have difficulty following directions and responding to questions. This difficulty is due primarily to their distractibility related to specific behavior traits (e.g., executive functioning deficits, ADHD, OCD). Development of these skills is facilitated when the child's attention is attained and the message is given with supporting cues (e.g., visual cues, touch cues). In environments adapted to meet the special needs of children with CHARGE, behavior and comprehension improves dramatically (Brown, 2005). Special adaptations may include the addition of picture cues, object cues, and words printed in Braille. Behavioral issues may be so challenging that the evaluation of language skills may be difficult or compromised significantly.

Language Production

Approximately 60% of children with CHARGE develop symbolic language skills (Thelin, Steele, & King, 2008). Most of these children, however, do not

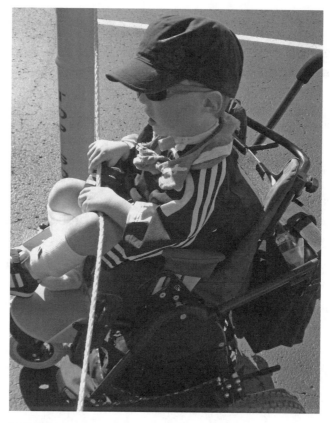

FIGURE 25–5. Children need opportunities to explore the world.

produce their first words until the late childhood years. Some school-age children and adolescents with CHARGE "catch up" on many of their language skills. They often have "functional" syntactic and semantic skills, but pragmatic skills continue to be delayed. During a recent investigation (King, 2009), communication samples were collected during clinician-child interactions. Twenty-one individuals (aged 20 months to 20 years) participated in this investigation. One third of these children were capable of producing multiword utterances using signs or speech. The mean length of utterance (MLU) for these children was short (mean: 4 words; range 1–9 words). They were capable of producing grammatical morphemes (e.g., plural -s, regular past tense -ed, articles, auxiliary verbs) but displayed difficulty with verb tenses and subject-verb agreement (They is going/They are going).

The mean type-token ratio (TTR) for these children was .355 (range: .25 and .59). This indicates that children with CHARGE have restricted vocabularies. In King's study (2009), the children were observed to use general, all-purpose (GAP) verbs (e.g., do, get) rather than specific verbs. They also lacked adjectives, which is not surprising given their visual and auditory deficits. Word-finding difficulties were also quite common.

Sidebar 25–1
Example Utterances from Two Participants with
Advanced Language (E = Examiner, C = Child)

Example utterances from Chloe (9 years):

E: I kind of know about chapter themes, but would you kind of explain it so everybody else will know what it is?

C: Um, you have to um um, well, here, I'll tell you one thing I learned from them brownie books well, here it is um, well, um, you can make like well cards like.

C: Like you know how puzzle pieces are like cardboard and stuff?

E: Uh-huh.

C: Like what you do is get a piece of construction paper cardboard.

E: Yeah.

C: And you what glue them together, and on the construction side you write like Happy Birthday or Congratulations or something like that?

E: Right.

C: And you cut it out into pieces, and you put it in an envelope, and send it to that person.

Examples from Trisha (17 years)

E: So, what happened when you took the baby home?

C: Uh, it woke me up at 4 o'clock one day, and I had to figure out why it was crying and all that, you know.

E: Well, what was the problem that made it cry?

C: It was either have to feed it or change the diaper, or . . .

E: Well, which one did you do?

C: I'd feed it first.

E: And did it quit crying after you finished?

C: Um, yeah like when it quit crying, then I don't have to feed again.

Note: Chloe exhibited sentence formulation problems with frequent use of mazes (false starts, revisions). However, Chloe's utterances did contain correct use of grammatical morphemes and some simple conjunctions and were 7.75 words in length. Trisha's utterances also contained some false starts, but they were not as interfering as Chloe's. Similarly, Trisha's utterances contained grammatical morphemes, simple conjunctions, but were shorter in length (MLU in words = 5.85) than Chloe's. Both of these children were beyond the stage of simple sentence construction.

In summary, children with CHARGE are late in acquiring first words, and their profile of language development is protracted. The same is true of their motor skills! Caregivers need to continue to target language skills well into the teen years. These children are capable of acquiring language skills beyond normal *critical periods* set for language acquisition in typical children.

Pragmatic Functions

Children with limited communication skills often learn to be passive (van Dijk & de Kort, 2005). Their parents and teachers fail to give them opportunities to initiate. On the rare occasion that these children do initiate, their subtle and often peculiar initiation attempts often go unnoticed. As a result, these children respond only when questions are directed to them. In King's study (2009), children with low communication skills were restricted to the use of earlier developing pragmatic functions (requesting objects and protesting) as opposed to more advanced functions (e.g., requesting clarification, making statements). They also had low rates of communication attempts.

Children with CHARGE who have conversational language skills are typically quite outgoing. These children are capable of teasing, humor, arguing, resolving conflicts, and negotiating with others, as evidenced by their YouTube videos, their participation at the CHARGE family conferences, and their writing on the CHARGE listserv. Some of these pragmatic skills are quite complex and only fully developed during the late school-age years in typically developing children. For example, one young adult with CHARGE is known to argue with his teachers about the answers to problems and tease them when he is correct. Similar to their typically developing peers, adolescents with CHARGE are interested in asking others on dates and experience the same pragmatic challenges as their typically developing cohorts. They often struggle with taking the perspective of others during conversations.

Children with more advanced language skills continue to struggle with topic maintenance due to their attentional problems. They fail to respond contingently to the comments and questions of others. They also have difficulty maintaining a topic while generating personal narratives.

Social Interactions

Children with CHARGE have immature social skills that correspond to their overall delayed development and sheltered lifestyles. Caitlyn's mother stated that "Social skills are among the most important for children, particularly a disabled child. . . . Yet these skills are often overlooked by doctors in the early years as being trivial compared with the severe medical problems these children face." Caitlyn missed participation in many community activities and play dates due to medical problems (McMullen, 2001, Sec I–D, p. 14).

As a result of immature social skills, many children with CHARGE are too friendly and trusting of others. For example, children who know how to

Sidebar 25–2
Example Utterances from Kiley (19 years)
(E = Examiner, C = Child)

E: Yeah, and I hear you like hair and makeup and lipstick, is that true?

C: I had a prom and got makeup.

E: Prom, you went to the prom?

C: I had my hair cut.

C: I had a doctor's appointment called orthodontist.

E: Orthodontist, for your teeth?

C: Yeah, teeth appointment.

C: And Alexis had her hair done.

E: At the orthodontist, you get your hair done?

C: No.

C: Teeth.

E: You're right, that was silly, wasn't it?

C: Your teeth.

E: So, where should I go to get my hair done?

C: Beauty shop.

C: I get my hair cut.

E: Hair cut.

C: A hair cut, it's short like that, and . . . style and it's short like that.

Note: The examiner made the topic shift from dental appointment to hair appointment apparent to the child. The examiner refused to carry the burden of the conversation!

introduce themselves may want to do so to everyone they come across. They tend to use close, even inappropriate, social distance when conversing due to their visual or hearing impairments. In contrast, other children with CHARGE are often anxious and reluctant to interact, perhaps as a result of their unusual behaviors (see Chapters 28 and 29, and for reviews, see Hartshorne, Grialou, & Parker, 2005; Wachtel, Hartshorne, & Dailor, 2007). Children with CHARGE who have normal intelligence face an enormous "social" challenge. Since many of these individuals have difficulty forming friendships with typically developing peers, they rely on listservs, Facebook, and other electronic inter-actions to maintain friendships, often with other individuals with CHARGE. One mother stated that the social needs of individuals with CHARGE become more difficult to fulfill as they mature. During the early years, her daughter was included in social groups because she was cute. But during adolescence, she was excluded actively or passively from social activities. It is important for parents to advocate for their child's social needs to prevent boredom and loneliness. Similarly, N. Hartshorne (2001/2002) stated that inclusion was "worth it" for her son, Jacob. Without inclusion, Jacob would not have achieved many goals because he would not have had his Circle of Friends and other opportunities to achieve them (see Chapter 24).

LITERACY

Although no formal data exists, middle school literacy probably is achieved by less than half of individuals with CHARGE. It may be important to note that physical development in CHARGE often is delayed very significantly (e.g., puberty may be reached at 20 years of age, see Chapters 16 and 24). During the early years, some delays in cognitive development are related to sensory impairment and delays in physical development. Among those who function at the highest levels, there is the ability to read and write, but rarely at age level. Many of those who have overcome the major challenges in learning to communicate often still have very significant delays in reading and writing. Nevertheless, many individuals with CHARGE are functioning as independent adults.

For specific techniques to facilitate reading and writing in children who are deafblind, see Bruce and colleagues (Bruce, & Conlon, 2005; Bruce, Randall, & Birge, 2008). The authors discuss the use of daily schedules and a home-school journal to provide opportunities to discuss past events. They describe pairing books with real objects to allow for meaningful experiential-based literacy. Finally, "child-guided" instruction is presented as a means to keep the student active in the learning process.

Children with CHARGE often are capable of a range of literacy activities. More than half of children with CHARGE are capable of reading and writing. The range of reading and writing skills is from single words, to simple sentences, to reading books for factual knowledge and pleasure. Among young adults with CHARGE, many are able to use computers and communicate online with the community of families who have children with CHARGE and with professionals interested in CHARGE. Interestingly, adolescents with CHARGE are frequent participants of the CHARGE listserv. They use the listserv to communicate with their peers with CHARGE, to provide information and support to parents, and to seek advice from professionals located throughout the world. Many have their own Websites and "blog" with others or are on Facebook. Children with CHARGE must be given the opportunity to develop literacy skills. From an early age, it should be assumed that they are capable of reading and writing. In a recent survey study (King, Schwarz, Steele, & Thelin, 2008), five of eight children who were at least six years old could read at least single words. Four of these five children (ages 6 to 18 years) participated in regular education classrooms, while the remaining child attended a special needs prekindergarten classroom. The highest reading level among these five children was grade four. This child's Website indicated that in grade four she participated in "most regular education curriculum with some modifications in math and language arts." She reported that her best subject was spelling and that she enjoyed singing in the choir. She used total communication as a young child but now uses speech as her primary mode of communication.

Many individuals with CHARGE (some of whom were mostly self-diagnosed) have graduated from college, and several have advanced degrees, responsible jobs, and families. The achievement of these individuals underscores the necessity to not limit expectations. One mother recounts a story of her child with CHARGE at age eight (but small for his age, appearing more like four). A lady asked her son if he would like her to read a book. Her son replied "Thanks, but I'm quite able to decipher written language." The mom states that the look on the woman's face was priceless. At 17 years of age, this young man was attending regular education classes in high school. He does not receive any modifications other than preferential seating (sits close to teacher). He passed the California High School exit exam in English as a sophomore and the exit exam in math as a junior. He was on the high school honor roll and plans to attend college without special accommodations.

CONCLUSIONS

Children with CHARGE present with a wide range of communication skills and potential communication skills. Communication development is affected dramatically by the multiple sensory deficits (e.g., vision, hearing, balance). Because it is impossible to fully or accurately assess the potential of children with CHARGE, it must be assumed from birth that every child with CHARGE is capable of typical language and literacy skills. The ability to develop symbolic language appears to be related to vision and mobility, successful audiologic management, early language stimulation, cognitive skills, and parent-child interactions. Speech-language pathologists need to provide each child with modes of communication early in life, with frequent evaluations and modifications of the language programs used. Intensive language services using multiple modalities are essential to establishing symbolic communication. Continued speech-language services throughout the child's protracted period of development typically is required to obtain and maintain age-appropriate communication and literacy skills.

Author Notes.   I want to thank Michael Harris, Meg Hefner, Emily King, Pamela Ryan, and James Thelin, for their valuable contributions to this chapter. I am grateful to the numerous individuals with CHARGE and to their families who have taught me about this syndrome.

REFERENCES

Abraham, S. S. (2003, March 18). Babies with tracheostomies: The challenge of providing specialized clinical care. *The ASHA Leader*, 4-5, & 26.

Blake, K. D., Hartshorne, T. S., Lawand, C., Dailor, A. N., & Thelin, J. W. (2008). Cranial nerve manifestations in CHARGE syndrome. *American Journal of Medical Genetics, 146A*, 585-592.

Bondy, A., & Frost, L. (2002). *The Picture Exchange Communication System training manual* (2nd ed.). Newark, DE: Pyramid Educational Consultants.

Brady, N., & Bashinski, S. M. (2009). Increased communication in children with complex communication needs. *Research and Practice in Severe Disabilities, 33*(1-2), 1-12.

Brown, D. (2005). CHARGE syndrome "behaviors": Challenges or adaptations? *American Journal of Medical Genetics, 133A*, 268-272.

Bruce, S. M., & Conlon, K. (2005). Colby's daily journal: A school-home effort to promote communication development. *TEACHING Exceptional Children Plus, 2*(1), Article 3. Retrieved June 1, 2009, from http://www.escholarship.bc.edu/education/tecplus/vol2/iss1/3

Bruce, S. M., Mann, A., Jones, C., & Gavin, M. (2007). Gestures expressed by children who are congenitally deafblind: Topography, rate, and function. *Journal of Visual Impairment & Blindness, 101*(10), 637-652.

Bruce, S., Randall, A., & Birge, B. (2008). Colby's growth to language and literacy: The achievements of a child who is congenitally deafblind. *TEACHING Exceptional Children Plus, 5*, 2-12.

Crais, E. R., Watson, L. R., & Baranek, G. T. (2009). Use of gesture development in profiling children's prelinguistic communication skills. *American Journal of Speech Language Pathology, 18*, 95-108.

Davenport, S. L. H. (1999). Influence of sensory loss on development. In M. Hefner & S. L. H. Davenport (Eds.), *CHARGE syndrome: A management manual for parents* (Section III-6). Columbia, MO: CHARGE Syndrome Foundation.

Davenport, S. L. H. (2002). Influence of sensory loss on development: The communication bubble. In M. Hefner & S. L. H. Davenport (Eds.), *CHARGE syndrome: A management manual for parents* (Version 2.1, Section IV-2C). Columbia, MO: CHARGE Syndrome Foundation.

Edwards, B. M., Kileny, P. R., & Van Riper, L. A. (2002). CHARGE Syndrome: A window of opportunity for audiologic intervention. *Pediatrics, 110*, 119-126.

Gregory, B. B. (2001). Physical therapy and occupational therapy in CHARGE syndrome. In M. Hefner & S. L. H. Davenport (Eds.), *CHARGE syndrome: A management manual for parents* (Version 2.1, Section IV-6C). Columbia, MO: CHARGE Syndrome Foundation.

Hartshorne, N. (Winter 2001/2002). It sounds nice, but is inclusion really worth it? *Deafblind Perspectives*, 12-13.

Hartshorne, N. (2002). Assessment of children with CHARGE. In M. Hefner & S.L.H. Davenport (Eds.), *CHARGE syndrome: A management manual for parents* (Version 2.1, Section IV-5A). Columbia, MO: CHARGE Syndrome Foundation.

Hartshorne, T. S., Grialou, T. L., & Parker, K. R. (2005). Autistic-like behavior in CHARGE syndrome. *American Journal of Medical Genetics, 133A*, 257-261.

Johnson, R. M. (2001). *The Picture Communication Symbols*. Solana Beach, CA: Mayer-Johnson.

King, E. A. (2009). *Communication Rate, Forms, and Functions in CHARGE Syndrome.* Unpublished master's thesis. University of Tennessee, Knoxville.

King, E., Schwarz, I., Steele, N., & Thelin, J. (2008, July 11-12). [Responses to literacy survey collected at Tennessee-South Carolina CHARGE Family Weekend]. Unpublished raw data.

Last, R. (2007, July). *CHARGE 103: Babies can't wait to communicate: The importance of communication in the early years and getting started early.* Presentation at the 8th International CHARGE Syndrome Conference. Costa Mesa, CA.

Lauger, K., Cornelius, N., & Keedy, W. (2005). Behavioral features of CHARGE syndrome: Parents' perspectives of three children with CHARGE syndrome. *American Journal of Medical Genetics, 133A*, 291-299.

McMullen, J. (2001). CHARGE stories: Caitlyn—A week in the life. In M. Hefner & S. L. H. Davenport (Eds.), *CHARGE syndrome: A management manual for parents* (Version 2.1, Section I-D, pp. 12-18). Columbia, MO: CHARGE Syndrome Foundation.

Paul, R. (2007). *Language disorders from infancy through adolescence: Assessment and intervention* (3rd ed.). St. Louis, MO: Mosby/Elsevier.

Peltokorpi, S., & Huttunen, K. (2008). Communication in the early stage of language development in children with CHARGE syndrome. *British Journal of Visual Impairment, 26*(1), 24-49.

Prouty, S. (2001). CHARGE stories: My son's influence on my life. In M. Hefner & S. L. H. Davenport (Eds.), *CHARGE syndrome: A management manual for parents* (Version 2.1, Section I-D, pp. 24-26). Columbia, MO: CHARGE Syndrome Foundation.

Reda, N. M., & Hartshorne, T. S. (2008). Attachment, bonding, and parental stress in CHARGE syndrome. *Mental Health Aspects of Developmental Disabilities, 11*(1), 1-12.

Roseberry-McKibbin, C. (2001, November 6). Serving children from the culture of poverty. *The ASHA Leader*, pp. 4-5, & 16.

Soper, J. (2006). Deafblind people's experiences of cochlear implantation. *British Journal of Visual Impairment, 24*, 19-29.

Souriau, J., Gimenes, M., Blouin, C., Benbrik, I., Benbrik, E., Churakowskyi, A., & Churakowskyi, B. (2005). CHARGE syndrome: developmental and behavioural data. *American Journal of Medical Genetics, 133A*(3), 278-281.

Stremel, K., & Malloy, P. (2006). Cochlear implants for young children who are deafblind. *Deafblind Perspectives, 13*(2), 1-5.

Strong, M., & Prinz, P. M. (1997). A study of the relationship between American Sign Language and English literacy. *Journal of Deaf Studies and Deaf Education, 2*(1), 37-46.

Taylor, E., Stremel, K., & Bashinski, S.M. (2005). *Outcomes for children who are deafblind after cochlear implantation.* OSEP Steppingstones of Technology, Grant #H327A050079.

Thelin, J. W., & Fussner, J. C. (2005). Factors related to the development of communication in CHARGE syndrome. *American Journal of Medical Genetics, 133A*(3), 282-290.

Thelin, J. S., Steele, N. K., & King, E. A. (2008). CHARGE syndrome: Developing communication in children with multi-sensory deficits [Webinar PowerPoint slides]. Retrieved December 21, 2009, from http://www.asha.org/eweb/OLSDynamicPage.aspx?Webcode=olsdetails&title=CHARGE.

Thelin, J. W., & Swanson, L. A. (2006). CHARGE syndrome. *The ASHA Leader*, *11*(14), 6-7.

van Dijk, J. P. M., & de Kort, A. (2005). Reducing challenging behaviors and fostering efficient learning of children with CHARGE syndrome. *American Journal of Medical Genetics*, *133A*, 273-277.

Wachtel, L. E., Hartshorne, T. S., & Dailor, A. N. (2007). Psychiatric diagnoses and psychotropic medications in CHARGE syndrome: A pediatric survey. *Journal of Developmental and Physical Disabilities*, *19*, 471-483.

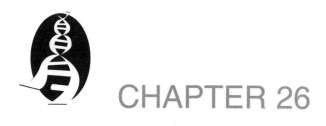

CHAPTER 26

Assessment of Prelinguistic Communication of Individuals with CHARGE

SUSAN M. BASHINSKI, ED.D.

*T*he communication skills of individuals who have CHARGE syndrome range from presymbolic, preintentional abilities to symbolic, intentional communication skills and all levels in between these extremes. Due to this incredible diversity, a variety of assessment strategies and tools must be utilized to profile reliably the communication abilities of individuals with CHARGE. Although communication profiles vary tremendously from individual to individual, it generally is accepted that development of both receptive and expressive communication abilities is delayed, in at least some areas, in all persons who experience CHARGE syndrome (Brown, 2005; Peltokorpi & Huttunen, 2008; Rowland, 2008; Thelin, Steele, & King, 2008).

The vast majority of young children with CHARGE very likely will demonstrate primarily prelinguistic skills at the time of their initial assessment and enrollment in an educational program. Many of these children over time will become competent language users; a significant proportion of them, however, are likely to *never* develop symbolic communication abilities. As noted in Chapter 27, Thelin and Fussner (2005) reported that approximately 40% of participants (11/28), all of whom had CHARGE, demonstrated essentially no symbolic communication skills. For these reasons alone, the identification of critical elements associated with prelinguistic communication, as well as robust strategies for assessing each of these elements, is essential knowledge for family members of individuals with CHARGE and the professionals who provide services to them.

CHALLENGES IN ASSESSING PRELINGUISTIC COMMUNICATION SKILLS

Professionals who implement communication programs are continuing to learn more about the full developmental progression from presymbolic and preintentional skills to symbolic, intentional communication abilities. Very few formal studies of the development of communication skills by individuals with CHARGE syndrome presently exist. Nevertheless, information relevant to evidence-based assessment practices can be gleaned from publications regarding the communication development of individuals with multiple disabilities due to etiologies other than CHARGE, as well as the practical experiences of professionals working in the field. Very few *unique* requirements exist for assessing the prelinguistic communication skills of a child, adolescent, or young adult with CHARGE. For the most part, assessment strategies implemented with individuals who experience multiple disabilities or concurrent vision and hearing losses due to other etiologies are not only applicable, but essential, to completing a thorough assessment of the prelinguistic communication abilities of an individual with CHARGE.

The challenge of reliably assessing any individual's prelinguistic communication skills must be met to the greatest extent possible. All individuals are entitled to "communicate using their chosen method" and deserve to have their own, idiosyncratic (i.e., nonconventional) communication "understood and heeded by others" (TASH, 2000). As opposed to formal, standardized tests that rely almost totally on an individual's use of conventional communication skills, the most informative strategies for assessing prelinguistic communication involve variations of informal and observational techniques (National Joint Committee for the Communicative Needs of Persons with Severe Disabilities, 1992). A rich description of the specific prelinguistic communication skills demonstrated by a child, adolescent, or adult with CHARGE is the targeted goal of any such assessment.

When gathering prelinguistic assessment data, it is critical that the person conducting the observation or informal assessment manage aspects of the physical environment—most especially, background noise and lighting conditions. Too much or too little light, glare, or unusual acoustic conditions dramatically can influence the results of an assessment. Adjustments of lighting and acoustic features of the assessment setting should be made in accordance with each individual's sensory skills and ability to attend. Most especially when conducting a prelinguistic skills assessment with an individual with CHARGE, the person conducting the assessment should use movement, vestibular activities, and physical contact as necessary in order to gain and maintain the individual's trust and engagement.

A thorough assessment of early communication skills should address each of the following critical elements associated with prelinguistic communication: the individual's symbolization ability, level of development of intentionality, rate of communication, the supportive nature of the individual's frequent communication contexts, and the level of gestural attainment.

Essential Elements of Prelinguistic Communication Skills To Be Assessed in CHARGE

Level of Symbolization Development

Van Dijk (as cited in Bruce, 2005b) "described the acquisition of symbolic understanding as 'the essential problem' of the prelinguistic stage" (p. 233). The ability to use symbols makes it possible for an individual to communicate about persons, places, or things beyond those in the "here" and "now." Symbols enable an individual to represent something in mind and refer to it with communicative behaviors.

The ability to use abstract symbols is regarded by many investigators as a very difficult achievement for individuals with CHARGE syndrome who have concurrent vision and hearing losses—an ability that many of these individuals will never attain (Bruce, 2005b; Siegel & Wetherby, 2006; Thelin, et al., 2008). Because the ability to use abstract symbols develops through a continuum of skills, however, symbolization abilities can be facilitated and improved. Expansion of presymbolic skills can have a significant impact on the quality of life of an individual, as well as the ability to communicate effectively. Advanced presymbolic forms have been demonstrated to be significant predictors of more positive language outcomes, not only in children who develop typically (Watt, Wetherby, & Shumway, 2006), but also in children with significant support needs (Brady, Marquis, Fleming, & McLean, 2004; Halle & Meadan, 2007), and children with CHARGE (Malloy & Bashinski, 2009).

In typical communication development, symbolization ability develops along a continuum, from signals that can be described only as presymbolic (nonsymbolic); through transitional, concrete symbolic forms; to ultimately fully symbolic, abstract forms (Figure 26–1). Although children with CHARGE often do not follow sequences of typical skill development, their communication skills do unfold in a manner consistent with the general levels of symbolization development described here (Bashinski, 2008; Brady & Bashinski, 2007; Bruce, Mann, Jones, & Gavin, 2007; Siegel & Cress, 2002).

When assessing an individual's prelinguistic communication, it is critically important to attempt to discern the level at which the *majority* of the individual's skills fall on the symbolization continuum. The challenge of assessing the individual's symbolization ability is exacerbated by the fact that the majority

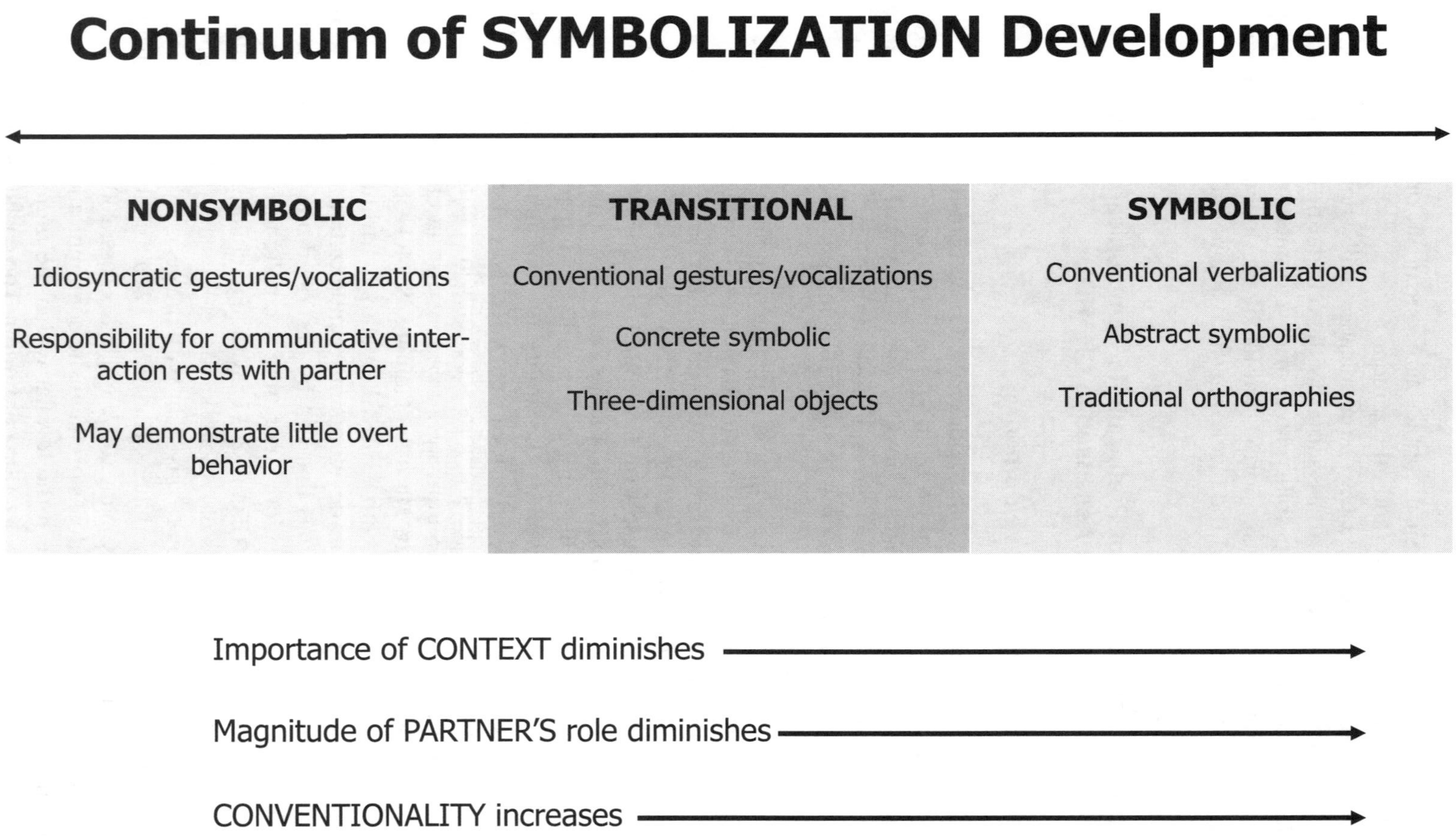

Continuum of SYMBOLIZATION Development

NONSYMBOLIC	TRANSITIONAL	SYMBOLIC
Idiosyncratic gestures/vocalizations	Conventional gestures/vocalizations	Conventional verbalizations
Responsibility for communicative inter-action rests with partner	Concrete symbolic	Abstract symbolic
May demonstrate little overt behavior	Three-dimensional objects	Traditional orthographies

Importance of CONTEXT diminishes ———→

Magnitude of PARTNER'S role diminishes ———→

CONVENTIONALITY increases ———→

FIGURE 26–1. Continuum of symbolization development.

of presymbolic communication forms are idiosyncratic—that is, unconventional and unique to the individual, making understanding and interpretation more difficult (Bruce, et al., 2007; Siegel-Causey & Bashinski, 1997). For an individual with CHARGE, these idiosyncratic behaviors are likely to involve vestibular activities and/or preferred patterns of movement. It is critical to note whether or not idiosyncratic behaviors constitute the *entire* body of the individual's communicative behaviors; if this is not the case, then the level of the individual's symbolization ability should be recorded as somewhat beyond the purely nonsymbolic stage.

With many individuals with CHARGE, it is a challenge to ascertain if, and to what degree, observed communication signals are a form of symbolic communication. Additional questions to help an assessor determine an individual's level of symbolization include the following: Can the meaning of the individual's communication be discerned somewhat independently of context, or is the context essential to understanding? What is the magnitude of the partner's role in a communicative interaction? Does this vary from situation to situation or partner to partner? Does the individual respond to specific touch cues (tactile contacts made directly on the individual's body in a consistent manner) in order to communicate (e.g., touching an adolescent's left elbow each time you approach to identify yourself and communicate, "I am here;" or tapping a child's right hip two times during diaper changing, to communicate, "Time to lift your hips; help me, please.")? How does the individual respond to specific object cues (objects, or parts of objects, consistently used to provide a concrete way of referring to a person, place, thing, or activity) used to facilitate communication (e.g., a plastic glass: "Lunchtime. Go to the table, please;" a bird's feather: "Let's go for a walk outside.")? To what degree are the individual's expressive communication forms conventional?

As part of a prelinguistic communication assessment of an individual with CHARGE, the evaluator is encouraged to use an instrument such as the form/function charts presented in Chapter 27 (which describe a wide variety of common prelinguistic elements), to record the individual's communications. In addition to noting the specific forms/functions used by a prelinguistic communicator, the assessor is advised to record the *frequency* of use of discrete signals, as well as their apparent or possible meanings, in order to yield the most reliable picture of an individual's symbolization ability. Although time-consuming and intensive, such evaluations may be the only way to accurately and thoroughly evaluate the communication ability of the individual and plan to build on those abilities with future therapies.

Level of Development of Intentionality

An important aspect of communication assessment for persons with CHARGE is the determination of intentionality. Intentionality is the deliberate pursuit of a goal; it cannot be observed directly, but rather must be inferred from an individual's observable behaviors. Behavior is interpreted as intentional if the individual performing the behavior "has an awareness of or a mental plan for a desired goal as well as the means to obtain the goal" (Siegel & Wetherby, 2006, p. 411). Applied to communicative behavior, these definitions support the notion that, in order for behavior to be *intentionally communicative*, an individual deliberately performs that behavior for the purpose of affecting a person with whom the individual is interacting, in some particular

The ability to demonstrate intentionally communicative behavior is regarded as an achievement that a significant percentage of individuals with CHARGE never attain; for many who do, intentional communication represents only a minority of their expressive communication abilities. In a study of three individuals with CHARGE syndrome, Peltokorpi & Huttunen (2008) found that only 15% to 18% of the communicative acts intentionally were communicative. It is important to acknowledge, however, that the communication abilities of individuals with CHARGE range from very early, nonintentional skills to a high level of purposeful, intentional conversational language abilities (Thelin, et al., 2008).

The skill to communicate intentionally, just as the ability to use symbols, emerges along a continuum. Intentionality skills can be improved; expansion of an individual's preintentional skills can have a significant impact on the individual's ability to communicate effectively with family, peers, and service providers.

In typical communication development, the level of intentionality develops along a continuum that begins with a stage in which behavior must be interpreted as communication (nonintentional). This initial stage is followed by a transitional stage, in which the individual's behavior is intentional, although not intentionally communicative (emerging intentional)—but can be *interpreted* as communication (Siegel-Causey & Bashinski, 1997). Individuals whose communication occurs primarily at this stage exhibit behavior that is under their control, but the behavior reflects only a general state of being (e.g., tired or thirsty); a person interacting with these individuals still must interpret the specific message (e.g., "I want you to get me something to eat." In the final stage of the intentionality continuum, an individual's behavior is both intentional *and* intentionally communicative (Figure 26–2).

Individuals with significant disabilities, including many persons with CHARGE, demonstrate lower rates of joint attention (Brady & Bashinski, 2008; Bruce, 2005b; Peltokorpi & Huttunen, 2008). This is significant because it is this ability, to jointly attend with another person, that serves as the basis for the development of intentional communication. The three participants in the Peltokorpi and Huttunen study of individuals with CHARGE (2008) did manifest general similarities to one another in their early communication development (i.e., low rates of initiation, low rates of intentionality, "protest" as the most commonly expressed function), although these varied from typically developing children. As with symbolization abilities, it generally is believed the communication skills of children with CHARGE syndrome do unfold in a manner consistent with the overall levels of intentionality development described here (Brady & Bashinski, 2007; Siegel & Wetherby, 2006).

Continuum of COMMUNICATIVE INTENTIONALITY Development

NONINTENTIONAL
Perlocutionary

Reflexive behavior

Random behavior

Behavior state

(partner must *interpret* behavior)

TRANSITIONAL
Illocutionary

Behavior is intentional

Behavior is NOT intentionally communicative

Behavior is meaningful *in context*

(some degree of partner interpretation may be involved)

INTENTIONAL
Locutionary

Behavior is intentional

Behavior IS intentionally communicative

Deliberate pursuit of goal AND means to obtain goal

Behavior is used to affect partner

FIGURE 26–2. Continuum of communicative intentionality development.

281

It is essential to attempt to discern at which level of the development of intentionality the *majority* of an individual's skills fall when assessing prelinguistic communication. Assessing the level of intentionality development in an individual with CHARGE is complicated by Yoder's (1987) finding that both the nonintentional and intentional communicative behaviors of persons with severe, multiple disabilities are more difficult to interpret than are the behaviors of individuals who experience less significant disabilities. In addition, the expressions of individuals with more complex communication needs have been observed to be qualitatively different from those of persons with less significant disabilities (Peltokorpi & Huttunen, 2008; Yoder, 1987).

To assist in the determination of an individual's level of intentionality development, an assessor is encouraged to watch for the use of any of the following as behavioral evidence of intentional communication: persistence of a behavior until a response is received; termination of a behavior when a response is received; display of satisfaction when a goal is met or dissatisfaction when it is not; change in the form or quality of a behavior until a goal is met (i.e., recasting the behavior); alternation of attention between the person with whom the individual is interacting and the goal; and/or reluctance to initiate any behavior (Brady & Bashinski, 2008; Bruce & Vargas, 2007; Fey, et al.,2006; Peltokorpi & Huttunen, 2008; Warren, et al., 2006). It is important to note, however, that particularly with individuals with CHARGE syndrome, termination of a behavior and/or reluctance to initiate might *not* be reliable indicators of communicative intentionality. With children and young adults with CHARGE, observations of prematurely terminating a behavioral signal or failing to initiate behaviors directed to others might be indicative of levels of cognitive function and/or social development.

As mentioned previously, an evaluator completing a prelinguistic assessment with an individual with CHARGE is encouraged to use the form/function charts included in Chapter 27, or a similar instrument. This information will contribute not only to an understanding of the individual's level of symbolization skills, but also to a reliable assessment of the individual's level of intentionality and inform plans for future therapies. As previously mentioned, although informal assessment is time-consuming and intensive, such evaluation may be the only way to accurately and thoroughly evaluate the communication abilities of an individual with CHARGE syndrome.

Communication Rate

Communication rate can be defined as the number of times an individual communicates over a specified period of time. Many professionals who study the emergence of early communication behaviors report communication rate as the number of communication acts per minute (Bashinski, 2008; Brady & Bashinski, 2008; Bruce & Vargas, 2007; Warren, et al., 2006), although they characterize what constitutes a "communication act" somewhat differently.

The most challenging aspect associated with determining an individual's communication rate is agreement upon exactly what constitutes an "intentional communicative act" (Bashinski, 2008; Bruce & Vargas, 2007; Warren, et al., 2006). Various professionals in the field of early communication development utilize different criteria for this purpose. Some definitions consist solely of a description of behaviors demonstrated by the communicator alone; others rely on the role of the communicator in an interaction with a partner.

Two taxonomies of elements comprising intentional communicative acts are referenced most frequently. The taxonomy developed by Wetherby and Prizant (1989) includes seven observable characteristics; the taxonomy of Bruce and Vargas (2007) utilizes nine characteristics to describe an intentional communicative act (ICA). Five elements are included in *both* of these taxonomies. The learner

- uses a message form the partner understands;

- persists in sending the message (i.e., continues to repeat the behavior) until the partner responds to it in some manner;

- pauses, in the middle of doing something overt, to wait for a response from the partner;

- changes the quality of the signal to repair the partner's misunderstanding;

- indicates satisfaction or dissatisfaction regarding achievement of a goal.

Wetherby and Prizant (1989) include two additional observable features to describe an (ICA). The learner

- terminates the signal when the goal is achieved,

- alternates gaze between the communication partner and the goal.

The remaining four characteristics which Bruce and Vargas (2007) use to identify an ICA, in addition to the common five (above), include the learner

- repeats a message when misunderstood,

- responds with pleasure or displeasure to the partner's communication,

- responds with a signal that indicates understanding of the partner's message,

- demonstrates joint attention with the partner.

In contrast, some professionals in the field determine what constitutes an ICA solely on the basis of whether an individual *initiates* the communication with a partner or *responds to* the partner. "Previous definitions of ICAs focus more on incidences when the child is the initiator of the interaction, even though most children with severe disabilities respond intentionally more often than they initiate" (Bruce & Vargas, 2007, p. 302); this same observation may be applied accurately to many individuals with CHARGE. A third criterion utilized in the determination of an ICA by some professionals is whether or not the individual directed the signal to another person (i.e., a partner), as opposed to demonstrating only object-directed behavior (Brady & Bashinski, 2008; Ogletree, Fischer, & Turowski, 1996).

These three contrasting criteria are not included here for the purpose of confusion. Rather, the various measures are described in some detail because each might legitimately be applied in an attempt to complete a comprehensive prelinguistic assessment with an individual with CHARGE syndrome. Some children with CHARGE will be very persistent and repeat a behavior over and over (e.g., attempt to get another person to take a toy and turn it back on), until the partner interprets and fulfills the "request." Other children will not persist, but rather respond to the other person's lack of "cooperation" with distinct displeasure, or no "other-directed" response at all (e.g., simply ceasing the behavior or responding by engaging in a stereotypic movement or behavior).

Generally speaking, individuals with disabilities, including many persons with CHARGE, demonstrate lower rates of communication, particularly intentional communication, than do their typically developing peers. When communication rate is calculated with ICAs that include responses to partner-initiated communication as well as self-initiations, however, children with CHARGE who communicate primarily at the prelinguistic level may be described as having relatively high communication rates (Brady & Bashinski, 2008; Bruce & Vargas, 2007). As demonstrated in the collection of Prelinguistic Milieu Teaching (PMT; see description in next section) model studies (Brady, et al., 2004; Fey, et al., 2006; Warren, et al., 2006), including Brady and Bashinski's Adapted PMT investigation (2008), children's rates of conventional gesture use and vocalizations can be increased, including the rates of children with CHARGE who communicate primarily at the prelinguistic level. The nine children who participated in Brady and Bashinski's Adapted PMT study all had complex communication needs, concurrent vision and hearing losses, and multiple disabilities—including one with CHARGE syndrome. At the outset, participants' overall mean rate of communication was 0.61 ICA/minute. Following individual sessions, during which the children were taught to use conventional gestures and/or vocalizations directed to a communication partner, the overall mean rate of communication increased to 1.92 ICA/minute. The participant with CHARGE generally kept pace with progress of the other children, demonstrating an increase in communication rate from .27 ICA/minute to 1.66 ICA/minute during the course of the study. (NOTE: These figures represent communication rates maintained for the duration of sessions averaging 45 minutes in length, for three consecutive weeks, prior to exit from intervention.)

Communication rate has been suggested as a significant predictor of more advanced linguistic skills (Brady, et al., 2004; MacCathren, 2000). Although at first this appears to be an oversimplification, research does suggest that an individual's rate of communication is correlated positively with the level of communicative skill development. It is reasonable to infer that such is the case in regard to individuals with CHARGE syndrome, as well.

When assessing an individual's prelinguistic communication, the evaluator is encouraged to record the occurrence of any of the eleven characteristics of ICAs, as explained previously. In addition, prelinguistic assessment with an individual with CHARGE should include the number of the individual's communicative responses and initiations and observations regarding whether or not the communicative acts were directed toward an object or a communication partner. Only through recording this variety of information can it be ensured that a prelinguistic assessment presents a comprehensive picture of the individual's communication rate.

ESSENTIAL METHODS TO BE UTILIZED IN PRELINGUISTIC COMMUNICATION ASSESSMENT WITH INDIVIDUALS WITH CHARGE

Structuring the Communicative Context

Setting a context for the assessment of an individual's prelinguistic skills is critically important to the success of the assessment. The Prelinguistic Milieu Teaching model (PMT) exemplifies one approach to the establishment of a communicative environment that has very successfully facilitated gesture and vocalization production by children in the earliest stages of communication development (Warren & Yoder, 1998), including those with CHARGE (Brady & Bashinski, 2008; Malloy & Bashinski, 2009). PMT combines the strategies of following the child's lead, delaying prompts, engaging in motivating routines, turn-taking activities, and purposefully arranging materials within natural contexts, to help children learn a variety of conventional gestures, vocalizations, and combinations of these. When structuring the context within which any prelinguistic assessment will occur through direct observation and/or communication probes (see later in this chapter), the assessor is well-advised to incorporate these five strategies, central to the PMT approach.

For individuals who do not use symbols for communication, the role a communication partner plays is critical. In order to elicit an individual's prelinguistic communicative skills, a responsive partner is required if an assessment session is to yield meaningful results (Fey, et al., 2006; Malloy, 2008). Communication skills assessment with an individual who communicates primarily at a prelinguistic level will, necessarily, also involve assessment of the partner's skills. Of particular importance is the communication *partner's* ability to demonstrate: sensitivity to the individual's behaviors and communication attempts, creativity, contingency of responses, and consistency of responses to the prelinguistic communicator's signals (Siegel-Causey & Bashinski, 1997). While gathering assessment data on an individual with CHARGE who demonstrates prelinguistic skills, the person conducting the assessment would be well-advised to simultaneously collect data regarding the degree to which the individual's communication *partner* utilizes these skills while interacting with the individual in the role of assessor.

Effectiveness of the PMT model has been well documented with children with developmental disabilities and significant communication delays, but had not been implemented with individuals with multiple disabilities, including CHARGE syndrome, prior to Brady and Bashinski's 2008 study. In their investigation, Brady and Bashinski sought to extend PMT strategies to make them appropriate for children with concurrent vision and hearing losses, multiple disabilities, and complex communication needs, including CHARGE. For their Adapted PMT study (A-PMT), all critical features of PMT were maintained; other aspects of the approach were modified to make them accessible to, and appropriate for, children with physical and/or sensory impairments.

Key features of A-PMT included, first, an emphasis on vestibular and tactile activities with all participants and the minimization of activities requiring typical hearing or vision skills. As might be predicted from knowledge of common preferences of children with CHARGE, movement and vestibular activities proved to be particularly motivating for Brady and Bashinski's (2008) participant with CHARGE. Because eight children in this study retained at least some residual hearing and/or vision, routines involving toys with loud sounds and/or flashing lights were also included—in accordance with each child's residual sensory abilities. All toys and available movement activities were kept in close proximity to the participant at all times to ensure the child's awareness of their continued accessibility. Second, during teaching sessions, Brady and Bashinski primarily used tactile prompts (instead of verbal prompts—the primary mechanism for support in PMT); their study participant with CHARGE responded particularly positively to tactile prompts. Third, a child's body orientation in the general direction of the partner and/or searching behaviors (e.g., reaching out a hand to find the partner), were utilized as indications of attention shift, in addition to directed eye gaze and shifting eye gaze from a desired object to the partner as utilized in previous PMT studies. Because Brady and Bashinski were able to effectively demonstrate improved prelinguistic communication outcomes for children with CHARGE syndrome and concurrent vision and hearing losses, a person conducting any prelinguistic assessment with an individual with CHARGE is strongly encouraged to incorporate these features of the A-PMT approach during all assessment activities.

Utilizing Functional Assessment Strategies

Few formal tools exist for assessing receptive or expressive communication skills at the prelinguistic level. Prelinguistic communication of individuals with multiple disabilities, including CHARGE syndrome, may be very difficult to interpret (Brady & Bashinski, 2008; Snell, 2002). To compensate for this challenge, communication assessment with individuals with CHARGE should ideally include: (1) direct observation of the individual, (2) interviews with family members and educational staff, and (3) "situational" or "structured" probes (Brady & Halle, 1997). Brady and Halle (1997) suggest that when utilized in combination, these strategies can yield a comprehensive analysis of an individual's functional communication skills. These three elements in combination are especially important when assessing an individual with CHARGE who has a repertoire of primarily prelinguistic communicative behaviors.

(1) Direct Observation

Direct observational assessment of individuals in their natural environments is likely to yield the most reliable information regarding their prelinguistic communication skills (Thelin, et al., 2008). This consists, simply, of the assessor observing the individual in natural environments, such as home or school, as opposed to an artificial, unfamiliar environment such as a testing room. Direct observation is the technique utilized by familiar partners (e.g., parents, intervenors) when they respond to interview protocols—either independently, or in conversation with the person responsible for the child's communication assessment. Direct observation, conducted by the person responsible for the assessment, makes possible an independent evaluation of communication skills reported via interviews with the family members of a child with CHARGE syndrome and the professionals who provide services to the child.

When observing a child with CHARGE, it is critical the assessor make note of the environmental conditions in which the observation is completed. Since vision and hearing losses are the norm in children with CHARGE, it is particularly important the observer ensure adequate lighting (e.g., reduction of glare, increase of contrast in materials, reduction of fluorescent lights, use of targeting lighting) and minimization of background/environmental noise (e.g., music, outside conversations, traffic, heat or AC blowers) as much as possible. The observer is well advised to allow the child to place/locate materials according to the child's own visual field preferences; this is especially true when assessing an individual with CHARGE, since visual field losses are common in this population. If the observation is completed under less-than-optimal sensory conditions, data from the observation should be interpreted very cautiously. In their Adapted PMT study, Brady and Bashinski (2008) found they collected their most reliable observational data with children with CHARGE in structured situations (as opposed to free time) that involved two or fewer children, and/or during routines that involved movement and vestibular or gross motor activities.

(2) Interviews

Interviews should be conducted with family members of the prelinguistic communicator, as well as service providers, to ensure that information from persons familiar with the child will be included in the communication assessment. It is important to gather information from a variety of familiar partners who interact with the individual being assessed in different settings or contexts. Four interview instruments appropriate for use when evaluating an individual's prelinguistic communication skills, including individuals with CHARGE, are: *Wisconsin Behavior Rating Scale* (Song, et al.,1984), *Inventory of Potential Communicative Acts* (Sigafoos, et al., 2000), *Home Talk* (Harris, et al., 2002), and *Communication Matrix* (Rowland, 2008).

The most formal of these instruments, the *Wisconsin Behavior Rating Scale (WBRS)*, is a rating scale comprised of 11 subscales. It is unique among the four instruments described here because it yields age-equivalent scores. One scoring option of this instrument allows for the recording of "emerging skill." Two of the *WBRS subscales*, though titled "receptive language" and "expressive language," include a variety of items regarding prelinguistic communication (0 months to 40 months [receptive skills] and 0 months to 54 months [expressive skills]); both of these subscales include special items and differential scoring for individuals with deafblindness (i.e., concurrent vision and hearing losses). Of particular interest regarding the *WBRS* is the fact that the norm group, with whom age-equivalents were determined, included individuals with multiple disabilities (64% of the total), nearly 7% of whom had concurrent vision and hearing losses (Song, et al., 1984), making this instrument especially appropriate for use with individuals with CHARGE.

The *Inventory of Potential Communicative Acts (IPCA)* is appropriate for assessing individuals with physical disabilities and severe communication challenges, including those who have vision and hearing losses, which so often is the case with individuals who have CHARGE. The inventory consists of 53 open-ended questions, categorized according to 10 distinct functions, yielding a graphic profile of results. The *IPCA* acknowledges the communicative potential of prelinguistic communicative skills, with the goal of gathering descriptive information regarding any behavior the individual might use for any communicative purpose (Sigafoos, et al., 2000)—for example, how the child responds to a favorite item being taken away or how the child seeks comfort. The *IPCA* includes many of the idiosyncratic, prelinguistic communicative behaviors demonstrated by many individuals with CHARGE.

Designed as a family-friendly booklet, *Home Talk* was developed collaboratively by parents of children with disabilities, including parents of children with CHARGE syndrome, and professionals. It "presumes that every child can accomplish every task" (Harris, et al., 2002, p. 1) with varying degrees of assistance (which are rated in various sections of the instrument). Family members may record, in narrative format, how their child demonstrates a variety of communication skills and functions, including many prelinguistic elements. Communication is one of five domains specifically assessed; other sections of *Home Talk* include "Habits and Routines," "People Skills," and "Exploring the Environment."

The *Communication Matrix* is an instrument originally designed in 1990, revised in 1996, and re-formatted as a web-based application (Rowland, 2008). It is available on the Internet, free-of-charge (http://www.communication matrix.org/). The *Matrix* was designed primarily for use by family members of individuals with significant communication disabilities; CHARGE syndrome is one of the specific categories of disability included in this instrument. The web-based application supports the notation of emerging skills; it branches, automatically, as family members record the body movements, early sounds, facial expressions, visual behaviors, simple gestures, conventional gestures, and combinations of these elements their child demonstrates. The *Communication Matrix* is designed to specifically describe an individual's current communicative skills, as well as provide a framework for developing communication goals. It yields a one-page summary profile, including seven levels of communication, from the earliest pre-intentional behavior through the level of abstract, symbolic communication; school professionals should find this profile extremely helpful in planning goals and objectives for incorporation in the individualized educational program (IEP) for a child with CHARGE.

(3) Situational/Structured Probes

A situational or structured probe is a tool utilized to assess an individual's communication skills in a pre-arranged context, through the systematic introduction and/or manipulation of elements in that context. Such probes offer the assessor the possibility to create opportunities for the individual to demonstrate specific forms/functions, use a particular communicative skill repeatedly, and for the observer to sample a variety of communicative skills in a relatively brief time period (Brady & Halle, 1997). Structured probes are recommended as a supplement to the information regarding a child's prelinguistic skills provided by family members and professionals acquired through interview/questionnaire formats, and to provide information regarding communication skills the assessor was unable to detect/assess through un-intrusive, direct observation. For example, the assessor might interact directly with a child with CHARGE, who has low vision skills or legal blindness, using a light box. The light box is turned on as the child and assessor approach the work station—but no materials appear to be available for use with the box. The assessor waits to see what the child will do. A second probe element might involve the assessor making brightly colored, translucent materials temporarily available on the light box, *or* available within the child's visual field—but out of reach. If the child does not discern how the box is activated, a third type of probe would have the assessor turn off the light box and again wait to see what the child will do.

Informal assessment of a child's prelinguistic skills is most likely to yield a comprehensive, reliable profile of the child's abilities if data gathered through direct observation, interview formats, and structured probes are viewed collectively.

Criticality of the Level of Gestural Attainment

Gestural communication meets the third criterion of intentionality as previously explained—an observable behavior (i.e., a gesture) which is both (1) produced intentionally and (2) is intentionally communicative. Level of gesture attainment has been demonstrated to be a strong predictor of more advanced linguistic skills in children who experience significant disabilities and severe communication delay (Brady, et al., 2004; McLean, Brady, McLean, & Behrens, 1999). The use of gestures in combination with vocalizations has consistently been cited as a critical marker in regard to later language development for children with communication delay (Fey, et al., 2006; Warren, et al., 2006), and for children with multiple disabilities, including CHARGE syndrome (Brady & Bashinski, 2008; Peltokorpi & Huttunen, 2008). Exhibition of conventional gestures, in studies of typically developing children, was shown to contribute significantly to positive receptive language outcomes (Watt, et al., 2006).

Gestural development proceeds in a progression from an individual's making direct *contact* with a person or object, to gesturing at some distance (i.e., *distal*) from the person or object of interest (Bruce, 2005a; McLean, McLean, Brady, & Etter, 1991; Werner & Kaplan, 1963). In typical communication development, this progression occurs naturally. Individuals with visual impairment or concurrent vision and hearing losses are more likely to continue to use contact gestures (Bruce, et al., 2007). For individuals who experience concurrent sensory losses, such as with CHARGE syndrome, this notion of distancing often must be directly taught. Progression in an individual's ability to functionally use distal (i.e., conventional, noncontact) gestures is, therefore, a key marker related to the development of symbolic communication skills (Bruce, 2005a; Bruce, et al., 2007; McLean, et al., 1991) and should be noted in any comprehensive assessment of prelinguistic communication abilities of an individual with CHARGE.

Gestures are influenced by culture and can be dependent on context. When assessing the gestural communication of individuals with CHARGE, it is important to remember that culture is defined not only by race/ethnicity, but also geographic location and the individual's membership in various communities (e.g., school, social club). Crais, Watson, and Baranek (2009) have suggested a general sequence of gesture development for the critical period that includes the transition from prelinguistic communication to the emergence of "true language." Nonetheless, it is recommended that the age-norms suggested by Crais, Watson, and Baranek be very cautiously applied to individuals with CHARGE, since these individuals are not likely to follow an exact, typical developmental sequence.

SUMMARY

Symbolization ability, level of intentionality, and communication rate should all be considered when assessing the prelinguistic communication skills of an individual with CHARGE. Assessment information should be collected by, and from, both family members of individuals with CHARGE syndrome and providers of their educational/habilitation services. It is strongly recommended that functional assessment information be collected through a variety of methods, including: direct observation; interview/questionnaire; and systematic probes in the authentic environments, in natural interactions with the individual who communicates without the use of symbols. Only by following such a comprehensive assessment of an individual's prelinguistic skills can decisions regarding design of a communication program, for an individual with CHARGE syndrome, be appropriately made.

REFERENCES

Bashinski, S. M. (2008, July). *Teaching communicative gestures to children with deaf-blindness through adapted prelinguistic milieu teaching.* Paper presented at the OSEP Project Directors' Meeting, Washington, DC.

Brady, N., & Bashinski, S. M. (2007, November). *Increased communication in deaf-blind children after adapted PMT intervention.* Paper presented at the American Speech-Language-Hearing Association (ASHA) Annual Convention, Boston, MA.

Brady, N. C., & Bashinski, S. M. (2008). Increasing communication in children with concurrent vision and hearing loss. *Research and Practice for Persons with Severe Disabilities, 33*(1-2), 59-70.

Brady, N. C., & Halle, J. W. (1997). Functional analysis of communicative behaviors. *Focus on Autism and Other Developmental Disabilities, 2,* 95-104.

Brady, N. C., Marquis, J., Fleming, K., & McLean, L. (2004). Prelinguistic predictors of language growth in children with developmental disabilities. *Journal of Speech, Language, and Hearing Research, 47,* 663-677.

Brown, D. (2005). CHARGE syndrome "behaviors": Challenges or adaptations? *American Journal of Medical Genetics, 133A,* 268-272.

Bruce, S. M. (2005a). The application of Werner and Kaplan's "distancing" to children who are deaf-blind. *Journal of Visual Impairment & Blindness, 99* 464-477.

Bruce, S. M. (2005b). The impact of congenital deafblindness on the struggle to symbolism. *International Journal of Disability, Development and Education, 52,* 233-251.

Bruce, S. M., Mann, A., Jones, C., & Gavin, M. (2007). Gestures expressed by children who are congenitally deaf-blind: Topography, rate, and function. *Journal of Visual Impairment & Blindness, 101*, 637-652.

Bruce, S. M., & Vargas, C. (2007). Intentional communication acts expressed by children with severe disabilities in high-rate contexts. *Augmentative and Alternative Communication, 23* 300-311.

Crais, E. R., Watson, L. R., & Baranek, G. T. (2009). Use of gesture development in profiling children's prelinguistic communication skills. *American Journal of Speech Language Pathology.*

Fey, M., Warren, S., Brady, N., Finestack, L., Bredin-Oja, S., & Fairchild, M. (2006). Early effects of prelinguistic milieu teaching and responsivity education for children with developmental delays and their parents. *Journal of Speech, Language, and Hearing Research, 49*, 526-547.

Halle, J., & Meadan, H. (2007). A protocol for assessing early communication of young children with autism and other developmental disabilities. *Topics in Early Childhood Special Education, 27*, 49-61.

Harris, J., Hartshorne, N., Jess, T., Mar, H., Rowland, C., Sall, N., . . . Wolf, T. (2002). *Home talk: A family assessment of children who are deafblind.* Portland, OR: Oregon Health & Science University.

MacCathren, R. (2000). Teacher-implemented prelinguistic communication intervention. *Focus on Autism and Other Developmental Disabilities, 15*, 21-29.

Malloy, P. (2008, August). The path to symbolism. *Practice Perspectives-Highlighting Information on Deaf-Blindness: Newsletter of the National Consortium on Deaf-Blindness, 1*(3). Retrieved December 21, 2009, from http://www.nationaldb.org/NCDBProducts.php?prodID=97

Malloy, P., & Bashinski, S. M. (2009, September). Teaching prelinguistic communication. *Practice Perspectives-Highlighting Information on Deaf-Blindness: Newsletter of the National Consortium on Deaf-Blindness, 1*(5). Retrieved December 21, 2009, from www.nationaldb.org/ISSelectedTopics.php

McLean, L., Brady, N., McLean, J., & Behrens, G. (1999). Communication forms and functions of children and adults with severe mental retardation in community and institutional settings. *Journal of Speech, Language, and Hearing Research, 42*, 231-240.

McLean, J. E., McLean, L. K. S., Brady, N. C., & Etter, R. (1991). Communication profiles of two types of gesture using nonverbal persons with severe to profound mental retardation. *Journal of Speech, Language, and Hearing Research, 34*, 294-308.

National Joint Committee for the Communicative Needs of Persons with Severe Disabilities. (1992). Guidelines for meeting the communication needs of persons with severe disabilities. *ASHA, 34*, March, Supp. 7, 1-8.

Ogletree, B., Fischer, M., & Turowski, M. (1996). Assessment targets and protocols for nonsymbolic communicators with profound disabilities. *Focus on Autism and Other Developmental Disabilities, 11*, 53-58.

Peltokorpi, S., & Huttunen, K. (2008). Communication in the early stage of language development in children with CHARGE syndrome. *The British Journal of Visual Impairment, 26*(1), 24-49.

Rowland, C. (2008). *The Communication Matrix.* Retrieved December 21, 2009, from the Communication Matrix website:http://www.communicationmatrix.org/

Siegel, E. B., & Cress, C. J. (2002). Overview of the emergence of early AAC behaviors: Progression from communicative to symbolic skills. In J. Reichle, D. R. Beukelman,

& J. C. Light (Eds.), *Exemplary practices for beginning communicators: Implications for AAC* (pp. 25–57). Baltimore, MD: Paul H. Brookes.

Siegel, E., & Wetherby, A. (2006). Nonsymbolic communication. In M. E. Snell & F. Brown (Eds.), *Instruction of students with severe disabilities* (pp. 405–446). Baltimore, MD: Paul H. Brookes.

Siegel-Causey, E., & Bashinski, S. M. (1997). Enhancing initial communication and responsiveness of learners with multiple disabilities: A tri-focus framework for partners. *Focus on Autism and Other Developmental Disabilities, 12*, 105–120.

Sigafoos, J., Woodyatt, G., Keen, D., Tait, K., Tucker, M., Roberts-Pennell, D., & Pittendreigh, N. (2000). Identifying potential communicative acts in children with developmental and physical disabilities. *Communication Disorders Quarterly, 21*(2), 77–86.

Snell, M. (2002). Using dynamic assessment with learners who communicate nonsymbolically. *Augmentative and Alternative Communication, 18*, 163–176.

Song, A., Jones, S., Lippert, J., Metzgen, K., Miller, J., & Borreca, C. (1984). Wisconsin Behavior Rating Scale: Measure of adaptive behavior for the developmental levels of 0 to 3 years. *American Journal of Mental Deficiency, 88*, 401–410.

TASH. (2000). *TASH resolution on augmentative and alternative communication methods and the right to communicate* (Rev.) [Resolution]. Retrieved December 21, 2009, from TASH: http://www.tash.org/IRR/resolutions/res02communication.htm

Thelin, J. W., & Fussner, J. C. (2005). Factors related to the development of communication in CHARGE syndrome. *American Journal of Medical Genetics, 133A*, 282–290.

Thelin, J. W., Steele, N. K., & King, E. A. (2008). *CHARGE syndrome: Developing communication in children with multi-sensory deficits* [Webinar PowerPoint slides]. Retrieved December 21, 2009, from http://www.asha.org/eweb/OLSDynamicPage.aspx?Webcode=olsdetails&title=CHARGE

Warren, S., Bredin-Oja, S., Fairchild-Escalante, M., Finestack, L., Fey, M., & Brady, N. (2006). Responsivity education/Prelinguistic milieu teaching. In R. McCauley & M. Fey (Eds.), *Treatment of language disorders in children* (pp. 47–77). Baltimore, MD: Paul H. Brookes.

Warren, S. F., & Yoder, P. J. (1998). Facilitating the transition from preintentional to intentional communication. In A. Wetherby, S. Warren, & J. Reichle (Eds.), *Transitions in prelinguistic communication* (Vol. 7, pp. 365–385). Baltimore, MD: Paul H. Brookes.

Watt, N., Wetherby, A., & Shumway, S. (2006). Prelinguistic predictors of language outcome at 3 years of age. *Journal of Speech, Language, and Hearing Research, 49*, 1224–1237.

Werner, H., & Kaplan, B. (1963). *Symbol formation: An organismic-developmental approach to language and the expression of thought.* New York, NY: Wiley.

Wetherby, A, & Prizant, B. (1989). The expression of communicative intent: Assessment guidelines. *Seminars in Speech and Language, 10*, 77–91.

Yoder, P. J. (1987). Relationship between degree of infant handicap and clarity of infant cues. *American Journal of Mental Deficiency, 91*, 639–641.

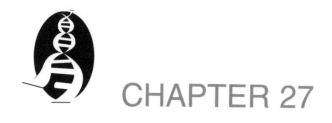

CHAPTER 27

Forms and Functions in Communication

EMILY KING MILLER, M.A., LORI A. SWANSON, Ph.D.,
NANCY K. STEELE, M.ED., SARA J. THELIN, M.A.,
AND JAMES W. THELIN, Ph.D.

COMMUNICATION SKILLS IN INDIVIDUALS WITH CHARGE SYNDROME

Communication abilities in children with CHARGE syndrome greatly vary, but expressive communication skills in all of these children are delayed. The abilities of the individual may range from preintentional to symbolic communication, regardless of age. Preintentional communication involves responding to pleasure or displeasure with expressions such as crying or laughing that is not directed towards a particular person. At the presymbolic level of intentional communication, behaviors such as reaching, pointing, crying, and vocalizing are directed toward a person to request, protest, or inform. Symbolic communication uses spoken or signed language to convey information to another person and receive information back. Though formal studies are not available, anecdotally, professionals believe that about 40% of individuals with CHARGE syndrome do not develop symbolic communication.

Individuals who do not develop any form of symbolic language may use gestures, pictures, touch cues, object cues, body movements, eye gaze shift, or, in frustration, maladaptive behaviors to communicate. Maladaptive or non-compliant behavior can include biting, hitting, screaming, and/or self-injury.

Many parents report that their children with CHARGE use noncompliant behaviors to communicate. These non-symbolic communicative forms may be highly idiosyncratic and interpretable only by members of the immediate family.

Individuals with CHARGE who develop symbolic language may use more than one form of communication: sign language, spoken language, voice output communication aid (VOCA), or a combination of the above. Among these individuals, delays are common in vocabulary recall, initiating communication, and abstract language forms (Brown, 2005). Thelin and Swanson (2006) reported that these children often show a delay in maintaining a topic and in turn-taking in a conversation. Because of the extreme diversity in communication styles and ability among children with CHARGE, generalizations about this group are of less value than descriptions of the capabilities of specific individuals (Figure 27–1).

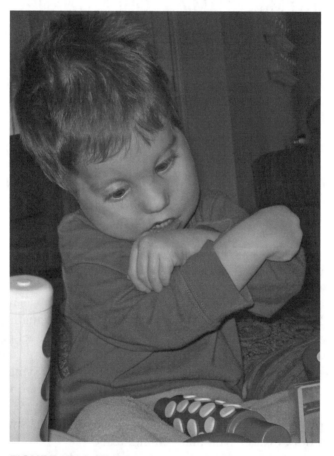

FIGURE 27–1. The development of symbolic communication varies a great deal among children with CHARGE. This boy is signing "bear."

CHALLENGES IN ASSESSING COMMUNICATION SKILLS IN CHARGE SYNDROME

Assessing communication abilities in individuals with CHARGE syndrome is challenging due to their delays in expressive communication and unconventional modes of communicating. Standardized language tests rely heavily on vocalizations, pointing, and functional vision and hearing to evaluate communication skills. Language tests exist which have been normed on children who are deaf or hard-of-hearing. However, these tests also rely on normal visual and motor abilities. For individuals with CHARGE who have some language ability but do not have these skills, test scores are likely to under-represent communication abilities. For individuals at the lowest levels of intentional communication, no useful information on the person's communication abilities is gained from standardized tests because the scores will likely fall several standard deviations below the mean. Even at the highest levels of symbolic communication, standardized test results may be skewed by the examiner's inability to understand the examinee, whose verbal communication may be affected by hearing and vision loss, craniofacial anomalies, and pragmatic abilities.

In lieu of standardized tests, some investigators support the use of observational assessment of individuals with deafblindness and multiple anomalies as the most effective way of assessing expressive communication skills (Brady, 2005; Wolf-Schein & Schein, 1998). The National Joint Committee for the Communication Needs of Persons with Severe Disabilities (1992) also suggests that assessment for individuals with severe disabilities should focus on a descriptive analysis of the individual's ability to use intentional communicative acts, including a description of the different communicative forms and functions rather than on scores from standardized tests.

COMMUNICATIVE FORMS, FUNCTIONS, AND RATE

There are few studies published specifically on communication development in CHARGE syndrome. However, investigators have reported information on language development and behavior in individuals with deafblindness and multiple disabilities that can be applied to the analysis of communication in individuals with CHARGE syndrome. Those analyses rely on the description of communicative forms, functions, and rate.

The term "communicative form" indicates the mode of communication used: pointing, reaching, vocalization, tantrum, self-injury, gesture, sign, speech, and so forth. There are two main categories of communicative forms: presymbolic (e.g., gestures, reaching, pointing) and symbolic (signed, spoken, or written language) forms. The term "communicative function" is used to refer to the reason or purpose for communication: a request, a response to a question, a comment, a greeting, an abstract thought, etc. The "communicative rate" is the frequency with which the individual communicates, calculated in communicative acts per minute (acts/min).

The types of communicative forms an individual uses at any point in development are important in predicting later language outcomes. Investigators have linked the acquisition of higher prelinguistic forms, such as distal pointing (index finger pointing without contact with the object), rate of communication, and the successful use of communicative functions, to higher levels of linguistic development in both typically developing children and individuals with disabilities (Brady, Marquis, Fleming, & McLean, 2004; Watt, Wetherby, & Shumway, 2006; Yoder, Warren, & McCathren, 1998). Crais, Watson, and Baranek (2009) proposed a general developmental sequence of gestures for typically developing children from age 9 months up to age 24 months. Pushing away objects and reaching for objects are described as the earliest developing gestures. Blowing kisses and head nodding are some of the later developing gestures described. These investigators suggest that careful analysis of specific communicative forms may be useful in distinguishing between certain disorders (e.g., autism, Down syndrome) in young children.

Development of communicative forms in individuals with deafblindness and/or multiple disabilities is nearly always delayed and may be limited to presymbolic forms of communication (e.g., direct behaviors, facial expressions). These individuals often use idiosyncratic presymbolic forms to communicate. Bruce, Mann, Jones, and Gavin (2007) describe seven children with deafblindness who used 44 different presymbolic forms to communicate. Each participant used a variety of gestures, which were mostly contact gestures and/or unconventional forms. Bruce, et al. (2007) suggest that contact gestures are common in individuals with visual impairment, and these individuals are less likely to use conventional gestures such as distal pointing. Symbolic forms of communication must be directly taught to individuals with deafblindness (Hagood, 1997). Brady and Bashinski (2007) suggest that the use of different communicative forms, such as touch cues, object cues, hand-under-hand strategies, are often required to facilitate functional communication in individuals with deafblindness. Other symbolic forms that individuals with deafblindness may use include finger spelling, signed English, Braille, Sign Language (which varies by country), lip-reading speech, Tadoma method of speech-reading, and Pidgin Signed English (Miles, 2005).

The use of communicative function requires an understanding of causality. At the level of preintentional communication, behaviors are reactions to environmental changes that are not dependent on the understanding of causality. Children with disabilities show lower rates of joint attention, which is the basis for developing intentional communication (Bruce, 2005). Communicative function begins when an individual moves on to intentional communication. Protesting, requesting objects, and requesting actions are some of the first communicative functions to develop in the presymbolic stage, in which gestures rather than speech are used for communication (Crais, Watson, & Baranek, 2009; Wetherby, Cain, Yonclas, & Walker, 1988). Behavioral regulation, social interaction, and joint attention are the three early categories of communicative function expressed by children (Crais, Watson, & Baranek, 2009). As the individual's language skills increase, these functions expand to include more specific purposes, like requests for information, responses to request for clarification and declarative statements. The ability to use communication for a variety of purposes is necessary in order to inform others of one's wants, needs, and opinions.

The ability to use a variety of communicative functions successfully is highly correlated with higher levels of presymbolic communication (e.g., distal pointing) and symbolic communication (Stephenson & Linfoot, 1996). The presence of multiple disabilities has an even greater impact on the acquisition of communicative functions and on the number of functions an individual utilizes (Bruce, Godbold, & Naponelli-Gold, 2004). Individuals with deafblindness often have difficulty understanding that communication has a purpose (Hagood, 1997). However, even when they have grasped this concept, they use relatively lower-level communicative functions such as to request or regulate others behavior for their own needs (Hagood, 1997). It has also been suggested that children with deafblindness are not only delayed or restricted in expressing different communicative functions but also show a unique pattern of development for communicative functions (Bruce, 2005). Bruce, et al., (2007) reported similar findings; most of the communication by their seven participants was to request action, request an object, or protest.

Peltokorpi and Huttunen (2008) studied the communication abilities of three children with CHARGE syndrome who differed in age (16 months; 3 years, 9 months; and 8 years, 4 months) but had similar communication skills. Communication samples were obtained from video tapes of the children interacting with their mothers. The analysis of the communication samples was conducted using modifications of the Tait Video Analysis for studying preverbal skills in children with hearing impairment and the Communicative Intention Inventory (Coggins & Carpenter, 1981). The investigators examined preintentional as well as intentional communication and described the communication in terms of mode, communicative function, and frequency of communicative initiations. The analyses revealed that these children were functioning at the presymbolic stage of communication. They most often used gestures and vocalizations, less often signs. The investigators also found that these children initiated communication less than half the time and that their rate of intentional communication was very low (less than 20% of communicative acts in sample). Protesting was the most common function used by the participants. Peltokorpi and Huttanen concluded that these three children with CHARGE showed similarities in the forms and purposes of communication in the early stages of communication development (mostly with gestures and to protest) even though their clinical profiles were very different. They also found that intentionality and communicative function were often difficult to determine in these children due to the combination of impairments and idiosyncratic forms of communication.

COMMUNICATIVE ANALYSIS OF INDIVIDUALS
WITH CHARGE: THE KING STUDY

A series of studies at the University of Tennessee was designed to describe and evaluate expressive communication skills across the communication spectrum for persons with CHARGE. A total of 21 individuals with CHARGE participated in the study. Preliminary results have been presented at conferences (King, Swanson, Thelin, & Steele, 2007; King Miller, Swanson, Steele, Thelin, Schwarz, & Thelin, 2009; Swanson, King, Thelin, & Steele, 2007), and the entire study was presented as a master's thesis (King, 2009).

The King (2009) study was similar to the Peltokorpi and Huttunen (2008) study; however, the University of Tennessee research included children with a wider range of communication abilities and focused on description of only intentional communication regarding communicative forms, functions, and rate. Some of the individuals in the study have abilities near the boundary between preintentional and intentional communication, while others are conversationalists. The objectives of the research were to discriminate between unintentional behaviors and the earliest presymbolic communication, describe intentional idiosyncratic communication modes, and provide useful descriptions of symbolic communicators that would not be described by standardized tests.

The most thorough description of the subjects' communication included forms, functions, and rate of communication. A coding scheme for communicative forms and functions was developed from coding systems developed by previous researchers (Fey, 1986; McLean & Snyder-McLean, 1999; Wetherby & Prizant, 2001; 2003).

An example of the coding scheme is shown in Table 27–1. Columns represent the communicative forms, proceeding from presymbolic (crying, tantrums, etc.) to symbolic communication (1-word or multiple-word). Signs, verbalizations, and voice output communication aids (VOCA) are the symbolic forms that were coded. Communicative functions are listed in rows and progress from the earliest developing communicative functions (requests for permission, greeting, etc) to higher developing functions (request for clarification, statement, etc.). Definitions of all forms and functions are in Table 27–2 and 27–3.

King's study is composed of the elements used in previous research on descriptive communication analysis of communicative forms and functions (Crais, Watson, & Baranek, 2009; Peltokorpi & Huttunen, 2008). Some adjustments were made to the type and method of analysis due to the large range of communication levels in the individuals included in the study. King's study included 21 individuals with CHARGE syndrome at multiple levels of communication and with 22 different communication modes and 20 different communicative functions that may be used by individuals with early presymbolic to symbolic communication. Fifteen-minute video-taped communication samples of each individual with a deafblind specialist were gathered, then analyzed according to communicative form, function, and rate.

TABLE 27–1. Sample Coding Scheme

COMMUNICATIVE FUNCTION		COMMUNICATIVE FORM																	
		Pre-Symbolic															Symbolic		
		CRY	TANT	AGRES	PM	GAZE	GIVE	SHOW	REACH	CP	DP	SHAKE	NOD	GEST	VOC	Pic X	1 word	Multi	VOCA
Behavioral Regulation	RQOB																		
	RQAC																		
	PROT																		
Social Interaction	RQSR																		
	RQCT																		
	GREET																		
	CALL																		
	RQPM																		
	SHOW																		
Conversational Act	COMT																		
	RQIN																		
	PRIN																		
	IMI																		
	RQCL																		
	ASST																		
	PERF																		
	RSAC																		
	RSCL																		
	RSAT																		
	RSAS																		

TABLE 27–2. Communicative Forms: Abbreviations and Definitions

Presymbolic Forms	Definitions
CRY Crying	Vocal cry directed towards an adult, either to protest, request an object or action, or gain attention. Reflexive cries, such as when infants are uncomfortable or sick, are not considered intentional.
TANT Tantrums	Kicking, screaming, and/or flapping arms that is communicative but that is not aimed to injure another person or self.
AGRES Aggression	Aggressive behaviors, such as hitting, kicking, pinching, biting, or any other injurious behavior that is directed towards self or another individual and shows communicative intent.
GAZE Gaze Shift	Change in eye movement and/or body position that has communicative intent.
PM Physical Manipulation	Manipulation of another person's hand or other body part in order to communicate a message.
GIVE Giving	Act of giving an object to another person for a communicative purpose.
SHOW Showing	Holding an object in the other person's view in order to communicate something about that object.
REACH Reaching	Extension of the arm/s and hand/s toward an object or person that is out of reach.
CP Contact Pointing	Use of index finger to point to an object or person while touching that object or person.
DP Distal Pointing	Use of the index finger to point towards an object or person that is out of reach.
SHAKE Head shake	Movement of head side to side to indicate a protest.
NOD Head nod	Movement of the head up and down in order to indicate affirmation.
GEST Gesture	Physical movement that is not a formal sign and is not included in the above list of gestures but communicates a message (e.g., waving hello or good-bye).
VOC Vocalizations	Vocal productions of vowels and/or consonants that are directed towards an adult and display communicative function.
PIC Picture Exchange	Exchange of visual pictures/symbols with another person in order to communicate.

TABLE 27–2. *continued*

Symbolic Forms	Definitions
s One-word signs	Recognizable one-word manual signs that are accompanied by communicative intent.
v One-word verbalizations	Recognizable spoken one-word utterances that are accompanied by communicative intent.
s+v One-word signs + verbalization	Combination of a spoken one-word utterance with its corresponding sign.
ss Multi-word signs	Combination of two or more recognizable signs that have communicative intent.
vv Multi-word verbalizations	Combination of two or more word utterances that have communicative intent.
ss+vv Multi-word signs + verbalizations	Combination of spoken multi-word utterance with its corresponding signs.
VOCA One or multi-word VOCA	Voice output communication aid (VOCA) on a computerized augmentative and alternative communication device that is used to communicate a message (e.g., Dynavox).

TABLE 27–3. Communicative Functions: Abbreviations and Definitions

Functions	Definitions
Behavioral Regulation	Communicative acts that attempt to affect another person's behavior.
RQOB Request Object	Request that the communicative partner give the desired object
RQAC Request Action	Request that the communicative partner perform an action.
PROT Protest	Indication of a disagreement with what the communicative partner is doing/not doing.
Social Interaction	Communicative acts seeking interaction with a partner.
RQSR Requesting social routine	Request that the communicative partner interact by performing a social routine (i.e., playing peek-a-boo).
RQCT Requesting comfort	Request that the communicative partner provide comfort (i.e., holding the child, providing favorite blanket).
GREET Greeting	Salutations to a communicative partner when he/she enters or exits (i.e. waving or saying hello and goodbye).

continues

TABLE 27–3. *continued*

Functions	Definitions
CALL Calling	Attempt to gain the attention of a communicative partner with the intent to communicate something.
RQPM Requesting permission	Request that communicative partner give permission to obtain an object or perform an action.
SHOF Showing	Communication with the intent to perform or show a skill or object so the communicative partner may praise or comment.
Conversational Acts	Communicative acts used to exchange information about an object or event.
COMT Comments	Identification or description of an object or event that is observable (i.e., "We went to the store today," "That's a ball").
RQIN Request information	Communicative acts that seek information or explanations about an object or event (i.e., rising intonation, palms up gestures, wh-questions).
PRIN Provide information	Communicative act that give information requested by the communicative partner.
IMI Imitation	Partial or complete imitation of the communicative partner's previous utterance, gesture, vocalizations, or action.
RQCL Requests for clarification	Request that the communicative partner provide clarification of a previous utterance either by repeating or rephrasing.
ASST Statements	Opinion, evaluation, or thoughts that are not directly observable (e.g., "I love ice cream," "I'm finished with that").
PERF Performative	Jokes, warnings, or teasing that are often accompanied by laughing and/or an expectant look.
RSAC Response to requests for action	Verbal or gestural communicative act that accompanies a requested action from the partner.
RSCL Response to requests for clarification	Attempt to repeat and/or clarify a previous utterance after the communicative partner directly or indirectly requests clarification.
RSAT Response to requests for attention	Utterances (i.e., "Yes," "What?") that signal to the partner that he/she is attending to the partner after the partner has requested attention.
RSAS Response to assertives & performatives	Responses (i.e., "uh-huh," "okay") that add no new information but let the partner know that he/she is paying attention and that the partner can continue; agreements.

Communication Categories

Results from the 21 participants in the study were sorted into three categories based on communication level as measured by rate, form, and function. Those in Category I were labeled "presymbolic communicators" and communicated at a low rate, using mostly presymbolic forms, and mainly behavioral regulation to communicate. Individuals in Category III, "symbolic communicators," communicated at a high rate, used mainly symbolic forms, and used primarily the function of conversational acts. Individuals in Category II, "transitional communicators," fell in between the presymbolic and symbolic communicators. Examples and descriptions of participants in each category are presented below with explanations on how the coding scheme can be utilized

Participant #1: Presymbolic Communicator

Participant #1 (P1) is a 9 year old female who communicates at the beginning levels of intentional communication. She has severe to profound mixed (sensorineural and conductive) hearing loss bilaterally and is aided by hearing aids. She has very limited vision in her right eye and reduced vision in her left eye due to coloboma and myopia. She wears corrective lenses. She is unable to walk independently, using a wheelchair for mobility. Her parent reported that she began receiving speech and language therapy by age 3.

P1's communication is intentional and presymbolic but very limited in the variety of communicative forms and functions used. Her parent reports that she communicates through emotional responses, direct behaviors, gestures, vocalizations, single word signs, and object symbols.

In the communication sample, P1 communicated at a very low rate (1.0 act/min). The number of communicative forms and functions she used are indicated by the gray shaded boxes in Table 27–4. All of her functions fall in the upper left area of the coding scheme, indicating that she is at a beginning level of presymbolic communication. All of her communicative acts are presymbolic, and she only uses four different forms. The majority of her communicative forms are two early-developing forms: physical manipulation and reaching. Her communicative functions were mostly behavioral regulations, with only one conversational act.

The analysis reveals that P1 is at a presymbolic level of intentional communication and is limited in expressing a variety of communicative functions. Most standardized testing protocols would indicate that she is several standard deviations below the mean for her age, which is true but unhelpful in determining how to advance her communication skills. This analysis provides specific information about what communicative skills P1 does utilize. It also shows that this child has the ability to use a higher developing communicative function (provide information), but needs assistance in increasing her rate of communication and developing higher-level communicative forms to

TABLE 27–4. Coding Scheme for Participant #1 (9:0 female): Pre-Symbolic Communicator

COMMUNICATIVE FUNCTION		COMMUNICATIVE FORM														Symbolic			
		Pre-Symbolic																	
		CRY	TANT	AGRES	PM	GAZE	GIVE	SHOW	REACH	CP	DP	SHAKE	NOD	GEST	VOC	Pic X	1 word	Multi	VOCA
Behavioral Regulation	RQOB				7				5										
	RQAC				1										1				
	PROT																		
Social Interaction	RQSR																		
	RQCT																		
	GREET																		
	CALL																		
	RQPM																		
	SHOW																		
Conversational Act	COMT																		
	RQIN																		
	PRIN					1													
	IMI																		
	RQCL																		
	ASST																		
	PERF																		
	RSAC																		
	RSCL																		
	RSAT																		
	RSAS																		

Communicative Rate = 1.0 acts/min

increase the range of her communication. Language therapy should focus on increasing her rate of communication, teaching the use of later-developing presymbolic forms, and increasing her communicative forms to include more social interaction and conversational acts.

Participant #2: Transitional Communicator

Participant #2 (P2) is a 13-year-old male with CHARGE syndrome. He has severe to profound hearing loss in his left ear and mild to moderate hearing loss in his right ear; both ears are aided with conventional hearing aids. His parent reports that his vision is stable, and he wears glasses. He is able to walk independently, with some balance problems due to low muscle tone in his upper body and likely disturbed vestibular function of the inner ear. P2 has a tracheostomy and is unable to vocalize. He currently attends middle school with a one-on-one aid. He receives speech and language therapy and occupational therapy at school.

P2 uses communication intentionally with a combination of presymbolic and symbolic forms of communication. His parent reports that he uses mainly sign language, emotional responses (facial expression, crying, looking), direct behaviors (reaching for objects, physically manipulating another person's hand), and gestures to communicate. He most frequently uses single words but also uses some 2–5 word sign language phrases to communicate. P2 uses symbolic communication but is not yet at a conversational level of communication.

P2 communicated more frequently than P1, but his rate of communication was still low for a symbolic communicator (4.1 acts/min). P2's communicative functions and forms fall mostly in the lower half of the table (Table 27–5). The table indicates that P2's development of symbolic communication is emerging, as he uses mostly 1-word signs along with several other presymbolic forms. In this sample, P2 often uses presymbolic forms of communication, such as distal pointing, showing, head nodding, gestures, and physical manipulation. He used a variety of communicative functions (10 different functions), most of which were the highest category of function, conversational acts. However, communicative acts were mostly responses (responses to requests for information or responses to assertives and performatives), which indicates that he rarely initiated communication.

This analysis shows that P2 is in a transitional stage between presymbolic and symbolic communication, and intervention should focus on expanding his expressive signs to 2–5 word combinations. Intervention should also target increasing his initiations, including increasing requests, protests, comments, and statements. Again, for this participant, standardized testing would only indicate age-related skills that he does not use, instead of indicating what communication skills he does use which can be expanded upon.

TABLE 27–5. Coding Scheme for Participant #2 (13:1 male): Transitional Communicator

COMMUNICATIVE FUNCTION		COMMUNICATIVE FORM																	
		Pre-Symbolic															Symbolic		
		CRY	TANT	AGRES	PM	GAZE	GIVE	SHOW	REACH	CP	DP	SHAKE	NOD	GEST	VOC	Pic X	1 word	Multi	VOCA
Behavioral Regulation	RQOB																		
	RQAC																s 1		
	PROT																		
Social Interaction	RQSR																		
	RQCT																		
	GREET																		
	CALL																		
	RQPM					1		1											
	SHOW																		
Conversational Act	COMT									2							s 4	ss 1	
	RQIN									8							s 9	ss 1	
	PRIN												13						
	IMI									1				1			s 1		
	RQCL																		
	ASST																		
	PERF					1		3											
	RSAC									1									
	RSCL									2								ss 1	
	RSAT												9						
	RSAS																		

Communicative Rate = 4.1 acts/min

Participant #3: Symbolic Communicator

Participant #3 (P3) is a 9½-year-old female who is at a conversational level of language development. She has a severe to profound bilateral hearing loss, which is aided by a Bone-Anchored Hearing Aid (BAHA) Divino Implant. She has several visual problems (far-sightedness, astigmatism, coloboma, amblyopia, extropia), but her parent reports that her functional vision is very good with corrective lenses. She is able to walk independently but has some balance problems.

P3 first received language therapy at age 12 months and is currently attending a regular education classroom. She communicates at a conversational level through spoken English. Her mother reports that she occasionally needs the support of manual signs along with spoken words for understanding.

In the communication sample, P3 communicated at a much higher rate than P1 or P2 (6.5 act/min). The shading in the table (Table 27–6) is mostly on the far right column, which indicates that she is a symbolic communicator at a conversational level. P3 utilized a variety of communicative functions (9 of 20), and most of them were conversational acts, such as responses to assertives and performatives and responses to requests for clarification. Her most frequent communicative functions were provide information, responses to requests for clarification, and requests for information. She rarely used communicative functions to initiate communication such as comments, statements, protests, and requests for action in this communicative sample.

The analysis indicates that while P3 is at a conversational level of communication, she still shows areas of weakness in her use of different communicative functions. Intervention should focus on increasing her initiations of communication, especially comments and statements.

SUMMARY

The forms of communication used by individuals with CHARGE are diverse, in part because each individual's patterns of anomalies are diverse. The development of communication in these individuals is nearly always very significantly delayed and may progress at a very slow rate because of these anomalies. Most standardized tests will indicate that the individual with CHARGE is performing well below age level but will not indicate what abilities are present and which are missing. The procedures described above provide a method for analyzing and describing the communication abilities that are specific to the individual and not related to chronological age.

The cases presented above illustrate the wide range of communication skills of individuals with CHARGE at similar ages. In two of the cases presented (P1 and P2), the individuals had grossly delayed communication development.

TABLE 27–6. Coding Scheme for Participant #3 (9:6 female): Symbolic Communicator

COMMUNICATIVE FUNCTION		Pre-Symbolic														Symbolic			
		CRY	TANT	AGRES	PM	GAZE	GIVE	SHOW	REACH	CP	DP	SHAKE	NOD	GEST	VOC	Pic X	1 word	Multi	VOCA
Behavioral Regulation	RQOB																		
	RQAC													1				vv 4	
	PROT														1		v 1		
Social Interaction	RQSR																		
	RQCT																		
	GREET																		
	CALL																	vv 1	
	RQPM																		
	SHOW																		
Conversational Act	COMT																	vv 4	
	RQIN							1									v 1	vv 14	
	PRIN																v 38	vv 10	
	IMI																		
	RQCL																		
	ASST																v 1	vv 2	
	PERF																		
	RSAC																		
	RSCL													1			v 8	vv 5	
	RSAT																		
	RSAS																v 3	vv 1	

Communicative Rate = 6.5 acts/min

At 9 and 13 years of age, each showed a limited ability to use symbolic communication with sign language. However, the analyses revealed that the communication abilities of these two individuals are very different with respect to their use of communication forms and functions. The 13 year old (P2) communicated at a much higher rate and with several symbolic forms, while the 9 year old (P1) used only presymbolic forms. P2 also showed a much better ability to communicate for a variety of purposes, like to make specific requests, comment, and respond to requests than did P1. While P3 was at a much higher level of communication, the analysis still revealed some specific areas of weakness in her expressive communication. Although this type of analysis is very time-consuming, it may be what is required to understand why one individual behaves very differently than another and to plan appropriate language and communication strategies for each child.

The communicative forms, functions, and rate included in the coding scheme for these analyses mainly targeted presymbolic and early symbolic communication. This was done because a very substantial percentage of individuals with CHARGE syndrome communicate at the presymbolic level and because there are few formal procedures for evaluating expressive communication at this level. For individuals with CHARGE who use a higher level of symbolic communication, standardized tests may be appropriate, but analysis with King's coding scheme may still have value in describing patterns of usage that are unusual in typically developing individuals. For each of the individuals described in this chapter, the value of the coding scheme was that it provided a *description* of capabilities and limitations of the individual that was useful as a tool to understand the individual's current communication abilities.

From this initial attempt, we know that communication in children with CHARGE syndrome ranges from little or no intentional communication to nearly age-appropriate symbolic communication. Regardless of their abilities, persistence in promoting development of communication skills is critical for the well-being of the child at all levels of communication.

REFERENCES

Brady, N. (2005). "Assessment strategies." In Communication services for individuals with severe disabilities: Current "best practices." National Joint Committee for the Communication Needs of Persons with Severe Disabilities. http://www.asha.org/ .../58B96E5A-012D-4A87-A416-C31EDE0451DB/0/ASHA2005NJCseminar.pdf

Brady, N., & Bashinski, S. (2007). *Increased communication in deafblind children after adapted PMT intervention.* Paper presented at meeting of the American Speech-Language-Hearing Association, Boston, MA.

Brady, N. C., Marquis, J., Fleming, K., & McLean, L. (2004). Prelinguistic predictors of language growth in children with developmental disabilities. *Journal of Speech, Language, and Hearing Research, 47,* 663–677.

Brown, D. (2005). CHARGE syndrome "behaviors": Challenges or adaptations? *American Journal of Medical Genetics, 133A,* 268–272.

Bruce, S. M. (2005). The impact of congenital deafblindness on the struggle to symbolism. *International Journal of Disability, Development and Education, 52*(3), 233–251.

Bruce, S. M., Godbold, E., & Naponelli-Gold, S. (2004). An analysis of communicative functions of teachers and their students who are congenitally deafblind. *Rehabilitation Education for Blindness and Visual Impairment, 36*(2), 81–90.

Bruce, S. M., Mann, A., Jones, C., & Gavin, M. (2007). Gestures expressed by children who are congenitally deafblind: Topography, rate, and function. *Journal of Visual Impairment & Blindness, 101,* 637–652.

Coggins, T. E., & Carpenter, R. L. (1981). The communication intention inventory: A system for coding intentions in infants eight to fifteen months of age. *Language and Speech 26*(Part II), 101–116.

Crais, E. R., Watson, L. R., & Baranek, G. T. (2009). Use of gesture development in profiling children's prelinguistic communication skills. *American Journal of Speech Language Pathology, 18,* 95–108.

Fey, M. E. (1986). *Language intervention with young children.* San Diego, CA: College Hill Press.

Hagood, L. (1997). *Communication: A guide for teaching students with visual and multiple impairments.* Austin, TX: Capital Printing Company.

King, E. (2009). *Communicative rate, form, and function in CHARGE syndrome.* Unpublished master's thesis, University of Tennessee, Knoxville, Tennessee.

King, E., Swanson, L., Thelin, J., & Steele, N. (2007). *An analysis of communicative intentions in children with CHARGE syndrome.* Presented at The 8th International CHARGE Conference, Costa Mesa, CA.

King Miller, E., Swanson, L., Steele, N., Thelin, S., Schwarz, I., & Thelin, J. (2009, July). *Communication assessment in CHARGE syndrome.* Paper presented at meeting of the 9th International CHARGE Conference, Chicago, IL.

McLean, J., & Synder-McLean, L. (1999). *How children learn language.* San Diego, CA: Singular Publishing.

Miles, B. (2005). Overview on deafblindness. *DB-Link,* 1–6.

National Joint Committee for the Communication Needs of Persons with Severe Disabilities. (1992). *Guidelines for meeting the communication needs of persons with severe disabilities* [Guidelines]. Available from www.asha.org/policy or www.asha.org/njc

Peltokorpi, S., & Huttunen, K. (2008). Communication in the early stage of language development of children with CHARGE syndrome. *British Journal of Visual Impairment, 26*(1), 24–49.

Stephenson, J., & Linfoot, K. (1996). Intentional communication and graphic symbol use by students with severe intellectual disability. *International Journal of Disability, Development, and Education, 43*(2), 147–165.

Swanson, L., King, E., Thelin, J., & Steele, N. (2007). *Communication skills of children with CHARGE.* Paper presented at meeting of the American Speech-Language-Hearing Association, Boston, MA.

Thelin, J. W., & Swanson, L. (2006). CHARGE syndrome. *The ASHA Leader, 11*(14), 6–7.

Watt, N., Wetherby, A., & Shumway, S. (2006). Prelinguistic predictors of language outcome at 3 years age. *Journal of Speech, Language, and Hearing Research, 49,* 1224–1237.

Wetherby, A. H., Cain, D. H., Yonclas, D. G. & Walker, V. G. (1988). Analysis of intentional communication of normal children from the prelinguistic to the multiword stage. *Journal of Speech and Hearing Research, 31*, 240–252.

Wetherby, A., & Prizant, B. (2001). *Checklist for communicative forms and means.* Presented at The 'SCERTS' Model for Enhancing Communicative and Socioemotional Competence from Early Intervention to the Early School Years" Conference, Cincinnati, OH.

Wetherby, A., & Prizant, B. (2003). *CSBS manual: Communication and symbolic behavior scales manual—Normed edition.* Baltimore, MD: Paul H. Brookes.

Wolf-Schein, E. B., & Schein, J. D. (1998, August). *The case for nonintrusive assessment of children who are deafblind.* Paper presented at meeting of the Canadian Conference on Deafblindness, Mississauga, Ontario.

Yoder, P. J., Warren, S. F., & McCathren, R. B. (1998). Determining spoken language prognosis in children with developmental disabilities. *American Journal of Speech-Language Pathology, 7*, 77–87.

PART V

Psychological Issues in CHARGE Syndrome

By the middle of the 1990s, it was becoming clear that many of the behavioral features observed in some children with CHARGE were actually common. Parents and professionals began to search for guidance in coping with some severely challenging behaviors. By the end of that decade, the use of psychotropic medication in children with CHARGE was fairly widespread. Although great strides have been made, there is much more to learn about behavioral issues in CHARGE. We begin with a look at the emerging behavioral phenotype (Chapter 28), followed by an examination of psychiatric issues and the use of medications in CHARGE (Chapter 29). The chapters on pain (Chapter 30) and stress (Chapter 31) address two sources of behavioral challenges. Finally, some considerations for parenting children with CHARGE are presented (Chapter 32).

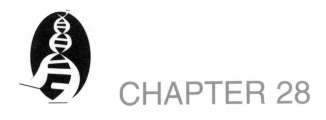

CHAPTER 28

Behavioral Phenotype

TIMOTHY S. HARTSHORNE, Ph.D.

*U*nusual behavior often is associated with genetic syndromes; therefore, it is not surprising that children with CHARGE syndrome exhibit characteristic behaviors. Sometimes, the behaviors of individuals with genetic syndromes are lumped into psychiatric categories such as autism or obsessive-compulsive disorder (OCD). An alternative approach is to attempt to identify the truly unique behavioral features associated with different syndromes. The identification and description of a behavioral phenotype helps parents and professionals focus on the specific and distinct behaviors of a particular syndrome.

A behavioral phenotype is "A pattern of behavior that is reliably identified in groups of children with known genetic disorders and is not learned" (Harris, 1995). In other words, if a person shows this unique behavior, "the behavior suggests the diagnosis" (Harris, 2006). For example, children with Down syndrome, as a group, will exhibit different behaviors or behavioral patterns than children with CHARGE syndrome or Prader-Willi syndrome. Interest in behavioral phenotypes has been increasing over the past 20 years. The field is populated by psychiatrists and other physicians, psychologists, special educators, and researchers, including those specializing in genetics, physiology, and neurology. For some disorders, aspects of a behavioral phenotype are well known. Overeating in people with Prader-Willi syndrome, sociability in persons with Down syndrome, and musical talent among those with Williams syndrome are common examples. There is always a danger in overgeneralizing among a specific group of people. Because of a shared genetic condition, similarities are likely. However, just as in the case of monozygotic twins, there will also be individual differences.

Two principles are important (Hodapp & Ricci, 2002). First, the effects of genetic disorders are "probabilistic," not "deterministic." Those with Prader-Willi syndrome are more likely than persons with other disorders to overeat, but there are exceptions. Second, every genetic syndrome will not necessarily have its own unique behavior. Even with these caveats, it can be helpful to know the range of behaviors that are likely to be encountered with any particular syndrome.

Research on a behavioral phenotype for CHARGE syndrome has been ongoing for a number of years (Hartshorne, Hefner, & Davenport, 2005). CHARGE is particularly challenging because of the large number of physical anomalies, the extreme variability among those with CHARGE, and historically a lack of clarity in diagnosis. However, progress on understanding the behavior is being made. All children behave, and really, all children misbehave. So, it is not surprising that children with CHARGE misbehave. But the concern in CHARGE is that behaviors often disrupt family and educational settings and at times, can even become so extreme or challenging that the persons with CHARGE can be a danger to themselves or others.

When a child with CHARGE has behavior challenges, the question frequently asked is whether this behavior is a manifestation of CHARGE or has other causes. There are four general sources of challenging behavior. First, the sensory and other physical problems in children with CHARGE affect how they experience and understand the world, and these perceptions in turn influence their behavior. Second, negative life experiences such as painful medical procedures or social relationship difficulties like bullying may lead to negative behavior. Third, environmental factors such as distractions, physical barriers, and poor acoustics can all influence behavior. Finally, some behavior patterns may be related to having a specific genetic disorder like CHARGE syndrome, independent of the sensory and physical difficulties. All four sources operate continuously and interact with each other. Sorting out the influences on the unique behaviors of a specific person can be complicated for any child. The variability among persons with CHARGE makes this task even more difficult.

So, is the behavior just CHARGE? It might be, but simply acknowledging that the behavior is part of CHARGE may imply that nothing can be done about it. This is not the case. Even though the behaviors may be to some extent due to features of CHARGE, that does not mean that intervention is useless or should not be attempted. On the other hand, saying "no, it is not CHARGE," is likely to lead to unrealistic expectations for the child's behavior. Every child is unique, and their behavior is unique. But as we study behavior in CHARGE, certain similarities and patterns are emerging. This chapter outlines seven features that together constitute a preliminary CHARGE Behavioral Phenotype. These are listed in Table 28–1.

TABLE 28–1. A CHARGE Behavioral Phenotype

Low normal cognitive functioning

Very goal directed and persistent with a sense of humor

Socially interested but immature

Repetitive behaviors that increase under stress

High levels of sensation seeking

Under conditions of stress and sensory overload, find it difficult to self-regulate and easily lose behavioral control

Difficulty with shifting attention and transitioning to new activities; easily lost in own thoughts

A PRELIMINARY BEHAVIORAL PHENOTYPE

1. Low Normal Cognitive Functioning

This may be the most controversial portion of the proposed behavioral phenotype. There is a wide range of abilities in children with CHARGE, including cognitive ability (see Chapter 20). Measuring or predicting cognitive ability in individuals with CHARGE is enormously challenging, if not impossible. But there is a distinction between "ability" and "functioning." There is a wide range of functioning among those with CHARGE. This can be attributed, in part, to many of the characteristics of CHARGE, especially the multi-sensory impairments. The few studies which have been done (see Chapter 20) have found a range of functioning, with a tendency toward the low normal range. As noted in Blake, et al., (1998), this is a major shift from earlier presumptions that children with CHARGE were all significantly cognitively impaired. Parents and educators should be optimistic about the ability of the child with CHARGE to learn and be successful in school and in life.

2. Very Goal-Directed and Persistent with a Sense of Humor

Children with CHARGE charge ahead. The following quote from David Brown nicely encapsulates this component of the phenotype: "I know of no identified subgroup within the population of people with multisensory impairment who have so many medical problems, of such complexity and severity, and with so many hidden or delayed difficulties, and yet no sub-group has shown such a consistent ability to rise triumphantly above these problems" (Brown,

1997). Children with CHARGE seem to know what they want and persist in their intentions. This stubborn persistence helps them to learn to walk, to eat, and to achieve beyond all expectations. It also creates difficulties for parents and educators, for when these children have an idea of what they want, they can have a lot of difficulty letting go of that idea. This is complicated by difficulties the child may have in expressing exactly what it is he or she wants. Parents and educators may recognize that there is something the child wants, but may not be able to identify it, and must simply watch helplessly as the child's behavior becomes more and more extreme until all control is lost. Fortunately, children with CHARGE also demonstrate a ready sense of humor which can be infectious (see Sidebar 28–1).

3. Socially Interested But Immature

Hartshorne and Cypher (2004) found that difficulty making same-age friendships was a frequent problem for children with CHARGE. When measured against children with autism or those who were deafblind from other conditions, Hartshorne, Grialou, and Parker (2005) found those with CHARGE were much more interested in relating to others and having friendships. However, making friends is difficult for children with CHARGE. They appear to have difficulty understanding other children and often miss or misunderstand social cues. Multisensory impairments are undoubtedly part of the problem, as is communication, but learning to play nicely, to take turns, and to back off when necessary, are all skills that seem to be hard for children with CHARGE to learn or grasp (see Chapter 21).

4. Repetitive Behaviors That Increase under Stress

Repetitive behaviors, or engaging in apparently purposeless behaviors, seem to be very common in CHARGE. Bernstein and Denno (2005) and Hartshorne and Cypher (2004) both found, for example, that ordering objects in a pattern was common. Other common repetitive behaviors observed by Bernstein and Denno included performing tasks in a certain order, eating specific foods at particular meals, following a set schedule, asking the same questions over and over, and being fascinated by numbers or dates. Bernstein and Denno found that these behaviors interfere with the daily life of some of the children and that it is extremely difficult to stop the behaviors once they have started. Frequently, the children will react aggressively when attempts to redirect their behavior are made. Individuals with repetitive behaviors are often diagnosed as having obsessive compulsive disorder (OCD). OCD is one type of anxiety disorder, with compulsions acting as a means to reduce anxiety. For example, when one particular young adult with CHARGE is anxious, she lines up her shoes.

Sidebar 28–1
CHARGE Sense of Humor

Parents of children with CHARGE know to start running when they hear that laugh or giggle coming from wherever their child might be. Is the cochlear implant flushed down the toilet? Have more treasures been stuffed down the floor air vent? Is the phone now hidden in the trash? The CHARGE sense of humor is a bit mischievous.

They also really enjoy setting people up. For example, Jeff loved math and was very good at it. "When he was still in high school his teacher would give him math worksheets to do. He could do them easily. Because he was so good at math, she would just skim the page and give him a happy face sticker. He got to where he would TEST the teacher. Every once in a while he would purposely put a wrong answer down. He'd wait as the teacher would go over his paper with him, and if she missed the one that was wrong, he'd just start laughing. Then he'd point to the one that was wrong. Once she caught on to his game, she made sure she didn't skim the paper anymore. But he still would test her and laugh." Jeff and another boy from his special needs class worked on job skills at McDonalds. "They were each given a McDonalds polo shirt to wear when they were working there. They were to change into their shirts before they left to walk to McDonalds. The other boy was usually later getting to the restroom to change than Jeff was. The shirts were kept in a cabinet in the restroom. Jeff would put on the other boy's shirt and come out just laughing away. When the other boy saw that Jeff had on his shirt, he'd get upset and tell the teacher Jeff was wearing HIS shirt, and Jeff would just bend over double laughing. Then he'd go change into his own McDonalds shirt. He just enjoyed teasing the other boy."

They can also be stand ups. "My 13 year old does not do well with surprises, even pleasant ones, and playing it by ear is just not in her repertoire. One day we were driving to see a children's play, and my husband asked if we were having dinner with my family afterwards, and if so, would they be bringing their friends. I hesitated before answering, and in that moment of silence, I hear my daughter from the backseat demand: 'Talk to me!' Tim once asked what time it was. I said, 'Look at the clock and tell me.' He said, 'I don't know that time I only know Verizon time!'" Another example, "We were at a doctor appointment today. After some questions and answers, Nate said to the doctor, 'I'm NOT a well-oiled machine'. I think this sums up his sense of humor AND his life!"

This behavior helps her to cope with her anxiety. Thus, under conditions of stress repetitive behavior may increase. Finding ways to reduce stress in children with CHARGE is one way to reduce repetitive behaviors. It is important to note that OCD very often occurs along with tic disorders and attention deficit hyperactivity disorder (ADHD) in children with CHARGE (Hartshorne & Cypher, 2004).

5. High Degree of Sensation Seeking

Light flicking, hand flapping, body shaking, and rocking are among the self-stimulatory behaviors that are common in children with CHARGE. Hartshorne, Grialou, and Parker (2005) found higher average scores on the Autism Behavior Checklist (Krug, Arick, & Almond, 1993) for these kinds of behaviors in children with CHARGE than in children who were deafblind from other conditions. Although increased over children with other forms of deafblindness, the levels still did not reach the level of children with autism. Brown (2005) attributes these behaviors in part to sensory integration difficulties, which he believes to be inherent in CHARGE. Not only are multiple senses impaired in CHARGE, sensory input is also not well processed and integrated, so that the child may find loud noises painful, may want to move away from lots of visual stimulation, or may just focus on a particular light source (Figure 28–1).

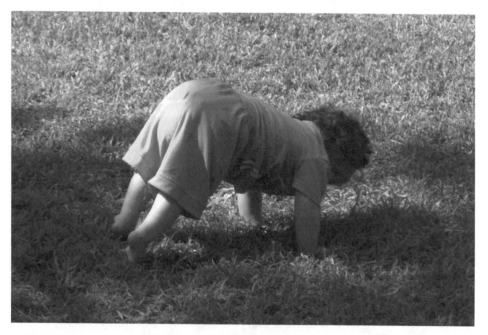

FIGURE 28–1. Due to tactile sensitivity, some children with CHARGE may find the touch of grass to be uncomfortable.

Although self-stimulatory behaviors can clearly interfere with other activities, they also may function as a means of receiving enough sensory stimulation during the course of the day to compensate for poor functioning of some of the sensory modalities. They also may be an important means of regrouping and reorienting. For example, a hard-working student might suddenly drop everything and shake his or her whole body for a moment, and then be able to go back to work (Figure 28–2).

6. Under Conditions of Stress and Sensory Overload, Find It Difficult to Self-Regulate and Easily Lose Behavioral Control

Every person has a different threshold for arousal. Some people need a lot of poking and prodding to get out of bed in the morning while others jump out in response to a soft tap. People also vary in their ability to tune out things in the environment. One person might be distracted by the background noise of a tapping pencil while others remain totally focused on work even in the presence of a loud television. Most of us find ways to maintain our equilibrium in the presence of varying activities and sensations around us. This is often difficult for individuals with CHARGE. At one moment they may crave some stimulation and actively seek it, for example by lying on a vibrating mat.

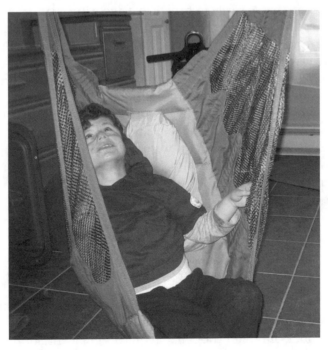

FIGURE 28–2. Lying in a swing might provide helpful sensory stimulation.

But at some point, the vibration might send them over the sensory edge and cause loss of behavioral control. They seem to experience a great deal of both too little and too much stimulation, and can seem to rapidly shift from one extreme to the other. At one moment the child is happily watching a spinning light, and then a split second later is pressing their face into the light and crying. It is important to point out that this loss of control may at times be due to physical pain the child is experiencing. Children with CHARGE may have difficulties expressing pain directly (see Chapter 30).

7. Difficulty with Shifting Attention and Transitioning to New Activities; Easily Lost in Own Thoughts

There are many reasons to become lost in one's own thoughts. For someone with sensory impairments, it takes intensive powers of concentration to stay focused on an external activity. But parents and educators have observed that sensory challenges do not seem to account for all of the difficulty children with CHARGE seem to have with managing their attention. Nicholas (2005) hypothesized that this was due to problems with the executive functions. These are the neurologically based functions that help to direct attention, memory, and the processing of information. Hartshorne, Nicholas, Grialou, and Russ (2007) found that children with CHARGE have many difficulties with executive function in general, and in three areas in particular. One is the ability to *shift*, or to move freely from activity to activity or situation to situation. Problems with shift are reflected in poor problem solving, rigidity, a need for consistent routines, and in extreme cases, repetitive behaviors. A second function that was impaired in CHARGE is *initiate*, or being able to start an activity or make a statement, and knowing how to respond or problem solve in new situations and transitions. An example of a mild difficulty with *initiate* is a child who wants to begin a task, but simply cannot get started. More extreme examples are difficulty clearly communicating what it is you want to say or the need for multiple cues for what you should do. The third function that was most impaired was *monitor*, or the ability to monitor one's own actions and their impact on other people. Examples include careless school work or not understanding how certain actions might bother other people.

RECOMMENDATIONS

Even though preliminary, this behavioral phenotype leads to some concrete recommendations. First, assume the child with CHARGE has enough ability to succeed in school, although they may require significant support and assistance. Second, recognize that it will not be easy to change the child's goals. Parents and teachers will do better by helping to develop appropriate behavioral goals on the part of the child. Third, the child most likely does not have a lot of social support (see Chapter 21) and this may be a problem in school and increasingly an issue in adolescence and beyond. Fourth, identifying possible sources of stress and anxiety and ways to limit them may reduce some of the repetitive behavior. Fifth, the child most likely needs considerable sensory input and stimulation, although not all of the time. Helping the child to learn to recognize and regulate their degree of sensory and emotional arousal is important. Sixth, watch out for emotional and behavioral meltdowns. When these occur, the child may need some time to regroup. Finally, children with CHARGE seem to thrive on schedules that are regular and predictable. Considerable preparation and advance warning can prevent problems when schedules and events change.

Behavioral Threshold

Many children with CHARGE have been observed to have abrupt changes in behavior, particularly to self-abusive or apparently aggressive behaviors. These can seem to come out of the blue. To understand this, consider the presence of a behavioral threshold. Below the threshold, the child is under control, but over the threshold behavioral control is lost. Children with CHARGE cross this threshold very abruptly and rapidly. One cause, as noted previously, can be the amount of sensory stimulation they are experiencing at the moment. This can change from pleasant or bearable to painful and upsetting very quickly. A second cause can be attributed to the buildup of stress in the child's environment to the point where they can no longer cope (see Chapter 31). Third, and perhaps most importantly, this can be due to the experience of pain (see Chapter 30). A change in health status such as ear infection (or fluid in the ears), sinus infection, intestinal gas, or migraine can cross the threshold from manageable pain to unmanageable very suddenly. Due to the communication difficulties often experienced by children with CHARGE, the behavior may actually be both a reaction to the pain or other change and a means of expressing or communicating that something is wrong. An underlying medical/pain situation should always be considered when dealing with sudden, challenging behavior. Because these medical conditions can be at times very difficult to diagnose, any sudden change in behavior should prompt a thorough evaluation for possible medical causes.

SUMMARY

The preceding is an initial and very preliminary description of a CHARGE behavioral phenotype. Because CHARGE is so variable, it is challenging to make statements that clearly apply to most people with the syndrome. However, even given this variability, the seven characteristics seem to describe a great deal of what we have observed and studied in persons with CHARGE. Work is needed to confirm and amend the profile.

REFERENCES

Bernstein, V., & Denno, L. S. (2005). Repetitive behaviors in CHARGE syndrome: Differential diagnosis and treatment options. *American Journal of Medical Genetics, 133A*, 232–239.

Blake, K. D., Davenport, S. L. H., Hall, B. D., Hefner, M. A., Pagon, R. A., Williams, M. S., . . . Graham, J. M. (1998). CHARGE association: Am update and review for the primary pediatrician. *Clinical Pediatrics, 37*, 159–173.

Brown D. (1997). CHARGE Association. *Talking Sense*, Summer, 18–20.

Brown, D. (2005). CHARGE syndrome "behaviors": challenges or adaptations? *American Journal of Medical Genetics, 133A*, 268–272.

Harris, J. C. (1995). *Developmental neuropsychiatry*. New York, NY: Oxford University Press.

Harris, J. C. (2006). *Intellectual disability: Understanding its development, causes, classification, evaluation, and treatment.* New York, NY: Oxford University Press.

Hartshorne, T. S., & Cypher, A. L. (2004). Challenging behavior in CHARGE Syndrome. *Mental Health Aspect Developmental Disability, 7(2)*, 41–52.

Hartshorne, T. S., Grialou, T. L., & Parker, K. R. (2005). Autistic-like behavior in CHARGE syndrome. *American Journal of Medical Genetics, 133A*, 257–261.

Hartshorne, T. S., Hefner, M. A., & Davenport, S. L. H. (2005). Behavior in CHARGE Syndrome: Introduction to the series. *American Journal of Medical Genetics, 133A*, 228–231.

Hartshorne, T. S., Nicholas, J., Grialou, T. L., & Russ, A. M. (2007). Executive function in CHARGE syndrome. *Child Neuropsychology, 13*, 333–344.

Hodapp, R. M., & Ricci, L. A. (2002). Behavioral phenotypes and educational practice: The unrealized connection. In G. O'Brien (Ed), *Behavioral phenotypes in clinical practice* (pp. 137–151). London, UK: Mac Keith Press.

Krug, D. A., Arick, J. R., & Almond, P. J. (1993). *Autism Screening Instrument for Educational Planning* (2nd ed.). Austin, TX: Pro-Ed.

Nicholas J. (2005). Can specific deficits in executive functioning explain the behavioral characteristics of CHARGE syndrome: A case study. *American Journal of Medical Genetics, 133A*, 300–305.

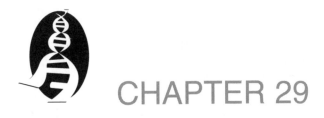

CHAPTER 29

Psychiatric Issues

LEE WACHTEL, M.D.

*T*his chapter aims to review our current knowledge of the psychiatric and behavioral challenges in CHARGE and proposes an organized method of assessment and treatment. Case examples are included.

After struggling in the early years of life with multiple medical problems affecting various organ systems, it certainly seems unjust that many children with CHARGE syndrome additionally demonstrate psychopathology in the form of various psychiatric diagnoses and challenging behaviors. Indeed, the presence of psychopathology in CHARGE syndrome has become a "hot topic" in recent years due to the significant negative impact of such on the overall functioning of many children, adolescents, and adults. CHARGE discussion groups are replete with desperate inquiries into psychiatric and behavioral symptomology, and children, adolescents, and adults with CHARGE have been diagnosed with various psychiatric illnesses and treated with multiple psychotropic and behavioral interventions, with varying success and many unanswered questions (Wachtel, Hartshorne, & Dailor, 2007). However, given the features of CHARGE syndrome, it is not surprising that psychiatric and behavioral issues are sometimes part of the phenotype.

PSYCHIATRIC DISTURBANCES IN PEOPLE WITH INTELLECTUAL DISABILITIES OR SENSORY DEFICITS

Numerous studies throughout the world have demonstrated significantly higher rates of *all known psychiatric illnesses* in the intellectually and developmentally disabled population as compared to those with typical development.

Estimates of the rate of psychiatric disturbance range from 10% to 80% in the intellectually disabled (ID) population, with a suggested prevalence 3–4 times that of the general population (Borthwick-Duffy, 1994; Kishore, Nizamie, Nizamie, & Jahan, 2004). Of course, not all children with CHARGE have intellectual impairments, but most will experience at least some form of developmental delay with decreased adaptive functioning (Salem-Hartshorne & Jacob, 2005), making it reasonable to conceptualize them within an intellectually and/or developmentally disabled population. Individuals with ID also are observed to have increased rates of "problem" or "challenging" behaviors. Prevalence rates in U.S. surveys of global ID suggest ranges from 2% to 28% for aggression, 10% to 31% for self-injury, and 7% to 30% for property destruction, with rates notably higher with more severe intellectual impairment and in institutional rather than community settings (Borthwick-Duffy, 1994; Eyman, Borthwick-Duffy, & Miller, 1981). Of course, some of the behaviors probably stem as much from situations as from the intellectual impairment or disorder.

Many genetic conditions are known to be associated with both psychiatric illness and aberrant behaviors (Einfeld, 2004; Harris, 2006). In fact, the study of psychopathology in genetic syndromes has led to the proposal of "behavioral phenotypes," or recognizable patterns of behavior associated with specific syndromes (Harris, 2006). CHARGE syndrome has a detailed somatic phenotype encompassing many organs, and the delineation of the CHARGE behavioral phenotype is actively under development (see Chapter 28).

Vision and hearing deficits are known to adversely affect social and interpersonal exchanges and also may have deleterious effects on behavior, resulting in reduced adaptive behavior and problem-solving abilities (Eaton & Menolascino, 1982; Matson & Sevin, 1994). The updated consensus guidelines for the treatment of behavioral disorders in the ID population includes sensory deficit as a "stressor" that may cause behavioral disturbance, with such being commonly reported in various blind and deaf-blind syndromes (Aman, et al., 2004; Carvill, 2005).

CHARGE FEATURES AND RISK FACTORS FOR PSYCHIATRIC ISSUES

Individuals with CHARGE have multiple risk factors for psychiatric illness and behavioral disturbance, including (1) intellectual and developmental disability, (2) presence of an underlying genetic syndrome, and (3) sensory deficits. Adding still the likely stresses of multiple chronic medical problems, hospitalizations, surgeries, and related early-age separations, educational, family, and service-related challenges, overwhelmed parents/caretakers and possible financial strain, it is actually difficult to imagine how an individual with CHARGE would *not* develop any psychological vulnerabilities.

PSYCHIATRIC DIAGNOSES IN INDIVIDUALS WITH CHARGE

CHARGE-specific research inquiries into behavioral and psychiatric pathology are illuminating. In a recent survey, Wachtel, Hartshorne, and Dailor (2007) asked parents to list diagnoses given for their child's "behavior." Of 87 children (ages 6 to 18), 32 (37%) had between one and five psychiatric diagnoses. The most common diagnostic category was anxiety disorders (17/87), including generalized anxiety and obsessive-compulsive disorder, followed by pervasive developmental disorders (PDD) (14/87), and attention-deficit-hyperactivity-disorder (ADHD) (11/87). Children with psychiatric diagnoses were found to have higher (more severe) scores on the Developmental Behavior Checklist, a scale designed to assess overall behavioral acuity (Einfeld & Tonge, 1995).

Additional CHARGE behavioral research echoes these findings, with evidence supporting the presence of both obsessive-compulsive and autistic-like features in individuals with CHARGE (Bernstein & Denno, 2005; Hartshorne & Cypher, 2004; Hartshorne, Grialou & Parker, 2005; Smith, Nichols, Issekutz, & Blake, 2005). Autism, a complex neuropsychiatric syndrome with likely multiple etiologies, is characterized in the current edition of the *Diagnostic and Statistical Manual (DSM-IV-TR)* by (1) deficits in social interaction, (2) communication impairment, and (3) repetitive, restricted, and stereotypical behaviors, interests and activities (APA, 2000). Many children with CHARGE easily fit anecdotally into such categories. Smith, et al. (2005) reported that the "majority of individuals with CHARGE syndrome show clinically significant symptoms associated with autism spectrum disorder." Hartshorne, et al. (2005) demonstrated autistic-like features in CHARGE, but also found that the CHARGE profile differs from both autism and deafblindness of other etiologies. Specifically, children with CHARGE were found to be more likely to make eye contact, allow touch, and be interested in friendships than those with autism or deafblindness; social impairment was overall seen as less in individuals with CHARGE.

In addition to the social and communicative challenges, the potential diagnosis of autism or a pervasive developmental disorder (PDD) frequently has been invoked based on the third category of autism diagnostic criteria (repetitive, restricted, and stereotypical behaviors, interests, and activities) to explain the repetitive behaviors including self-injury and aggression, often seen in children with CHARGE. Self-injury and aggression are well-known in CHARGE, with studies reporting prevalence rates from 40% to 54% for self-injury and 38% to 46% for aggression (Souriau, et al., 2005; Thelin & Fussner, 2005).

The issue of such repetitive behaviors, including self-injury and aggression, leads as well into the potential diagnosis of obsessive-compulsive disorder (OCD). The DSM-IV-TR diagnosis of OCD requires the presence of obsessions or compulsions that cause distress, are time-consuming, or significantly impair overall functioning (APA, 2004). These are frequently discussed problems in

CHARGE, with many families fully exasperated with their children's repetitive behaviors, particularly those that cause bodily injury and impair daily functioning. Bernstein and Denno (2005) found that not only did repetitive behaviors consume a large portion of their students' day, but blocking the behaviors often led to further self-injury and aggression.

Many parents, educators, and individuals with CHARGE themselves have described the overall challenges with OCD in CHARGE. One parent described her son "as if his mind got stuck in a rut," with various sorting, lining, and checking behaviors (Lauger, Cornelius, & Keedy, 2005). This author has worked with children with CHARGE with various obsessions, including vacuums, cameras, balloons, string, various toys, videos, repeated questioning regarding time and schedule, rigid arranging rituals, and categorical refusal to eat anything green. An adult with CHARGE described ongoing difficulties with worrying and rumination, alleviated only with antidepressant medication. Such challenges easily can overpower an individual's life; indeed, one young boy with CHARGE literally would have discussed various makes, models, and colors of vacuums during all waking hours if allowed.

It is extremely helpful that we are becoming more aware of some commonly encountered psychopathology in CHARGE. However, this is but the first step toward resolution. Indeed, the next question is "what in the world can be done?"

ASSESSMENT AND TREATMENT

Many individuals with CHARGE currently are not accessing the mental health services they need. The author has encountered individuals with CHARGE who have been dismissed by mental health-care providers as "just disabled," and given myriad psychiatric medications based on unclear indications and with poor evaluation of efficacy, side effects, or potential drug interactions. "Diagnostic overshadowing," or the tendency to simply ascribe psychopathology to the underlying disability, is a significant challenge throughout the field of ID (Reiss, 1993). The challenge becomes how to perform a comprehensive assessment of the child's overall psychiatric presentation and come up with an accurate diagnosis.

Ideally, psychiatric assessment of an individual with CHARGE should be undertaken by a mental health professional familiar with developmental disabilities, including CHARGE. However, even the psychiatrist who has never heard of CHARGE can arrive at an accurate assessment when offered an overall understanding of the challenges of the syndrome.

Assessment should include patient and parent interviews, as well as information from treating physicians, therapists, educators, caregivers, and service providers to gain a more complete picture of the patient. Best practice dictates that the developmentally disabled patient, *like any psychiatric patient*, be assessed for the full range of psychiatric illness (Reiss, 1993). Individuals with CHARGE utilize a wide variety of communication methods (see Chapter 25), and so someone familiar with their method, such as a sign language interpreter (not the patient's parent), should be present. The patient ideally should be observed in various settings, particularly as the office setting is artificial and not representative of daily situations. Multiple rating scales for psychiatric assessment in people with developmental disabilities exist (O'Brien, Pearson, Berney, & Barnard, 2001). These may provide further insight into the issues.

In addition to a review of "pure" psychiatric symptomology, a functional behavioral assessment generally should be pursued, especially in the case of prominent negative behaviors like self-injury and aggression. Classic psychiatric diagnoses may scratch only the surface of a disabled child's psychiatric and behavioral presentation. Indeed, many children with ID may have problem behaviors that are under operant, or environmental, control. Some behaviors may occur after specific events and have a history of producing reinforcing consequences that further strengthen the problem behaviors (Iwata, et al., 1994; Derby, et al., 1992). Operant functions for negative behavior can be assessed by a behavioral psychologist or analyst trained in the field of applied behavior analysis (ABA). Although a given negative behavior *may* be part of a psychiatric syndrome, it is also possible that the behavior has become a learned entity with known results for the individual. Collaboration between psychologist and psychiatrist then should occur to tease apart the psychiatric and operant/environmental causes for a given behavior. Common operant causes for negative behaviors in ID include access to desired tangible items such as food and toys, access to attention, and escape from demands. With CHARGE, sensory issues and the need for stimulation also should be considered. The following case example is demonstrative.

CASE 1

M is a 15-year-old boy with CHARGE. He is profoundly deaf, has a tracheostomy, and swallowing dysfunction. M is reported as physically overactive, very stubborn, wanting only to do "what he wants when he wants to do it," and to have frequent aggressive outbursts, particularly at school. M is fixated on schedules and lists and can spend hours arranging balloons in the market. He is the youngest of three children, and his family openly admits "spoiling" him after his multiple serious medical interventions and hospitalizations. M has been diagnosed with OCD and ADHD and is on medications for both (sertraline and clonidine). Behavioral assessment at the school and home confirm the suspected "escape from demands" function of M's aggression. Medication will not make M less aggressive toward his teacher when he knows that she will respond by removing tasks and he will no longer have to work! However, a behavioral program whereby M can earn reinforcement for compliance is highly effective in decreasing school aggression and improving learning. Guaranteeing that the school always has a signing aide for M and removes "mandated" curricula for which M does not have sign vocabulary is also crucial in improving his overall school functioning.

Psychiatric assessment of a person with CHARGE should not neglect potential somatic and drug-related causes for a patient's psychiatric presentation, particularly with the known physical vulnerabilities in CHARGE. Even therapeutic and recreational drugs may be implicated and should be assessed.

CASE 2

S is a 12-year-old girl with CHARGE. She has significant vision impairment and has required multiple GI surgeries. She usually demonstrates low-frequency and low-intensity self-injurious behaviors that are readily managed with a behavioral program. A previous increase in self-injury followed a urinary tract infection. Self-injury suddenly escalates again, including deep skin picking and scratching to the point of extensive bleeding and tissue damage. Usually a happy and energetic young lady, S also begins crying incessantly. A GI work-up is pursued based on history, and S is found to have an actively bleeding stomach ulcer. Self-injury resolves with treatment of the ulcer.

CASE 3

P is a 32-year-old man with CHARGE. He has bilateral partial hearing loss, attention and executive function impairments, reduced communication skills, and a beer-drinking history since age 14. He lost his older brother at age 17 in an accident and, subsequently, had three suicidal overdose attempts using alcohol and over-the-counter medications. P was dismissed from psychotherapy "because he didn't talk" and had similar communication challenges in drug and alcohol abuse recovery groups. He had been prescribed multiple psychotropic medications without benefit but with the development of multiple side effects. P had truly "fallen through the cracks" due to his disability. Not amenable to standard "talking" treatments for his substance abuse and flagrant depression following the loss of his brother, he had been shuffled through the system only to continually relapse. Recommendation was made for an inpatient admission for full drug and alcohol detoxification, followed by comprehensive psychiatric assessment once free of mind-altering substances. Recommendations were also made for supervised living as well as structured and supervised work and leisure programming once psychiatrically stable.

LESSONS FROM CASE STUDIES

The preceding cases emphasize the need for full review of a patient's social and family history. Drug use may not be rampant in individuals with CHARGE, but it certainly can exist, particularly with higher-functioning individuals who have the resources and cognitive capacity to access recreational substances. The author has encountered two adults with CHARGE with significant substance abuse leading to legal difficulties including incarceration. Similarly, the impact of one's social and living environment, including losses, strains and stressors, affects *all people* and certainly should not be minimized or ignored because a patient is disabled. On the contrary, patients with disability likely have reduced coping skills to manage life's challenges. P certainly could have benefited from an alternative mental health approach to the loss of his brother before his suicide attempts.

When a psychiatric diagnosis is made, it should be clear to the treating professional, as well as the patient and caregivers, what specific symptoms are to be targeted in treatment. Patient understanding may vary according to cognitive level, but in the same way that attempts should be made to explain the cardiac, gastrointestinal or ENT surgery a child must undergo, similar attempts should be made to place psychiatric issues in an understandable context. Visual information and social stories may be very helpful depending on age and overall level of functioning. Clear delineation of symptoms and plans for objective monitoring allows treatment interventions to be pursued.

TREATMENT CONSIDERATIONS

The myriad of psychotropic, behavioral, and other interventions available for specific psychiatric and behavioral conditions is beyond the scope of this chapter. However, some important principles place a framework for understanding the options.

(1) First and foremost, although psychotropic drugs may be true life-savers in some cases, they are not always necessary and usually are not sufficient. If a child with CHARGE with obsessions and repetitive behaviors is diagnosed with OCD, for example, the child *may* benefit from medication with a selective serotonin reuptake inhibitor or tricyclic antidepressant, agents with proven efficacy in OCD in the general population, and whose usage in ID populations has also been studied (Janowsky, Barnhill, Shetty, & Davis, 2005). However, the same behavioral interventions for OCD that are well-established best practices in the general child population (AACAP, 1998a) also should be pursued and perhaps as the first-line intervention. Similarly, best practices in the management of pediatric mood disorders and

ADHD that urge combined medication and behavioral interventions for maximal benefit (AACAP, 1997; AACAP 1998b), should apply to individuals with CHARGE as well.

(2) Indeed, drugs come with a big CAUTION sign in the ID population, as individuals with disabilities are known to be much more likely to suffer side effects and unusual, idiosyncratic reactions to psychotropic drugs, often limiting their efficacy and tolerability (Aman, et al., 2004). Many of the families the author has worked with have reported negative reactions to antipsychotics in their children with CHARGE. Current consensus guidelines make a "start low, go slow" recommendation in their best practices for psychotropic usage in ID (Aman, et al., 2004). If a medication is started, it becomes crucial to assess its efficacy for the given target symptoms. Response should be assessed regularly, and the benefit of any medication weighed against the development of side effects. If a medication is ineffective, it should be discontinued. Although this seems obvious, individuals with ID are at an increased risk of having multiple drugs prescribed simultaneously, sometimes out of simple fear of "rocking the boat" in discontinuing a medication, and often in an attempt to simply sedate the patient for behavioral control (Stolker, Heerdink, Leufkens, Clerkx, & Nolen, 2001). Such polypharmacy is rarely beneficial, except when it is clear what each drug is doing, and each drug's efficacy demonstrated.

(3) Actual drug choice is dictated by diagnosis. Specific medication recommendations for the major psychiatric illnesses identified by an expert consensus panel for those with intellectual disability are *identical* to those received in surveys for psychiatric illness without disability (Aman, et al., 2004). If a child with CHARGE is depressed, the child should receive an antidepressant; if truly psychotic, an antipsychotic. If there is not a clear consensus of target symptoms, one should be wary of medications.

(4) Psychotropic medications may be chosen to target specific behavioral symptoms without a psychiatric diagnosis. Again, there is research in the ID population supporting the usage of classic and atypical antipsychotic medications, as well as serotonin-enhancing antidepressants and opioid antagonists in the resolution of *some* cases of self-injury and aggression (LaMalfa, Lassi, Bertelli, & Castellani, 2006). Lithium, anticonvulsants, and antihypertensive agents have also shown efficacy in aggression (Kowatch & Bucci, 1998). Wachtel, et al. (2007) found that the most frequently prescribed psychotropic classes for people with CHARGE were antidepressants, antihypertensives, and antipsychotics, yet actual efficacy of these agents in CHARGE is yet to be systematically researched. Best practices would dictate medications being used as parsimoniously as possible, and in tandem with a comprehensive behavioral assessment and behavioral treatment implementation (Mace & Mauk, 1995; Wachtel & Hagopian, 2006).

The following cases demonstrate the efficacy of comprehensive assessment and treatment in CHARGE behavioral and psychiatric disturbance:

CASE 4

Z is a 4-year-old male with CHARGE. He has profound hearing loss, bilateral retinal colobomas, respiratory concerns, and gastrostomy-tube feeding since infancy. He was admitted to an in-patient facility for assessment of self-injury and disruption, including head banging, self-biting, scratching, and head punching, and throwing items at others. He refused needed daily nebulizer treatment, and would not wear his glasses or hearing aides. Z further demonstrated excessive physical hyperactivity, insomnia, and frequent tantrums. Prior trials of two antipsychotics had led to emergency room visits due to development of sustained contractures (dystonia) of ocular muscles, and usage of a third antipsychotic had led to concerning EKG changes.

Functional assessment of Z revealed that self-injury was maintained by sensory reinforcement and access to adult attention. Disruptions were directly related to escape from demands. Low-dose fluvoxamine led to reduction in repetitive self-injurious behaviors, and clonidine sharply reduced hyperactivity. Behavioral treatment of Z included preferred items identified as successfully competing with self-injury, functional communication training, and a token system that allowed access to reinforcement for compliance with demands without disruption. Desensitization was pursued to gain compliance with nebulizers and wearing hearing aides and glasses.

CASE 5

R is a 15-year-old male with CHARGE. He has swallowing dysfunction with gastrostomy tube, bilateral moderate hearing loss, retinal and optic nerve colobomata, hypogonadism, growth retardation, and developmental delay. R's multiple challenges had led him to be placed in an institution for most of his life, and he was admitted to an in-patient unit for self-injury and aggression. Self-injury included finger biting as well as banging of his head, arms, and teeth against hard surfaces. Aggression consisted of grabbing, scratching, clawing, head butting, and kicking. R also had severe insomnia and rigid compulsions, including needing to carry a filled cup and his shoes at all times, holding his helmet (although not wearing it) and wearing his coat zipped to a certain point. At admission, R was on five psychotropic medications, including an agent normally used by anesthesiologists for conscious sedation (to treat his insomnia). He was highly sedated on admission.

All medications were serially weaned without any change in R's behavior, but with much-improved alertness. Functional behavioral assessment demonstrated that aggression and self-biting were maintained by escape from demands, while head and body self-injury behaviors were maintained by sensory stimulation. A program of functional communication training and access to reinforcement was developed, with compliance of demands improving from 0% to 75%. The self-injury behaviors were addressed with alternative sensory toys identified as effective competitors with head and body self-injury. Trazodone effectively treated insomnia, and very low-dose escitalopram worked in tandem with behavioral interventions to reduce self-injury. Residual negative behaviors were addressed with response reduction procedures including a 30-second facial screen and contingent demands.

CONCLUSIONS

Psychiatric and behavioral disturbances are common in individuals with CHARGE and may present significant challenges in multiple areas of functioning. Although the presence of a developmental and/or intellectual disability certainly increases the risk of psychiatric and behavioral pathology, these difficulties can be addressed effectively. Comprehensive assessment and treatment development are crucial. Accurate psychiatric and behavioral diagnoses must be established and treatment interventions tailored to each patient's specific needs. Behavioral interventions are usually indispensable, and concomitant medication benefits should be maximized while avoiding the pitfalls of psychotropic medication usage in disabilities. The consistent application of such an approach can often afford significant amelioration of psychiatric and behavioral challenges in CHARGE syndrome.

REFERENCES

Aman, M. G., Crismon, M. L., Frances, A., King, B. H., & Rojahn, J, (Eds). (2004). *Treatment of psychiatric and behavior problems in individuals with mental retardation: An update of the Expert Consensus Guidelines® for mental retardation/developmental disability populations.* Englewood, CO: Postgraduate Institute for Medicine.

American Academy of Child and Adolescent Psychiatry. (1997). Practice parameters for the assessment and treatment of children, adolescents and adults with attention-deficit/hyperactivity disorder. *Journal of the American Academy of Child and Adolescent Psychiatry, 36*(10 Supplement), 85S–121S.

American Academy of Child and Adolescent Psychiatry. (1998a). Practice parameters for the assessment and treatment of children and adolescents with obsessive-compulsive disorder. *Journal of the American Academy of Child and Adolescent Psychiatry, 37*(10 Supplement), 27S–45S.

American Academy of Child and Adolescent Psychiatry. (1998b). Practice parameters for the assessment and treatment of children and adolescents with depressive disorders. *Journal of the American Academy of Child and Adolescent Psychiatry, 37*(10 Supplement), 63S–83S.

American Psychiatric Association. (2004). *Diagnostic and Statistical Manual of Mental Disorders (DSM-IV-TR)*. Washington, DC: Author.

Bernstein, V. & Denno, L. S. (2005). Repetitive behaviors in CHARGE syndrome: differential diagnosis and treatment options. *American Journal of Medical Genetics*, *133A*, 232-239.

Borthwick-Duffy, S. (1994). Epidemiology and prevalence of psychopathology in people with mental retardation. *Journal of Consulting and Clinical Psychology*, *62*(1), 17-27.

Carvill, S. (2005). Sensory impairments, intellectual disability and psychiatry. *Journal of Intellectual Disability Research*, *45*(6), 467-483.

Derby, K. M., Wacker, D. P., Sasso, G., Steege, M., Northup, J., Cigrand, K., & Asmus, J. (1992). Brief functional assessments techniques to evaluate aberrant behavior in an outpatient setting: a summary of 79 cases. *Journal of Applied Behavior Analysis*, *25*, 713-721.

Eaton, L. F. & Menolascino, F. J. (1982). Psychiatric disorders in the mentally retarded: types, problems and challenges. *American Journal of Psychiatry*, *139*(10), 1297-1303.

Einfeld, S. L. (2004). Behavior phenotypes of genetic disorders. *Current Opinion in Psychiatry*, *17*, 343-348.

Einfeld, S. L. & Tonge, B. J. (1995) The Developmental Behavioral Checklist: the development and validation of an instrument to assess behavioral and emotional disturbance in children and adolescents with mental retardation. *Journal of Autism and Developmental Disorders*, *25*(2), 81-104.

Eyman, R. K., Borthwick-Duffy, S. A. & Miller. C. (1981). Trends in maladaptive behavior of mentally retarded persons placed in community and institutional settings. *American Journal of Mental Deficiency*, *85*(5), 473-477.

Harris, J. C. (2006). *Intellectual disability*. New York, NY: Oxford University Press.

Hartshorne, T. S., & Cypher, A. D. (2004). Challenging behavior in CHARGE syndrome. *Mental Health Aspects of Developmental Disabilities*, *7*(2), 41-52.

Hartshorne, T. S., Grialou, T. L., & Parker, K. R. (2005). Autistic-like behavior in CHARGE syndrome. *American Journal of Medical Genetics*, *133A*, 257-261.

Iwata, B. A., Pace, G. M., Dorsey, M. F., Zarcone, J. R., Vollmer, T. R., Smith R. G., . . . Mazalesk, J. L. (1994). The functions of self-injurious behavior: An experimental-epidemiological analysis. *Journal of Applied Behavior Analysis*, *27*, 215-240.

Janowsky, D. S., Barnhill, L. J., Shetty, M., & Davis J. M. (2005). Minimally effective doses of conventional antipsychotic medications used to treat aggression, self-injurious and destructive behaviors in mentally retarded adults. *Journal of Clinical Psychopharmacology*, *25*(1), 19-25.

Kishore, M. T., Nizamie, A., Nizamie, S. H., & Jahan, M. (2004). Psychiatric diagnosis in persons with intellectual disability in India. *Journal of Intellectual Disabilities Research*, *48*(1), 19-24.

Kowatch, R. A., & Bucci, J. P. (1998). Child and adolescent psychopharmacology: mood stabilizers and anticonvulsants. *Pediatric Clinics of Northern America*, *45*(5), 1173-1186.

LaMalfa, G., Lassi, S., Bertelli, M., & Castellani, A. (2006). Reviewing the use of antipsychotic drugs in people with intellectual disability. *Human Psychopharmacology*, *21*, 73-89.

Lauger, K., Cornelius, N., & Keedy, W. (2005). Behavioral features of CHARGE syndrome: Parents' perspectives of three children with CHARGE syndrome. *American Journal of Medical Genetics, 133A,* 291-299.

Mace, F. C., & Mauk, J. E. (1995). Bio-behavioral diagnosis and treatment of self-injury. *Mental Retardation and Developmental Disabilities Research Review, 1,* 104-110.

Matson, J. L., & Sevin, J. A. (1994). Theories of dual diagnosis in mental retardation. *Journal of Consulting and Clinical Psychology, 62*(1), 6-16.

O'Brien, G., Pearson, J., Berney, T., & Barnard, L. (2001). Measuring behavior in developmental disability: a review of existing schedules. *Developmental Medicine & Child Neurology, 43*(Suppl. 87), 1-72.

Reiss, S. (1993). Assessment of psychopathology in persons with mental retardation. In J. L. Matson, & R. P. Barrett (Eds.), *Psychopathology of the mentally retarded* (2nd ed.). Boston, MA: Allyn & Bacon.

Salem-Hartshorne, N., & Jacob, S. (2005). Adaptive behavior in children with CHARGE syndrome. *American Journal of Medical Genetics, 133A,* 262-267.

Smith, I. M., Nichols, S. L., Issekutz, I., & Blake, K. D. (2005). Behavioral profiles and symptoms of autism in CHARGE syndrome: preliminary Canadian epidemiological data. *American Journal of Medical Genetics, 133A,* 248-256.

Souriau, J., Gimenes, M., Blouin, C., Benbrik, I., Benbrik, E., Churakowskyi, A., & Churakowskyi, B. (2005). CHARGE syndrome: Developmental and behavioral data. *American Journal of Medical Genetics, 133A,* 278-281.

Stolker, J. J., Heerdink, E. R., Leufkens, H. G. M., Clerkx, M. G. M., & Nolen, W. A. (2001). Determinants of multiple psychotropic drug use in patients with mild intellectual disabilities or borderline intellectual functioning and psychiatric or behavioral disorders. *General Hospital Psychiatry, 23,* 345-349.

Thelin, J. W., & Fussner, J. C. (2005). Factors related to the development of communication in CHARGE syndrome. *American Journal of Medical Genetics, 133A,* 282-290.

Wachtel, L. E., & Hagopian, L. P. (2006). Psychopharmacology and applied behavioral analysis: tandem treatment of severe problem behaviors in intellectual disability and a case series. *Israeli Journal of Psychiatry and Related Sciences, 43*(4), 265-274.

Wachtel, L. E., Hartshorne, T. S., & Dailor, A. N. (2007). Psychiatric diagnoses and psychotropic medications in CHARGE syndrome: A Pediatric Survey. *Journal of Developmental and Physical Disabilities, 19,* 471-483.

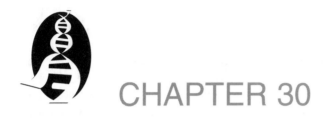

CHAPTER 30

Experiencing Pain

JUDE NICHOLAS, PSY.D.

INTRODUCTION

Pain is ultimately a subjective experience, as illustrated by the definition of the International Association for the Study of Pain: "an unpleasant sensory and emotional experience associated with actual or potential tissue damage, or described in terms of such damage" (Merskey & Bogduk, 1994). Although everyone comes equipped with the same basic nerve fibers, neurotransmitters and brain structures, pain systems of different people behave in radically different ways depending on the cognitive, motivational, and emotional features of the pain experience. Pain now is described as "a symphony," a complex dynamic involving not only pain sensors but hormones, emotions, and thoughts, rather than as a simple, specific or discrete entity.

ACUTE AND CHRONIC PAIN

In its most basic and acute form, pain can be a force for good. Sip a cup of burning coffee, and the tongue fires off a message to the brain, causing the person to wince and then slow down, sparing cells further damage. Acute pain, also known as warning pain, often signals injury or disease, such as infection, injury, hemorrhage, tumor, or metabolic or endocrine problems. It produces a wide range of actions to mitigate it and treat its causes. Memories of earlier pain warn to avoid potentially dangerous situations. Another effect of pain, especially after serious injury or surgery, is to make a person rest, thereby promoting the body's healing process. Chronic pain, which can linger for months, years, even a lifetime, is a very different matter. Chronic pain has been defined as repeated or persistent episodes of acute pain (e.g., headache, abdominal pain) that are experienced as a component of a medical disorder, or experienced by otherwise healthy children in the absence of a well-defined organic etiology (McGrath, 1990). Chronic pain clearly is not a warning to prevent physical injury or disease, and it is not just a prolonged version of acute pain. The very system that works on behalf of the individual however, also can break down. This is where the symptoms of pain become the disease of pain. Chronic pain is a chronic condition with its own pathological changes, its own set of clinical and behavioral characteristics, and its own subset of effective approaches to treatment (Whitten & Cristobal, 2005).

PAIN IN NEWBORNS AND CHILDREN

For many years, it was believed incorrectly that newborns were incapable of experiencing or expressing pain (Figure 30–1). But, today, medical professionals are responding with strategies for managing discomfort in their youngest

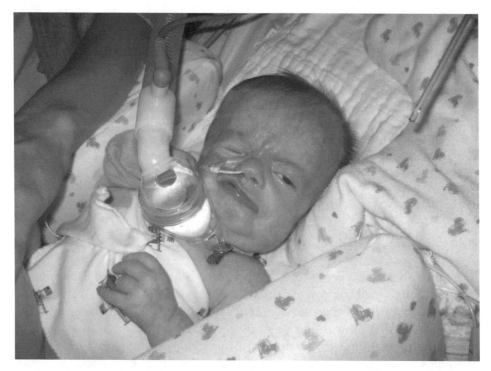

FIGURE 30–1. Infants with CHARGE may experience considerable pain.

patients. Acute or chronic pain is a common experience in children and adults without disabilities. However, acute and chronic pain in children and adults with developmental disabilities has received very little scientific attention. There is good reason to believe that pain is much more a part of the daily lives of children with physical or developmental disabilities and neurological impairments than is the case for children without disabilities or impairments. Nevertheless, pain research has been limited in these populations, in large part as a result of the inherent difficulties associated with the assessment of pain in these individuals, as well as the widespread and pernicious belief that they do not experience pain (Bottos & Chambers, 2006). The development of pain in children with a genetic disorder and multisensory impairment occurs, as it does for all children, in a dynamic web of exchange.

This chapter focuses on understanding pain in persons with CHARGE syndrome and provides a brief overview of the current knowledge regarding neurobiological and neuropsychological processes involved in pain transmission within a biopsychosocial model.

NEUROLOGY OF PAIN

Pain processing requires an intact nervous system linking the peripheral sensory nerve fibers that first detect pain stimuli to the somatosensory cortex and other areas of the brain where this information is processed. Six major components are involved in pain processing: transduction, inflammation, conduction, transmission, modulation, and finally perception (Whitten & Cristobal, 2005). A change that occurs in the organization of the CNS pathways is likely a major contributing factor in the development and perpetuation of chronic pain. In addition to peripheral sensitization, tissue injury can lead to increased sensitivity of the central neurons, called central sensitization. Central sensitization (also termed "central windup") is an increase in the excitability of neurons within the central nervous system, so that normal inputs begin to produce abnormal responses causing all pain to become more painful.

In the short term, these changes allow healing by forcing protection of the injured area. "Central windup" usually resolves as the injury heals; in chronic pain patients, however, these changes persist. The more severe the pain and the longer it persists, the more likely the change will become permanent (Brookoff, 2000). Sensitization is a typical feature of pain pathways: pain produces pain. This neural sensitization concept of pain may give us a better understanding of pain arising from innocuous stimulation and the withdrawal behaviors seen in children with CHARGE syndrome when touched. This kind of tactile defensiveness and sensitivity in CHARGE has been reported frequently by parents (Brown, 2005).

In some individuals with CHARGE syndrome with chronic pain, the ability to block incoming pain messages may be lost, causing the pain signals to fire unheeded and magnifying the pain of once harmless sensations. In addition to the physical status, thoughts or cognitive features, mood states, communication skills, and the social context of the individual with CHARGE need to be considered if the pain perception and response to pain are to be fully understood. Pain cannot be understood without an appreciation of the interpersonal nature of the experience. The biopsychosocial model of pain has potential to assist in understanding the challenges of controlling pain in people with CHARGE syndrome.

PAIN IS A COMPLEX MULTIDIMENSIONAL AND BIOPSYCHOSOCIAL EXPERIENCE

The biopsychosocial approach now is accepted widely as the most heuristic perspective to the understanding and treatment of chronic pain disorders (Gatchel, 2004), and pain in CHARGE syndrome is best conceptualized within this framework. In order to fully understand perception and response to pain of a person with CHARGE, the interrelationships among biological changes, psychological status, and the social cultural context all need to be considered.

Biological

Medical Issues

Research during the past decade indicates that certain conditions are particularly prevalent among individuals with developmental disabilities. Common medical conditions occurring in CHARGE include chronic recurrent otitis media and/or sinusitis, chronic constipation, feeding problems, cranial nerve anomalies, and sleep problems. Some of these chronic medical conditions may be associated with pain. For instance, cranial nerve abnormalities may be involved in specific pain experiences. Cranial Nerve V (CN V; also known as the trigeminal nerve) anomaly has been implicated in migraine headaches (Hargreaves, 2007). A recent study has shown evidence for CN V anomaly in CHARGE (Blake, Hartshorne, Lawland, Dailor, & Thelin, 2008) and migraine symptoms as adolescent concerns have been reported in CHARGE syndrome (Blake, Salem-Hartshorne, Daoud, & Gradstein, 2005). Other trigeminal autonomic headaches with pain and autonomic involvement in the area supplied by the trigeminal nerve may prove to be a phenomenon in CHARGE given problems with CN V (Blake, et. al., 2008).

Sleep Disturbance

Sleep disturbances (sleep loss or interrupted sleep) can cause changes in pain perception. Many patients with chronic pain conditions experience more pain at night because the surroundings are quiet and there are fewer stimuli to compete with the pain. Clearly, pain in the presence of certain chronic medical conditions might make sleep difficult. A recent study found significant sleep disturbances in children with CHARGE, and a relationship was found between disturbed sleep and ear infections (Hartshorne, et al., 2008, see also Chapter 23).

Developmental Disabilities

The presence of a chronic medical condition in a person with developmental disabilities, along with communication challenges, is a primary means by which pain can cause discomfort that results in a greater probability of aggression, destructive behavior, or self-injury. Considerable evidence from both clinical and preclinical studies of chronic pain and its behavioral sequelae supports the hypothesis that some self-injurious behavior may be regulated by altered pain mechanisms (Symons, 2002). Children with CHARGE present a unique array of behaviors that are reported frequently as "challenging" (Hartshorne & Cypher, 2004; also see Chapter 28). Obviously, some of these "challenging" behaviors the child exhibits may be an expression of pain. In some instances, the challenging behavior may arise only in the presence of a medical condition (e.g., ear or sinus infection), while in other instances, the challenging behavior may have been precipitated initially by the medical condition, but it may have evolved to be maintained by social reinforcement contingencies (i.e., positive reinforcement in the form of access to attention).

Nonresponse to Painful Stimuli

The nonresponse to or under-registration of pain stimuli technically is called decreased sensitivity. Children with decreased sensitivity often react less than others to a pain stimulus, and many of these children do not seem to perceive the pain of a minor injury, or may laugh in response. The incidence of documented pain insensitivity in children is rare (Oberlander, O'Donnell, & Montgomery, 1999); however, it often has been reported in the developmental disability population, including children with autism (Nader, Oberlander, Chambers, & Craig, 2004). Gilbert-MacLeod, Craig, Rocha, and Mathias (2000) noted differences in the pain reactions of young children with developmental delays in daycare as compared with typical children. However, it is not clear whether the observed pain insensitivity is due to real decreased sensitivity or to other factors such as socio-communicative impairments (Gilbert-MacLeod, et al., 2000), problems with decoding the pain reactions of children (Nader, et al., 2004), or the ability to comprehend and communicate pain (Oberlander, et al., 1999). It is hypothesized that children with sensory integration dysfunction may appear to be unaware of pain and put themselves in dangerous situations (Allison, Gabriel, Schlange, & Fredrickson, 2007). Parents, professionals, and some young adults with CHARGE have reported a high tolerance for pain in children with CHARGE. Further empirical work is needed to clarify whether this reflects true decreased sensitivity or is a reflection of other factors. Children with CHARGE certainly have a great deal of experience with pain. It is possible that due to sensory integration issues (Brown, 2005), communication problems, social-emotional experiences, or having simply accommodated to the experience of pain, children with CHARGE do not express more typical reactions to pain. As Bottos and Chambers (2006) note, "Indeed, a disrupted *expression* of pain does not necessarily imply that these individuals are pain insensitive" (p. 71).

Psychological

The psychological factors of the biopsychosocial model of pain involve both emotion and cognition. Emotion is the more immediate reaction to noxious stimuli, whereas cognition attaches meaning to the emotional experience and can then trigger additional emotional reactions and thereby amplify the experience of pain.

The ability of psychological factors to influence the development of chronic pain by shaping behavior and amplifying peripheral sensations is well supported by research. Cognitions and emotions are intimately associated with interpretation of pain. The experience of pain includes an important affective component and incorporates many different emotions, but they are primarily negative. The relationship between pain and negative affect varies both between individuals and within the same individual over time. Negative affects include the states of tension, distress, nervousness, and irritability, whereas negative moods include the clinical manifestations of fear and anxiety, depression, anger, and chronic stress. As pain becomes more chronic, emotional factors play an increasingly dominant role in the maintenance of dysfunction and suffering. Ploghaus, Beccerra, Borras, and Borsook (2003) noted that fear and the anticipation of pain are seen commonly in patients with chronic pain. Anxiety, depression, chronic stress, pain, and pain modulation are all intertwined. From a clinical standpoint, it often is difficult to ascertain the precise boundary between chronic pain, depression, and poor stress management. They interact and augment each other over time.

Pain is also a specific form of stress and recognizing the role of the stress system in the pain process is important. Clearly, deficits in emotion regulation, depressed mood, anxiety and chronic stress can exert a significant impact on pain tolerance in persons with CHARGE. Impairments in emotion regulation in the form of poorly regulated negative affect play a crucial role in the interpretation of pain. Many older individuals with CHARGE syndrome exhibit behaviors such as social detachment, aggression, emotional outbursts, and depression (Abi Daoud, Gradstein, & Blake, 2002). Children with CHARGE are reported to be affected by anxiety (Souriau, Gimenes, Blouin, Benbrick, & Churakowskyi, 2005), repetitive behaviors, and obsessive-compulsive disorder (OCD). OCD tendencies are seen in many children and young adults with

CHARGE (Hartshorne, Hefner, & Davenport, 2005). A dramatic increase of repetitive behaviors in times of stress and illness also has been observed in some individuals with CHARGE (Bernstein & Denno, 2005). Thus, it is important to be aware of the impact stress and high levels of negativity in emotional expressions have on the perception of pain in persons with CHARGE (see Chapter 31).

A reciprocal relationship exists between affective-emotional states and cognitive interpretive processes. Thinking affects mood, and mood influences appraisals, and, ultimately, the experience of pain (Gatchel, Bo Peng, Peters, Fuchs, & Turk, 2007). The experience of pain may initiate a set of extremely negative thoughts or cognitions and arouse fears—fear of inciting more pain and injury or fear of their future impact. Pain cognitions are shaped largely by the individual's learning history, either through direct experience, observational learning or modeling by others. Pain appraisal, pain beliefs, and pain catastrophizing are cognitive factors that can have a strong impact on an individual's affective and behavioral response to pain. "Pain appraisal" refers to the meaning ascribed to pain by an individual; whereas "pain beliefs" refers to assumptions about reality that shape how one interprets painful events. For example, if a pain signal is interpreted as harmful (threat appraisal) and is believed to be associated with actual or potential tissue damage, it may be perceived as more intense and unpleasant and may evoke more maladaptive behavior. "Pain catastrophizing" is defined as an exaggerated negative orientation toward actual or anticipated pain experiences. This negative anticipation of pain exacerbates fear-beliefs and negative interpretation of bodily sensations, which in turn leads to enhanced pain experience and a wide array of psychological reactions and problems (e.g., depression, pain related threat-anxiety, distress-anger, etc.). The role of pain catastrophizing may indeed be causally implicated in maladaptive pain cognitions and poor behavioral and psychological adjustment to pain (Smeets, Vlaeyen, Kester, & Knottnerus, 2006). Pain cognitions are most likely to be observed in the ability of persons with CHARGE to deploy adaptive cognitions and cognitive coping skills to understand, predict, and control circumstances associated with the painful event.

Recently, neuropsychological deficits, such as executive function deficits, have been proposed as factors that could influence pain perception and pain tolerance. Executive functions are the abilities needed to monitor, to control and to regulate thought and action and they include strategic planning, decision making, self-monitoring, and mental flexibility. Children with CHARGE have been reported to have deficits in executive functions (Hartshorne, Nicholas, Grialou, & Russ, 2007). A study by Karp, et al., (2006) found a relationship between pain severity and impaired mental flexibility. This finding suggests that mental flexibility deficits or inhibition deficits (the ability to block or ignore information) may diminish the individual's ability to suppress the influence of pain. Neuropsychological deficits may have an impact on the qualities of pain experience and pain tolerance in CHARGE syndrome. However, the challenge is to understand the underlying neurocognitive mechanisms involved in the uncommon patterns of pain display. Some persons with CHARGE may not be able to "shut down" the cognitive interference from pain due to executive function deficits. Further research is needed in identifying the involvement of these neurocognitive factors on pain in CHARGE syndrome.

Social

Pain cannot be fully understood without considering the social contexts that shape the experience and expression of pain. The social factors of the biopsychosocial model involve the environmental stressors, the setting in which pain is experienced, what pattern of pain expression is socially appropriate, the presence and reactions of others, social relationships and the interpersonal communication dynamics. The interpersonal communication dynamics of pain expression involve behavioral complexities such as body language, vocalization, facial expression, posture, body movement, and physiological changes. These pain behaviors are overt communications of pain and distress. However, the major challenge we face with individuals with CHARGE syndrome is trying to understand and interpret their expressions of pain, especially when the individual lacks a formal communication system.

PAIN IN INDIVIDUALS WITH CHARGE SYNDROME

Comorbid Medical Conditions

Individuals with CHARGE may be particularly vulnerable to both acute and chronic forms of pain because they frequently have comorbid painful medical conditions and may be more frequently subjected to a variety of potentially painful medical procedures to treat their underlying disorders. Children with CHARGE are exposed to far more surgeries, hospitalizations and other medical procedures that are painful than are typical children (Hartshorne & Cypher, 2004). Although all children with CHARGE experience acute pain at many points in their development, not all will develop chronic pain conditions. However, being able to effectively communicate information about painful distress to others is an important step in the path to pain relief.

Poor Communication

Poor communication ability is common in individuals with CHARGE syndrome, with many using primarily gestures in combination with some vocalizations (Thelin & Fussner, 2005; Peltokorpi, & Huutunen, 2008; see also Chapter 27). They are likely to be delayed in acquiring the language used by typically

developing children to describe painful distress. Therefore, we need to identify the bodily and gestural affective expressions and understand the patterns of
communicative and interactive systems that are unique to each individual with
CHARGE. The limited "communication bubble" in individuals with CHARGE
severely restricts opportunities of learning about pain regulation through typical social channels. They may be less likely to display a social response (like
seeking help), or they may be less able to engage in self care following episodes
of pain. Finding alternative ways to educate children with CHARGE to understand and communicate about pain is an important component of pain management for this population. However, many challenges exist in trying to help
a child with limited vision and hearing and limited communication abilities
build up a mental image of pain. The degree of success depends largely on the
ways in which the environment is supportive and involved in sharing emotions and communicating pain. That means one has to build up shared events
and shared meanings around specific pain experiences. The sensory and communicative development of persons with CHARGE is heavily dependent on
the quality of their social experiences (Souriau, et al., 2005). When attending
to the needs of people with CHARGE, it is important for professionals and
family members to attend to reflexive and spontaneous bodily-emotional
expressions of distress and try to understand the available behavior as a sign
or expression of pain.

Chronic Pain in CHARGE

Some individuals with CHARGE truly have chronic pain, from continuous ear
infections, sinus infections, abdominal bloating, gastrointestinal problems,
jaw discomfort, migraines, etc. However, specific physical anomalies such as
facial palsy (which can mask a grimace or other expression of pain) and the
reduced ability to communicate about pain create a barrier to the identification
and recognition of pain. It has been reported that individuals with CHARGE
seem to be insensitive to some types of pain (Souriau, et al., 2005) and have
an increased threshold for acute pain. These studies are based on parent or
informant report and may not truly reflect the individual's pain experience
and may lead to the belief that individuals with CHARGE have a high pain
threshold. Children and adults with CHARGE may fail to display typical pain
behaviors one would expect when in contact with a noxious stimulus or
when a painful chronic condition is present. They may process information
and respond more slowly to painful incidents and may have difficulties in
detecting or localizing pain specifically. They also may communicate their
pain experiences differently, fundamentally through changes in behavior and
other forms of nonvocal communication. Thus, a major challenge is to be able
to accurately identify and recognize pain signals in persons with CHARGE.
The failure to display typical pain behaviors may put a person at risk for sub-
standard healthcare and pain management (Oberlander, et al., 1999).

ASSESSMENT

Pain must be assessed to be managed. The "gold standard" in pain measurement often is said to be self-report (Merskey & Bogduk, 1994). One tool used for self-report is the Visual Analogue Scale (VAS). The VAS consists of a horizontal line 10 cm long, with "no pain" at one end and "worst imaginable pain" at the other end, and patients are asked to mark the position on the line that best reflects the intensity of their pain. Assessment of pain utilizing self-report measures in individuals with CHARGE often is hindered by limited expressive repertoire, difficulty with verbal expression of pain, and/or inability to self-report the level of discomfort. Pain assessment procedures focusing on non-verbal signs and behaviors that are reliably associated with pain states may help assess pain in a person with CHARGE. Several standardized pain rating scales incorporating these nonverbal behaviors have been developed. One form of nonverbal pain assessment tool is the measure of facial reaction to pain, which would not be useful in the presence of bilateral facial palsy. Multi-dimensional pain assessment tools have been used with individuals with developmental or cognitive impairments. These involve evaluating behavioral characteristics such as vocalization, facial expression, body and limb movements during disturbed sleep, self-injurious behavior and physiological changes. Two multidimensional pain assessment tools are the Pediatric Pain Profile (PPP; Hunt, et al., 2004) and the Non-Communicating Children's Pain Checklist-Revised (NCCPC-R; Breau, McGrath, Camfield, & Finley, 2002). The NCCPC-R has good properties for specificity and sensitivity to pain and scores appear to be consistent over time (Breau et al., 2003). Breau et al. (2003) examined the validity of the NCCPC-R in children who displayed self-injurious behavior and the results suggested that children with chronic pain showed a different pattern of self-injury, suggesting that self-injurious behavior might be a reaction to pain in some children, rather than evidence of insensitivity to pain. Research investigating the NCCPC-R as an appropriate pain assessment tool in individuals who have CHARGE syndrome is underway in several countries (USA, the Nordic countries).

LONG-TERM CONSEQUENCES

Little is known about the possible long-term consequences of prolonged pain in individuals with CHARGE. There is increasing evidence that pain, or stressful events early in life that can cause pain, may change subsequent responses to pain, contribute to maladaptive behavior such as self-injury, and increase the risk of developing a Post-Traumatic Stress Disorder (PTSD). PTSD is a specific form of anxiety that comes on after a stressful or frightening event.

Those who have endured more stress in life are considered more susceptible to PTSD. Many individuals with CHARGE experience severe stress and trauma early in life since they undergo many surgical procedures and illnesses that require long-term hospital stays and long recovery periods. This stress and trauma early in life might make them more susceptible to PTSD. They may underreport or not report their pain to avoid further medical examinations and hospitalizations or they may display behaviors of "learned helplessness," in that, as the pain experience becomes more persistent and uncontrollable, behaviors directed at avoiding the noxious stimulus become less frequent. The symptoms of PTSD and helplessness behavior overlap considerably. Learned helplessness theory proposes that helplessness behavior is the result of people's expectations about events which they perceive to be uncontrollable. The way a person explains or attributes cause to events which occur influences these expectations. It has been proposed that perceived control attenuates pain because it changes the "meaning" of pain, making it less threatening. In other words, voluntary and consciously controlled forms of reinterpretation can weaken aversive emotional reactions to pain. Although cognition and emotion are components of pain behavior, specific pathways linking cognition and emotion to particular pain behavior in persons with CHARGE need to be identified. Given that memory and certain neurocognitive functions are vital for individuals to understand treatment programs and goals, it is likely that this too is an under recognized area of research and potential treatment for individuals with CHARGE and chronic pain.

In conclusion, the biopsychosocial model of pain has the potential to assist in understanding the challenges of controlling pain in people with CHARGE syndrome. This model emphasizes an integrative approach that considers not only biological or psychological features of pain, but also the social contexts and communicational dynamics that shape the experience and expression of pain.

REFERENCES

Abi Daoud, M. S., Gradstein, J., & Blake, K. D. (2002). CHARGE in the adolescent and adult decades. *Pediatric Child Health*, 7, 27A.

Allison, C. L., Gabriel, H., Schlange, D., Fredrickson, (2007). An optometric approach to patients with sensory integration dysfunction. *Optometry*, 78(12), 644–651.

Bernstein, V. & Denno, L. S. (2005). Repetitive behaviors in CHARGE syndrome: differential diagnosis and treatment options. *American Journal of Medical Genetics*, 133A, 232–239.

Blake, K. D., Hartshorne, T. S., Lawland, C., Dailor, A. N., & Thelin, J. W. (2008). Cranial nerve manifestations in CHARGE syndrome. *American Journal of Medical Genetics*, 146A, 585–592.

Blake, K. D., Salem-Hartshorne, N., Daoud, A., & Gradstein, J. 2005. Adolescent and adult issues in CHARGE syndrome. *Clinical Pediatrics*, 44(2), 151–159.

Breau, L. M., Camfeild, C., Symons, F. J., Bodfish, J. W., McKay, A., Finley, G. A., . . . McGrath, P. J. (2003). Pain and self-injurious behaviour in neurologically impaired children. *Journal of Pediatrics, 142,* 498–503.

Breau, L. M., McGrath, P. J., Camfield, C., & Finley, G. A. (2002). Psychometric properties of the Noncommunicating Children's Pain Checklist—Revised. *Pain, 99,* 349–357.

Bottos, S., & Chambers, C. T. (2006).The epidemiology of pain in developmental disabilities. In T. F. Oberlander & F. J. Symons (Eds.), *Pain in children & adults with developmental disabilities* (pp. 67–87). Baltimore, MD: Paul H Brookes.

Brookoff, D. (2000). Chronic Pain: 1. A new disease? *Hospital Practice, 35* (7), 45–52.

Brown, D. (2005). CHARGE syndrome behaviors: Challenges or adaptations? *American Journal of Medical Genetics, 133A,* 268–272.

Gatchel, R. J. (2004). Comorbidity of chronic pain and mental health: The biopsychosocial perspective. *American Psychologist, 59,* 792–794.

Gatchel, R. J., Bo Peng Y., Peters M. L., Fuchs, P. N. & Turk, D. C. (2007). The biopsychosocial approach to chronic pain: Scientific advances and future directions. *Psychological Bulletin, 133*(4), 581–624.

Gilbert-MacLeod, C. A., Craig, K. D., Rocha, E. M., & Mathias, M. D. (2000). Everyday pain responses in children with and without developmental delays. *Journal of Pediatric Psychology, 25,* 301–308.

Hargreaves, R. 2007. New migraine and pain research. *Headache, 47*(Suppl 1), S26–S43.

Hartshorne, T. S., & Cypher, A. D. (2004). Challenging behavior in CHARGE syndrome. *Mental Health Aspects of Developmental Disabilities, 7*(2), 41–52.

Hartshorne, T. S., Hefner, M. A., & Davenport, S. L. H. (2005). Behavior in CHARGE syndrome: introduction to the special topic. *American Journal of Medical Genetics, 133A,* 228–231.

Hartshorne, T. S., Heussler, H. S., Dailor, A. N., Williams, G. L., Papadopoulos, D., & Brant, K. K. (2008). Sleep disturbances in CHARGE: types and relationships with behavior and care-giver well-being. *Developmental Medicine & Child Neurology, 51*(2), 143–150.

Hartshorne, T. S., Nicholas, J., Grialou, T. L., & Russ, J. M. (2007). Executive function in CHARGE syndrome. *Child Neuropsychology, 13,* 333–344.

Hunt, A., Goldman, A., Seers, K., Crichton, N., Mastroyannopoulou, K., Moffat, V., . . . Brady, M. (2004). Clinical validation of the Pediatric Pain Profile. *Developmental Medicine and Child Neurology, 46,* 9–18

Karp, J. F., Reynolds, C. F., Butters, M. A., Dew, M. A., Mazumar, S., Begley, A. E., . . . Weiner, D. K. (2006). The relationship between pain and mental flexibility in older adult pain clinic patients. *Pain Medicine, 7*(5), 444–452.

Kehl, L. J. & Goldetsky, G. (2006). Overview of pain mechanisms: neuroanatomical and neurophysiological processes. In T. F. Oberlander & F. J. Symons (Eds.), *Pain in children & adults with developmental disabilities* (pp. 41–64). Baltimore, MD: Paul H Brookes.

Merskey, H., & Bogduk, N. (Eds.). (1994). *Classification of chronic pain: descriptions of chronic pain syndromes and definition of pain terms* (2nd ed). Seattle, WA: IASP Press.

McGrath, P. A. (1990). *Pain in children: Nature, assessment and treatment.* New York, NY: Guilford Press.

Nader, R., Oberlander, T. F., Chambers, C. T., & Craig, K. D. (2004). Expression of pain in children with autism. *Clinical Journal of Pain, 20,* 88–97.

Nicholas, J. (2005). Can specific deficits in Executive functioning explain the behavioural characteristics of CHARGE syndrome? *American Journal of Medical Genetics*, *133A*, 300-305.

Oberlander, T. F., O'Donnell, M. E., & Montgomery, C. J. (1999). Pain in children with significant neurological impairment. *Developmental and Behavioral Pediatrics*, *20*, 235-243.

Oshiro, Y., Quevedo, A. S., McHaffie, J. G., Kraft, R. A., & Coghill, R. C. (2007). Brain mechanisms supporting spatial discrimination of pain. *The Journal of Neuroscience*, *27*(13), 3388-3394

Peltokorpi, S., & Huutunen, K. (2008). Communication in the early stage of language development in children with CHARGE syndrome. *The British Journal of Visual Impairment*, *26*(1), 24-49.

Ploghaus, A., Beccerra, L., Borras, C., & Borsook, D. (2003). Neural circuitry underlying pain modulation: expectation, hypnosis, placebo. *Trends in Cognitive Sciences*, 7, 197-200.

Smeets, R. J. E. M., Vlaeyen, J. W. S., Kester, A. D. M., & Knottnerus, J. A. (2006). Reduction of pain catastophizing mediates the outcome of both physical and cognitive-behavioral treatment of chronic low back pain. *The Journal of Pain*, 7, 261-271.

Souriau, J., Gimenes, M., Blouin, C., Benbrick, I., & Churakowskyi, A. (2005). CHARGE syndrome: developmental and behavioural findings. *American Journal of Medical Genetics*, *133A*, 278-281.

Symons, F. J. (2002). Pain and self-injury: Mechanisms and models. In S. Schroder, T. Thomson, & M. L. Oster-Granite (Eds.), *Self-injurious behaviour: Genes, brain and behaviour* (pp. 223-234). Washington, DC: American Psychological Association.

Terman, G. W., & Bonica, J. J. (2001). Spinal mechanisms and their modulation. In J. D. Loeser (Ed.), *Bonica's management of pain* (pp. 73-152). Philadelphia, PA: Lippincott Williams & Wilkins.

Thelin, J. W., & Fussner, J. C. (2005). Factors related to the development of communication in CHARGE syndrome. *American Journal of Medical Genetics*, *133A*, 282-290.

Tracey, I. (2008). Imaging pain. *British Journal of Anaesthesia*, *101*(1), 32-39.

Whitten, C. E., & Cristobal, K. (2005). Chronic pain is a chronic condition, not just a symptom. *The Permanente Journal*, *9*(3), 43-51.

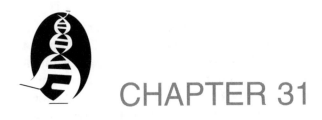

CHAPTER 31

Experiencing Stress

KASEE K. STRATTON, PH.D. CANDIDATE AND
TIMOTHY S. HARTSHORNE, PH.D.

INTRODUCTION

In the early years of the life of an individual with CHARGE, there are seemingly endless invasive medical procedures, hospital stays, and doctor visits. In the preschool years, there are fewer surgeries, but still many medical visits, with therapies added on. Through grade school, children experience an increasing emphasis on complex academics and demands for more time on task. And, yet, the medical visits and therapy appointments still continue, disrupting the academic day. Due to the physical, communication, and sometimes cognitive challenges, peer experiences are limited, and peer social support may be lacking. Individuals with CHARGE experience considerable chronic and episodic pain, probably throughout their lives. Thus, there is every reason to expect that all individuals with CHARGE experience a great deal of stress throughout their lives.

POST TRAUMATIC STRESS DISORDER

Virtually nothing has been published on the experience of stress in children with disabilities. Much of the literature on stress in children focuses on Post-Traumatic Stress Disorder (PTSD). PTSD is thought to occur when an individual has experienced a threat to his or her own life or the life of another or a threat to physical integrity. PTSD often is thought of in relation to war-related trauma and, more recently, following natural disasters such as earthquakes or hurricanes. PTSD, however, has been documented in children with life-threatening diseases such as cancer or liver failure (Pelcovitz, et al., 1998; Saxe, Vanderbilt, & Zuckerman, 2003; Stallard, 2006). PTSD symptoms in children often are expressed behaviorally; for example, by loss of emotional regulation, poor attention, physical complaints, and self-injurious behavior (Cohen, 1998; Stallard, 2006). Trauma also may interfere with an individual's capacity to integrate sensory, emotional, and cognitive information as a comprehensive whole (van der Kolk, 2005).

Several potential sources of PTSD for individuals with CHARGE syndrome are possible. Beginning in infancy, many have life-threatening medical conditions requiring multiple surgeries and frequent, often long-term, hospital stays. Such procedures often have a protracted recovery period, with poorly managed chronic pain. Infants and many children do not have the communication skills by which to self-report their pain experiences. In social situations, children with CHARGE may be exposed to more physical and emotional bullying than children without the developmental delays and physical issues associated with CHARGE. In addition, as with all individuals with a development disability, children with CHARGE may be at increased risk for physical or sexual abuse (Hershkowitz, Lamb, & Horowitz, 2007). Individuals with CHARGE may not exhibit symptoms severe enough to warrant a PTSD diagnosis, either because they do not have full PTSD, or because their disabilities mask their symptoms. In either case, their experiences may be very similar to PTSD and have an impact on their well-being and behavior.

Although it is likely that individuals with CHARGE experience a great deal of stress, and may in fact develop symptoms of PTSD, it is difficult to document. In order to investigate the degree to which individuals with CHARGE might experience stress, interviews were conducted with high-functioning young adults with CHARGE. Of particular interest were the behavioral reactions the individuals described having during stressful situations. Although these interviews were conducted with young adults with high-functioning communication skills, it is reasonable to generalize the results to those who are less able to communicate their needs and stressors, as they face many of the same challenges.

INTERVIEWS

Ten individuals with CHARGE from the United States, Canada, Australia, and New Zealand participated in the interviews (six female, four male, ages 15 to 27). Interview questions covered school experiences, social relationships and friendships, family relationships, work experiences, and reactions to stressful situations. Themes that emerged from each of the topic areas are summarized in Table 31-1.

School Themes

Communication

One of the first themes to emerge was problems with communication. One interviewee commented on how she did not know how to let school personnel know when she was tired and needed a break, "I get tired easily at school and I find it hard to concentrate. Sometimes my behavior is bad. I don't know why I do it and I hate it when that happens." Another young adult explained how she had an FM amplification system in the classroom to help hear the teacher and classmates, but the school took the FM system away during lunch, between her classes, and at other free times. As a result, she missed out on all nonacademic aspects of the school day, making it difficult to socialize with classmates.

TABLE 31-1. Themes Emerging from Interviews with Young Adults

Themes	
School	• Communication challenges • School staff understanding of multisensory impairments • Emotional immaturity • Quickly tiring from concentration—a need for breaks • Physical and emotional bullying
Friendships/ Social Relationships	• Need for social interaction and core group of friends • Communication challenges • Difficulty understanding appropriate social behavior
Family	• Importance of positive relationship between parents and school • Acceptance of physical characteristics of CHARGE • Families provide important support when needed
Abuse	• Incidences of physical and sexual abuse
Obsessive Compulsive Disorder	• Understanding needed from family, peers, and school staff regarding the individual's obsessions and compulsive behaviors and why they are performed

Sensory Impairment

A second school theme involved the school personnel not appreciating the student's multisensory impairments (especially combined hearing and vision loss). One student commented, "I had an FM system to help with my hearing but I found that I didn't have the adequate services for my vision . . . for whatever reason I found it hard to communicate what I was being taught." "Teachers had no clue how to make accommodations for me; they often just gave up entirely," stated another young adult. Interviewees noted that although staff might understand one sensory difficulty, such as hearing loss, they often did not understand the vision loss, other sensory difficulties, or the effects of multiple sensory impairments. For example, one student said her teacher was wonderful at enlarging materials so they could be read more easily; however, this teacher used an open learning style with several individual stations around the classroom. The chaotic nature of this arrangement and the increased noise level often produced aggressive reactions from this student due to sensory overload and difficulty concentrating.

Emotional Immaturity

The third school theme was emotional immaturity. Many of the interviewees reported crying in their classes in junior high and high school. One young man said, "In high school, I would cry a lot, I would just get so upset." Such behavior is not commonly seen at the high school level; therefore, this student also had to deal with the social impact of his behavior.

Exhaustion

Exhaustion was the fourth school theme. All interviewees discussed how quickly they became tired at school from the effort involved in concentrating with hearing and vision losses and other sensory deficits. They were exhausted when they returned home. One stated she "often came home and just wanted to lie down on the sofa after school." She was so tired after the long school day that it became difficult to get up and complete her homework in the evenings, much less participate in extracurricular or other social activities. A second young adult agreed: "The teacher refused to acknowledge that the amount of work that was expected of me was way too much. There was not enough time to get it all done. It wasn't ever fully explained to me so I could understand the material they were teaching . . . they just ignored the fact that I needed help . . . I needed a break." Interviewees repeatedly expressed a need for *schedules that included breaks* to avoid sensory overload and exhaustion. Many interviewees admitted that at some point during their school years they had lost control and been aggressive toward others, including teachers and best friends.

Emotional Bullying

Unfortunately, a fifth school theme identified was physical and emotional bullying. Interviewees were made fun of for their appearance, such as being shorter and smaller than same age peers. One stated she was often bullied physically at her school bus stop and felt like an easy target.

Friendships and Social Relationships

Friendships and social relationships are very important to all children, and yet for children with CHARGE, they can be incredibly challenging to initiate and maintain. Individuals interviewed wanted a core group of friends and social interaction. One young man said, "I hate being sick and missing out on school. I want to be at school everyday. I want more people like me around." Although the desire for interaction is there, one interviewee noted, "Friendships were always hard to make and they still are . . . I don't know how to strike up one." Individuals with CHARGE communicate in several different ways (speech, sign language, gestures, etc.), often not in the same way as their peers. Communication challenges are evident in the following quotes: "I get frustrated especially when friends won't play with me. I don't know how to tell them what I mean (when we play)" and "It's hard to be at the mall and hear and see my friend at the same time. I can't follow our conversations well; it just makes it hard to communicate." Finding an environment that is conducive to establishing and maintaining friendships can be challenging.

Individuals with CHARGE have significant concerns regarding social behavior. After one interview, a young woman with CHARGE and the interviewer went shopping in the city. Throughout the shopping excursion she continuously asked whether she was "bothering [the interviewer]," or "Is it okay that I follow you around?" The shopping experience was dominated by her concerns about possibly behaving inappropriately. Such comments may drive away friends who do not realize this hyper-vigilance is a reaction to wanting to perform the right behaviors to fit in. All interviewees expressed a need for friends who will remain their friend despite behavior that is unpredictable at times.

Family

Nearly all interviewees commented on the importance of a positive relationship between parents and the school system. Many parents who sat in on the interviews were surprised to realize their child had noticed the conflicts between the parents and the school. Feeling responsible for poor relationships between school and parents can cause additional stress for the individual with CHARGE.

A desire for acceptance of their physical characteristics also was expressed. One stated that she would not have been so self-conscious about her looks if her family had not always focused on how her physical characteristics made her different from her sibling. On the other hand, a very positive family theme identified was how incredibly supportive their families were: "they fought a lot for me." Efforts from parents to provide supports, especially within the school system, did not go unnoticed.

One unfortunate theme was the mention of physical and/or sexual abuse. Research shows children with communication and learning disabilities are perhaps two to three times more likely to be victims of abuse than typically developing peers (Hershkowitz, et al., 2007). As many incidents go unreported, actual figures may be higher. Victims of such abuse often have associated conduct disorders or difficult behavior. Such statistics should be kept in mind when educating children about reporting abuse and what is appropriate and inappropriate behavior.

A final family concern was the acceptance of obsessive-compulsive disorder (OCD) or OCD-like behaviors by family and educators. OCD behaviors are sometimes techniques individuals with CHARGE use in an attempt to deal with anxiety and stress. OCD is a type of anxiety disorder in which the individual experiences involuntarily thoughts or impulses that are unwanted, persistent, and repeated. Such obsessions may appear senseless to others, for example, a fear of germs. Compulsions are repetitive behaviors that the individual performs to rid themselves of the unwanted obsessions or thoughts, such as washing, counting, checking, and repeating actions. The obsessions and compulsions then continue in a cycle.

Some examples of OCD behaviors that were observed or described during the interviews included changing clothing several times a day, gelling hair continuously until it was stiff—sometimes using an entire container of hair gel, picking at skin, and lining up objects. One individual kept dialing a pattern on the telephone and calling randomly until she felt she had a satisfying conversation. Another would browse the Internet for a particular musical group/band or until some action occurred. The purpose of these behaviors appeared to be to distract from the real issue; for example, when one interviewee was worrying about work, she lined up her shoes. The lining up of shoes is not as productive as solving the issue at work. Although these behaviors may seem pointless, they serve as a form of control and release of anxiety for the individual performing them. Parents and educators should be aware that when these behaviors are performed, the child may be under intense stress. Reducing sources of stress may be more effective than medication in reducing OCD behaviors.

In conclusion, individuals with CHARGE have many stressors with which to cope. When communication is limited or reduced, it is especially important to remember that behavior serves as a form of communication. Aggressive outbursts, loss of emotional control, and self-destructive behaviors may indicate the individual is under intense stress. They should be indicators to parents and educators that the individual is experiencing high levels of stress.

REFERENCES

Cohen, J. A., (1998). Practice parameters for the assessment and treatment of children and adolescents with posttraumatic stress disorder. *Journal of the American Academy of Child and Adolescent Psychiatry: Special Issue, 37*, 4s-26s.

Hershkowitz, I., Lamb, M. E., & Horowitz, D. (2007). Victimization of children with disabilities. *American Journal of Orthopsychiatry, 77*, 929-635.

Pelcovitz, D., Libov, B. G., Mandel, F., Winblatt, M., & Septimus, A. (1998). Posttraumatic stress disorder and family functioning in adolescent cancer. *Journal of Traumatic Stress, 11*, 205-221.

Saxe, G., Vanderbilt, D., & Zuckerman, B. (2003). Traumatic stress in injured and ill children. *PTSD Research Quarterly, 14*, 1-8.

Stallard (2006). Post-traumatic stress disorder. In C. Gillberg, R. Harrington, & H. C. Steinhausen (Eds.), *A clinician's handbook of child and adolescent psychiatry* (pp. 221-245). New York, NY: Cambridge University Press.

Van der Kolk, B.A., (2005). Developmental trauma disorder. *Psychiatric Annuals, 35*, 401-408.

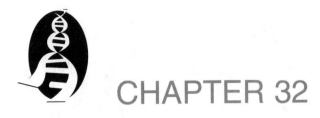

CHAPTER 32

Parenting

TIMOTHY S. HARTSHORNE, Ph.D.

Very little in the parenting literature addresses the experiences surrounding raising a child with significant disabilities, let alone conditions as complex as CHARGE syndrome. Although this is understandable given the small size of this population, these are parents very much in need of help and support to deal with the challenges of parenting.

Several aspects of raising a child with CHARGE make parenting particularly challenging (Figure 32–1). First, some parenting techniques are very difficult to implement with a child with significant disabilities. Talking about the behavior is problematic if your child has poor or limited communication skills. You may not want to isolate a child who is medically at risk and needs continuous observation and monitoring. Time out may not be effective if the child prefers to be by themselves. Food as a reinforcer is not helpful if your child is tube fed.

Second, there may be a tendency on the part of parents to excuse the child's behavior because they have a disability and already have been through so much; especially if there have been serious medical complications. If the child has a heart defect, for example, the parent may be tempted to give in to demands and temper tantrums out of caring for the challenges the child experiences. Some parents may have had to invest a great deal of time and energy during the early years of their child's life to keep the child alive, and the consequence of that may be to have lower standards for the child's behavior. In other words, there may be a tendency to spoil a child with CHARGE. The parents themselves may be exhausted from the shock of having a child with

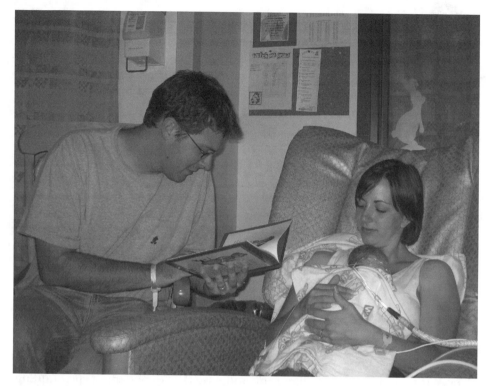

FIGURE 32–1. Even from the beginning, figuring out how to parent a child with CHARGE can be challenging.

disabilities and the struggle just to keep their child alive (and in a house, and with medical insurance), and find little energy left over for teaching their child to behave.

Third, parents may experience problems relating with their child. Due to deafblindness, developmental delay, or autistic-like features to their behavior, some children with CHARGE may not be very responsive to their parents, which can lead to difficulties with attachment and bonding. Parents may feel rejected by their child and their child's behavior.

Parents of children with CHARGE syndrome struggle on two fronts. They often experience guilt about their failure to produce and to advance a "normal" child, along with their self image of not doing a good enough job raising their child. A second challenge is trying to understand and make sense out of the rather unusual and challenging behaviors many children with CHARGE display. Very challenging behavior often is associated with genetic syndromes, and CHARGE is no exception (Moss, Oliver, Arron, Burbidge, & Berg, 2009). For example, when faced with severe aggression on the part of the child, parents may not know whether to attribute it to their own failures as parents, to the personality of the particular child, or to the syndrome itself.

GUILT AND THE COURAGE TO BE IMPERFECT

Many parents experience significant guilt over their ability, or lack of ability, to meet the needs of their child. One parent remarked, "How do you know if you have the right doctors and therapists doing the right things and enough of them? How do you know if you're doing all the right things and enough of them? I have been avoiding phone calls and insurance stuff, etc., because I just want us to be normal."

During the first four years or so of the child's life, parents of children with CHARGE typically are busy working with the medical establishment. Over a short period of time, they have to develop a huge medical vocabulary, deal with dozens of medical specialists at several different locations and act as case manager for their child. Some parents reported being asked quite frequently whether they are nurses. Yes, parents have to develop sophisticated nursing skills to cope with all of the various medical procedures and conditions; but it is hard to ever feel truly adequate, particularly when their child's life is at stake.

Soon after the medical difficulties have stabilized, parents prepare to send their child to school, but this is not the school they themselves experienced. Like the medical world, the world of special education is replete with its own vocabulary, rules, laws, and procedures. The process of evaluations, plans, and schedules with a variety of specialists adds another layer to the time commitment. Parents often find themselves embroiled in conflicts with the schools and having to stay in constant touch with advocacy organizations to preserve their child's rights. After trust between school personnel and parents is lost, it is very difficult to re-establish.

The challenge for parents is to learn to do two things simultaneously. They need to be able to love their child with no need or expectation that their child will get any better or make any progress. If a child is loved only for what the parent hopes they will become, he or she can never be appreciated for who they are. It is not easy for parents to give up expectations for what they "need" their child to become. But failure to do so can mean lack of acceptance for who the child is. At the same time, parents must never give up hope that with lots of focused effort and energy, their child can progress and develop and improve. If parents give up on their child, the child is unlikely to make a great deal of progress. But it is very hard to do these two simultaneously: to accept and be content with where the child is and yet to work as hard as possible to help the child progress.

Hartshorne (2002) has described how parental behavior, as they reconcile these two goals, sometimes may appear to professionals as denial. "Why does that parent fail to insist that their deaf child wear a hearing aide at all times? Have they given up?" "Why does that parent insist we keep using sign language with their child when there has been no progress? Are they in denial?" In fact, courage is not denial, and parents of children with significant disabilities have to have the courage to know their limits and accept their child's potential. And all the while, parents worry that they may not have enough of what their child needs. Parents benefit from and appreciate professionals who understand not only the struggle of parents to figure out how to enjoy their child while they push their child and everyone else to do better, but also the constant guilt that they experience over not doing enough of either. Parents are hard enough on themselves. They do not need their shortcomings pointed out to them by professionals. Parents need help to develop the courage to be imperfect; the courage to recognize that they are doing the best that they can and it is enough.

BEHAVIOR AS COMMUNICATION

Part of the normal parenting challenge is coping with difficult behaviors. This is what sends many parents to parent education programs; so that they can come to understand some of the behaviors and develop skills and ideas for disciplining their children and shaping their behaviors. Developing effective discipline strategies is often difficult even with children who do not have disabilities. It can be overwhelming when the child's behavior is labeled as autistic-like, or obsessive-compulsive, or indicative of attention deficit disorder. A dearth of strategies for disciplining children and feeling overwhelmed by the challenge of coping with a child's behavior (at home and at school) may be one reason so many children with CHARGE end up on psychotropic medications (Wachtel, Hartshorne, & Dailor, 2007).

Parents need a means by which to make sense out of their child's apparently bizarre behavior in order to feel somewhat empowered to cope with it. Understanding that *behavior is communication* can help. Two major principles help one to understand behavior. First, all behavior has a purpose. Behavior is not random. Sometimes, the purpose may be very simple, like scratching an itch, but it is goal-oriented. The behavior demonstrated by children with CHARGE is not random. They engage in it for a reason. The second principle is equally important: behavior serves a communicative function. This means that behavior is used to communicate something. If we can understand the communication, and if we can determine the purpose of the behavior, then any behavior can make sense.

Learning to "read" behaviors can seem challenging at first, but most parents rapidly can become very skilled at it. They do this naturally with their healthy babies as they notice what kind of behaviors or vocalizations suggest hunger, dirty diaper, a need for sleep, boredom, not feeling well, etc. The behavior of their child with CHARGE may be more unusual: wrenching their neck against objects might be indicative of an ear infection in a particular child, loud giggling might mean a bowel movement is imminent, walking around turning on and off light switches might mean "I need something—figure it out." There is no dictionary for these, and the meaning behind many behaviors can be obscure. But with time, patience, and careful observation, parents and others often can make remarkable discoveries.

CASE EXAMPLE

To illustrate the problems of assisting parents of children with severe disabilities, we offer the following case example from a parent: "I have a question. I struggle with this. My daughter's OCD obsessions are our biggest battles. One is water. She has to get her clothing wet before she can take them off. And she needs to change her clothes often. I have tried making her stop both behaviors, but she just goes over the edge. I have finally come to the realization that I can't stop her, but maybe I can control the amount of water she gets when she soaks her clothes. If we take the water away completely, she will pee on them, so we have our choice of water supply there. Is it wrong to help her with the water? I am saying it is ok and maybe that is feeding the obsession. But I have little hope of getting her to stop, and so I don't know what to do. What harm I am doing by allowing it? Her obsessions seem to have come from routines. The routines turn into habits, rituals and then true obsessions. If I had noticed that earlier in life, do you think that I could have prevented some of this?"

This is not the kind of problem typically addressed in parent education groups. In approaching this problem, we should first consider that the behavior is somehow the child's adjustment to her life situation. In other words, it was developed for a reason, and it most likely communicates something to us. All behavior is communication. What might needing to be wet in order to change clothes possibly be communicating? Here are a few possibilities:

- Look what I know how to do!
- I really enjoy the feel of wet clothes.
- If I change my clothes, I can avoid something I don't like.
- I am in pain, and this really helps reduce the pain or distract me from it.
- I am anxious, and this helps reduce my anxiety.
- I like having you engage with me, and this accomplishes that.

Understanding the purpose of the behavior helps it to make sense and suggests possible parenting practices to perhaps modify the behavior.

The mother has some unique questions and problems that also need to be considered. She wants to know whether it is okay to participate in the ritual.

The answer may depend on the purpose of the behavior. If the behavior is evidence of an obsessive-compulsive disorder, it may be very hard to change even knowing the purpose. Any attempt to stop compulsive behavior could intensify a power struggle and possibly lead to aggression (Bernstein and Denno, 2005). This mother also communicates guilt about not having prevented the behavior in the first place. Any parenting intervention program needs to address parental guilt. Parents need reassurance that they did everything they could. Finally, it is important to note that this is an exhausted mother. She needs immediate assistance and time to regenerate her energy.

SPECIFIC RECOMMENDATIONS FOR CHILDREN WITH CHARGE

When a child with CHARGE presents with challenging behaviors, especially if there has been a change in behavior, pain and health issues should be immediately pursued as possible (even most likely) causes. Some children with CHARGE cannot directly communicate that they experience pain. Others may be so accustomed to living with pain that they themselves are not aware that it is affecting their behavior. One young man with CHARGE syndrome stopped sleeping at night, which created a great deal of distress for the parents. The pediatrician could not find anything amiss except some wax in the ear. He suggested a psychotropic medication to facilitate sleep. The parents finally took the boy to the emergency room where the piece of "wax" was found to be a foreign object imbedded in the ear and rubbing against the ear drum. After it was removed, the young man started sleeping again. When drugs are used to change behavior, a major form of communication is lost.

Because of the high incidence of regulatory disorders in CHARGE (see Chapter 28), parents and caregivers must be sensitive to issues related to sensory overload. With a regulatory disorder, some children can shift from a very low state of arousal to a very high state in a matter of seconds, depending on the kind of sensory input they are experiencing. Even something as apparently innocuous as music sometimes can overwhelm a child and lead to behavioral outbursts.

Most people respond better when they are given choices. However, if choices are offered, they must be respected. "You don't seem to want to do this task. You can either do it or go to your room." If the child chooses their room, you must honor that choice. A variation is requesting that the child postpone something they want to do until after he or she performs what the adult has requested. An adolescent with CHARGE wanted to use the computer in his classroom. After challenging the teacher repeatedly, he agreed to complete a language task first, with the promise of using the computer afterwards. After completing the task, the boy turned to the computer but then was told by the teacher he had a second task to perform before he could use it. The boy lost behavioral control at that point.

Another example of sensory overload and its effect on behavior is a 12-year-old girl who had extreme temper tantrums when asked to remain in her seat during classroom time. An expert observer recognized that the girl was communicating her need for a break. He suggested that her team teach her an alternative and more appropriate way to ask for a break from seat work. Although some team members agreed that this was something that could be done, they worried that the girl would now "win" if they honored her request for a break. It was pointed out to them that communication is based on a regular response to communicative attempts; it is not a game with winners and losers.

Stress is pretty much a constant in the world of a child with CHARGE (see Chapter 31). Reducing stress should be a major goal. One way to help reduce stress is to provide as much routine and consistency in the child's life as possible. Predictability and routine reduces stress. When changes in routine are coming, repeated advanced warning in anticipation of the change can help reduce stress. Children with CHARGE need as much information as possible about what is going to happen next. This is typical of children who are deaf-blind, who often find themselves whisked off from one place to another without really knowing why or where. A child may be put into the car without knowing whether they are going on a five-minute ride to the store or a10-hour drive to a relative's house. The typical OCD tendencies in children with CHARGE on top of deafblindness exacerbate the need for routine. Calendar systems can be extremely useful and should be encouraged.

Even though behavior is communication and must be respected, sometimes limits simply must be imposed. A child cannot be permitted to destroy a room because he or she is upset. There need to be routine consequences that can be imposed in as calm a manner as possible. It will be easier to impose limits during a crisis if there has been a history of limits having been imposed with the child in previous noncrisis situations. As noted earlier, it is easy to spoil a child with significant disabilities, and it is essential that this be limited as much as possible.

Parents often experience moments when they question their ability to go on: "Tonight, I am so very tired of being the person figuring out what's going on. It's been awhile since I've felt so isolated, scared, on and on. Right now it's as though nothing is enough to really help. I'm damned tired of this. I would like some help, too. I need it now. My daughter needs it now." Professionals should be prepared to offer support to parents in their struggles to provide appropriate parenting for their children. It helps just having someone to vent to. Helping identify respite programs so the parent can get a break could be useful. Professionals do not have all of the answers, but they can model and participate in a problem solving process to help the parent regain their sense of courage in the face of raising a child with CHARGE.

REFERENCES

Bernstein, V. & Denno, L. S. (2005). Repetitive behaviors in CHARGE syndrome: Differential diagnosis and treatment options. *American Journal of Medical Genetics, 133A*, 232–239.

Hartshorne, T. S. (2002). Mistaking courage for denial: Family resilience after the birth of a child with severe disabilities. *Journal of Individual Psychology, 58*, 263–278.

Moss, J., Oliver, C., Arron, K., Burbidge, C., & Berg, K. (2009). The prevalence and phenomenology of repetitive behavior in genetic syndromes. *Journal of Autism and Developmental Disorders, 39*(4), 572–588.

Wachtel, L. E., Hartshorne, T. S., & Dailor, A. N. (2007). Psychiatric Diagnoses and Psychotropic Medications in CHARGE Syndrome: A Pediatric Survey. *Journal of Developmental and Physical Disabilities, 19*, 471–483.

PART VI

Conclusions and Questions for Future Research

*A*lthough the first cases of what is now known as CHARGE syndrome were published in 1979, knowledge of CHARGE grew slowly, with only a few articles published each year until 1985, when there were six. In 2005, there were 33, thanks in part to a special issue of the *American Journal of Medical Genetics 133A*(3), which was devoted to CHARGE syndrome. It is apparent to the editors of this book that we have come to know a great deal about this syndrome. It is also clear to us that much more is yet to be learned. In this brief section, we list some of these areas, especially medical questions. This list is by no means meant to be exhaustive.

- Understanding of the functions of the CHD7 gene is advancing at a rapid pace, thanks in part to the development of at least two animal models (mouse and zebra fish). Further study may elucidate significance of particular mutations within the gene, interaction of the CHD7 protein with other genes, and their effects on the huge variety of clinical and developmental outcomes seen in individuals with CHARGE. Other genes likely will be identified, which either influence the expression of CHD7 or result in similar clinical findings.

- Infections are a constant factor in the lives of children with CHARGE. Very little is known about possible immunological factors that influence these infections.

- The relationship between enlarged adenoids (and sometimes tonsils) and breathing obstruction has been noted in many cases and has even caused seizure-like episodes. However, as adenoids and tonsils are the first line of defense against infective agents that arrive through the nose and throat, a careful investigation of the benefits and risks of removing adenoids or tonsils should involve both otolaryngologists and immunologists.

- Hypotonia of the shoulder girdle and trunk has not yet been explained. Are there weak muscles that can be strengthened, or are some muscles abnormal in size or internal structure or even missing? Is scoliosis caused by the weakness of particular muscle groups? Can progression of scoliosis be avoided by appropriate preventive physical therapies or exercises? How do hypotonia, scoliosis, and vestiblular anomalies interact?

- Congenital vestibular dysfunction clearly causes major balance issues. Dizziness is not involved: Is this because the sensory cells have never formed and, therefore, are not causing dizziness as they are attacked by infections or agents, or are other factors involved? What are the best methods to promote and encourage motor development and upright and balanced posture? How does the vestibular dysfunction interact with the other sensory impairments? How does vestibular dysfunction affect cognition, the acquisition of symbolic language, and behavior?

- Why is osteoporosis such a major problem beginning in adolescence (or even earlier)? Is there a problem with bony mineralization involving not just the lack of sex hormones or even growth hormone but also a problem with calcium, magnesium, and vitamin D? Or is it related more to nutrition and exercise?

- What is the effect of growth hormone on both skeletal growth and muscle strength over time? Can it stave off the early development of osteoporosis?

- Sleep disturbance is a major issue. Although some of the problem is related to lack of sensory input and/or obstructive sleep apnea, disturbances in diurnal rhythm need further investigation.

- Neurologic questions abound:
  - Which structural brain abnormalities correlate with seizures, intellectual functioning, and/or behavioral changes?
  - What kinds of seizures are the most prevalent, and is treatment any different from treatment of seizures in children with other syndromes?
  - Why are some cranial nerves involved and not others, or are they all involved, but not as clearly manifested?
  - Are the cranial nerve nuclei in the brain malformed, or is the problem the connection with the end organ, e.g., vestibule and

cochlea, or does the malformation of the end organ cause retrograde destruction of the connecting nerves?

- ◼ Is the autonomic nervous system (ANS) malfunctioning? This system controls muscle functions not under voluntary control such as breathing and peristalsis. Peristalsis is the neurologically based propulsion of food down the esophagus and gut, the regulation of voiding, and other functions. Is the persistent troublesome constipation more related to peristalsis or diet and exercise?

- ◼ Are the pain sensors of the body malformed or not functioning properly? Is there a high threshold for pain in this population, or is there a difference in response to painful stimuli or both?

- ◼ What brain factors predict central auditory or central visual processing issues?

◼ Why does enuresis (urinary accidents) persist into childhood and even teenage years?

◼ Why is the cartilage of the ear soft in many cases and cartilage in the trachea soft in some?

◼ When is tracheostomy a necessity? For instance, if excessive secretions are avoided or breathing obstruction treated, can tracheostomy be avoided?

◼ Excess salivary secretions in infancy and early childhood have been controlled successfully with Botox injections in one child we know of and not in another. This is another area that needs further investigation.

◼ When is cochlear implantation truly contraindicated? What are the otologic criteria that accurately predict surgical success or failure? What is the relationship between presurgical diagnostic criteria and the range of auditory outcomes—including no benefit, awareness of environmental sounds, and ability to use the auditory channel as the primary mode for communication? What cochlear anatomy predicts when implants will be helpful for environmental awareness and when for speech detection and/or acquisition? What are appropriate expectations from a cochlear implant?

◼ What is the range of sex hormone production over adolescence and adulthood? Do the levels follow normal patterns, or is there something distinctive about CHARGE?

◼ What is the fertility rate in males? In females? What factors predict success in childbearing?

◼ We know that there are many adults with CHARGE who have not been diagnosed. How many are there? How are they functioning? What kinds of developmental and educational support did they receive?

■ Is there truly a behavioral phenotype that is part of CHARGE, or is it a result of the multiple sensory impairments, inability to communicate adequately, and medical issues?

■ When are psychotropic medications truly indicated? What about drug–drug interactions?

■ What is the typical life span for individuals with CHARGE, and what unique medical issues emerge in adolescence, adulthood, and old age?

■ How can case management in medical, educational, and rehabilitation settings be optimized?

COMMUNICATION, COMMUNICATION, COMMUNICATION

In addition to the genetic and medical questions, many questions remain unanswered regarding best practices for helping individuals with CHARGE to reach their full potential. The editors feel that the key to CHARGE is **communication**. Without communication, individuals with CHARGE will *not* reach their full potential, whatever that may be. At this juncture, it is critical for professionals working with individuals with CHARGE, as well as parents and the individuals with CHARGE themselves, to observe, publish, and otherwise communicate with one another to add to the growing body of knowledge about all the possible strategies for helping facilitate the communication skills of people with CHARGE.

Index

W